WAYFARING

Wayfaring

A Christian Approach to Mental Health Care

Warren Kinghorn

WILLIAM B. EERDMANS PUBLISHING COMPANY

GRAND RAPIDS, MICHIGAN

Wm. B. Eerdmans Publishing Co.
4035 Park East Court SE, Grand Rapids, Michigan 49546
www.eerdmans.com

Published 2024

Book design by Leah Luyk

Printed in the United States of America

30 29 28 27 26 25 24   1 2 3 4 5 6 7

ISBN 978-0-8028-8224-0

Library of Congress Cataloging-in-Publication Data

A catalog record for this book is available from the Library of Congress.

To Susan, Ava, and Mills

Contents

Foreword

The field of mental health care is complex and often controversial. This complexity deepens as we develop novel technologies, new forms of medication, and fresh knowledge about the biological location of people's languishing. All of these developments are important and have the potential to bring healing and relief to people going through very difficult times. We wouldn't want to go back to a time when such understandings and the treatments that have emerged from them were not available. Nevertheless, the allure of such powerful, shiny things can easily distract us from other important aspects of mental health care. The pull of technology, genetics, pharmacology, and neurobiology tempts us to focus our attention on problems rather than people. But the fullness of people matters.

Mental health problems may well turn out to have biological elements that require biological treatments. But mental health is never a straightforward internal process that can be understood without paying attention to the wider dimensions of a person's life. I recently read an article that suggested that we are very close to finding a pill that can reconfigure our biology to avoid the experience of loneliness. This may happen, but to reduce loneliness to a biological process is to miss something vital about human beings. We are exocentric beings, made for relationships. Simply palliating our loneliness with medication may make us feel better, but it strips something of our humanness from us. Likewise, turning our sadness and unease about the world into categories such as depression and anxiety and then treating them without thinking through what people's experiences are saying about them and the world around them may be pragmatically effective, but is it faithful to the vision of flourishing that we encounter in the Scriptures? Biomedicine is important, but a rigid adherence to it as the primary or even sometimes the only explanatory framework by which we come to understand mental health issues risks turning persons into machines and confining the task of the carer to making sure the machine runs well and people remain as close to being symptom free as possible.

Human beings are creatures who live, breathe, love, cry, find sadness and joy. All of these dimensions are important for our mental health. Recognition of this is the beginning point for *Wayfaring: A Christian Approach to Mental Health Care*. With wisdom, grace, humility, and compassion, Warren Kinghorn invites us on a journey within which we are called unrelentingly to recognize and protect the personhood of people in the midst of difficult situations that refuse to yield to simplistic explanations. Kinghorn takes the science of mental health very seriously. His is not an approach that tries to downplay the role of psychiatry or psychology. Nevertheless, he recognizes that when viewed through a theological lens, people living with mental health challenges deserve more than what science alone can offer. They deserve strategies and approaches that ensure they know that they are loved. Struggling people are not simply objects to be fixed. Rather, they are intricate creatures, formed for relationship and love; persons who need a certain kind of attention, which will remind them of their irrefutable status as made in the image of a God who is love. Through stories and insights combined with the deep theology of Thomas Aquinas, Kinghorn reframes mental health care in a theological vein, guiding us away from isolation and shame toward the embrace of community and the divine love of Jesus. At its heart, the book reminds us of the therapeutic power of faithfulness to God, but not in a way that claims "religion is good for your mental health." Rather, Kinghorn calls us peaceably, gracefully, and humbly to follow Jesus in our caring practices. He reminds us of who and whose we are and urges us to hold onto the healing knowledge that, in God's eyes, it is good that we are here. God is glad that we exist. Central to the model of faithful mental health care that Kinghorn presents is the desire to help people see, hear, and feel this affirming love of God. This book is a beautiful contribution to theology, a gift to the church, and a powerful reminder of the soulfulness that all good mental health care should aim for.

John Swinton

Of Stories and Symptoms

If I take the wings of the morning
  and settle at the farthest limits of the sea,
even there your hand shall lead me,
  And your right hand shall hold me fast.
                              —*Psalm 139:9-10*[1]

Sweetest Jesus, Body and Blood most holy,
  be the delight and pleasure of my soul,
  my strength and salvation in all temptations,
  my joy and peace in every trial,
  my light and guide in every word and deed,
  and my final protection in death.
                              —*Saint Thomas Aquinas,*
                    "Short Prayer after Communion"[2]

Ann was in her forties when she first realized that she was depressed, but she was no stranger to mental health challenges. Her mother's life was "colored by cycles of mania and depression." When Ann was four years old, she was summoned to her family's living room. She saw her mother dressed in a nightgown

---

1. All quotations of Scripture, unless indicated otherwise, are from the New Revised Standard Version.

2. Thomas Aquinas, "Short Prayer after Communion," in *The Aquinas Prayer Book: The Prayers and Hymns of St. Thomas Aquinas,* trans. and ed. Robert Anderson and Johann Moser (Manchester, NH: Sophia Institute Press, 2000), 78-79.

and sitting on a sofa and crying. Her pastor told her and her three older siblings that her mother was going to be hospitalized in an institution. Her mother was hospitalized several more times over the course of Ann's childhood, receiving treatments that included tranquilizers and electroconvulsive therapy (ECT). When Ann's mother was up, she would buy things or take the children on a trip. When she "began to crash on the other side," she would "drink, and talk, and cry." She died when Ann was just entering adulthood.[3]

Growing up in a small town in North Carolina, Ann and her siblings did their best to cope, but "most often we were left alone to do so. In that time, there was little conversation or education." In her neighborhood and in her Presbyterian church, plenty of families, including many Second World War veterans, were struggling. "You knew which houses you could go into, and which you couldn't, because you didn't know what was going on or who wasn't 'feeling well.'" But no one talked about it—especially at church. "For me," Ann says, "the result was a lot of fear, anger, and shame that built up over the years. I developed a mantra rooted in a belief system that said, 'I must and I can take care of myself.'"

In retrospect, Ann sees that "most of my young adult and middle years were colored by bouts of depression." Depression became, in Winston Churchill's phrase, her "black dog."[4] "There were times," she says, "it felt like I had been banished to a dark and small dungeon or forced to drag a wagon of rocks with me at all times." Then, in her forties, things broke. She was married and juggling the demands of a career, family life, and a move. Her children were dealing with their own mental health challenges. At a church women's retreat, she found herself lying on the floor, sobbing, unable to move or talk. A group of friends sat with her, witnessing her pain, comforting her, not judging her. "You've opened the door," one said to her, gently but firmly. "Now you have to walk through it."

Ann began to see a counselor and grew to realize that "I entered my adult years with a measure of unresolved issues. My baggage was packed full. My

---

3. I am grateful to Ann and her husband Dave for telling their story to me and for giving permission to include their story in this book. Direct quotations are from a personal interview with Ann and Dave on June 3, 2022, as well as from an address that Ann and Dave gave to a church Sunday school class on May 1, 2016. Direct interview quotations are occasionally lightly edited for syntax and style.

4. Churchill himself borrowed this phrase from Samuel Johnson and used it most memorably in a 1911 letter to his wife. For further context, see Anthony M. Daniels and J. Allister Vale, "Did Sir Winston Churchill Suffer from the 'Black Dog'?," *Journal of the Royal Society of Medicine* 111 (2018): 394–406.

belief system needed an overhaul." She tried multiple medications, but they never seemed to help much. Seeing a therapist helped more. But her greatest "light through those years" was that "I was blessed by people who loved me well and drew alongside and offered their presence." She also recovered a hunger for Scripture, "where I discovered the stories of God and his people to be my own." "I was blessed to be led and taught and changed and healed through those years of circling," she says.

> I unpacked my baggage from my childhood and learned to dress myself in forgiveness and grace and mercy. I, like Lazarus, was called out of my tomb. My grave clothes were removed and I got used to the bright light. The Scriptures were alive to me and within me and I came to understand I couldn't and shouldn't "do it myself."

Ann clung to the promise of Isaiah 62:

> You will be a crown of splendor in the LORD's hand,
>   a royal diadem in the hand of your God.
> No longer will they call you Deserted,
>   or name your land Desolate.
> But you will be called Hephzibah.[5]

Now in her late sixties, recently retired from a career in business, Ann still lives with the "black dog." She has learned to live with it, but that does not mean that things are easy. She remains a "glass-half-empty kind of person," and bouts of depression continue to plague her at times. But some challenges have been too great, and some losses have been beyond fixing. Ann's son, a talented artist and musician, died young after a struggle with depression and addiction that was complex and never fully resolved. Ann and her husband Dave are still grieving. There is blessing in their lives, and also pain. And in the midst of the blessing and the pain, they live in hope.

Mental Health in an Anxious Age

Mental health problems all too often reflect a fragmented and anxious age.
Some headlines and reports are personal. News organizations have reported

---

5. Isaiah 62:3–4 NIV. Hephzibah means "my delight is in her."

on the deaths by suicide of public figures such as Robin Williams, Kate Spade, Naomi Judd, Anthony Bourdain, and David Foster Wallace. They report on the many leaders and public figures who have stepped forward courageously to tell their stories of living with psychological struggle and mental illness: professional basketball players Kevin Love and Jeremy Lin, gymnast Simone Biles, actor Carrie Fisher, and many others.

Some headlines and reports reflect concerning population trends. The rate of deaths by suicide in the United States, stable for decades, rose over 35 percent between 2000 and 2018 before trending slightly down since then. Over 47,600 Americans died by suicide in 2021.[6] An even higher number of Americans, approximately 100,000, died of drug overdose in 2021, largely from opioids like heroin and fentanyl.[7] Despite substantial investment in mental health services for US military veterans, US veterans continue to die by suicide at higher rates than the general population: although veterans comprise 6 percent of the US population, veterans comprised 13.4 percent of deaths by suicide in 2020 (6,146 veteran deaths by suicide, or nearly seventeen per day).[8] On US college and university campuses, students are seeking mental health services at record levels and self-reporting mental health problems more and more each year. In a national survey, the percentage of American college students who reported on a national survey that they had "seriously considered suicide" doubled from 6 percent to 12 percent between 2011 and 2019.[9]

These troubling trends fit into a larger narrative of a mental health crisis in our contemporary culture. Research in both the United States and other countries suggests that mental health challenges are pervasive and costly. In

6. S. C. Curtin, M. F. Garnett, and F. B. Ahmad, "Provisional Numbers and Rates of Suicide by Month and Demographic Characteristics: United States, 2021," National Center for Health Statistics, Vital Statistics Rapid Release 24, September 2022, https://dx.doi.org/10.15620/cdc:120830.

7. "Vital Statistics Rapid Release Provisional Drug Overdose Death Counts," Centers for Disease Control and Prevention, https://www.cdc.gov/nchs/nvss/vsrr/drug-overdose-data.htm.

8. "2022 National Veteran Suicide Prevention Annual Report," Office of Mental Health and Suicide Prevention, Department of Veterans Affairs, September 2022, https://www.mentalhealth.va.gov/docs/data-sheets/2022/2022-National-Veteran-Suicide-Prevention-Annual-Report-FINAL-508.pdf. Number of US deaths from suicide in 2020 (45,979) obtained from Curtin, Garnett, and Ahmad, "Provisional Numbers."

9. Data are from the "National College Health Assessment," American College Health Association, https://www.acha.org/NCHA/ACHA-NCHA_Data/Publications_and_Reports/NCHA/Data/Publications_and_Reports.aspx?hkey=d5fb767c-d15d-4efc-8c41-3546d92032c5.

2016, over sixteen million American adults met psychiatry's diagnostic criteria for an acute major depressive episode.[10] Over ninety million Americans have met the criteria for an anxiety disorder over the course of our lives.[11] The World Health Organization has stated that depression is the "single largest contributor to global disability."[12] Around 46 percent of the American population—over 150 million people—will meet the criteria for a mental disorder at some point in our lives.

Two Ways of Speaking about Mental Health Problems

Our culture has two distinct ways of speaking about mental health problems. The first takes the form of narrative and story. It involves stories of people like Ann making their way amid challenge, heartache, promise, and grace. This way is rich in nuance and lived experience. The second way, in contrast, takes the form of statistics, data, and labels. This is the language of psychiatric diagnosis, epidemiology, and public health reports.

To be sure, the language of statistics, data, and diagnostic labels has its uses. It allows us to group together people with similar experiences in order to offer them particular treatments. It also sheds powerful and unsentimental light on how many people suffer and struggle in our culture. In the United States, nearly one in three women and one in six men have experienced some form of sexual violence involving physical touch,[13] and 20 percent of these

10. "Key Substance Use and Mental Health Indicators in the United States: Results from the 2016 National Survey on Drug Use and Health (HHS Publication No. SMA 17-5044, NS-DUH Series H-52)," Substance Abuse and Mental Health Services Administration (Rockville, MD: Center for Behavioral Health Statistics and Quality, Substance Abuse and Mental Health Services Administration, 2017), https://www.samhsa.gov/data/.

11. This number is extrapolated from a current US population of 325,000,000 and a *DSM-IV* lifetime prevalence rate for all anxiety disorders of 28.8 percent in Ronald C. Kessler et al., "Lifetime Prevalence and Age-of-Onset Distributions of DSM-IV Disorders in the National Comorbidity Survey Replication," *Archives of General Psychiatry* 62 (2005): 593-60, using the assumption that anxiety disorder prevalence has not decreased since the NCS-R was conducted in 2001-2003.

12. See p. 5 of "Depression and Other Common Mental Disorders: Global Health Estimates," World Health Organization, 2017, http://apps.who.int/iris/bitstream/handle/10665/254610/WHO-MSD-MER-2017.2-eng.pdf.

13. S. G. Smith et al., *The National Intimate Partner and Sexual Violence Survey (NISVS): 2010–2012 State Report* (Atlanta: National Center for Injury Prevention and Control, Centers for Disease Control and Prevention, 2017).

survivors live with post-traumatic stress disorder (PTSD).[14] Around 23 percent of US combat veterans of the wars in Iraq and Afghanistan live with PTSD.[15] These statistics should warn us against any glorification of American childhood, family life, or war. Understanding that one in twenty-five American adults meets criteria for bipolar disorder should unsettle any presumption that depression and mania are rare. Numbers like these make clear that human suffering and human challenges riddle the everyday world, though often behind closed doors and known only to a few others, if at all. They also tell those living with mental illness, "You are not alone."

But there is a cost to prioritizing the language of data, diagnosis, and symptoms over the language of context and story. Terms like *major depressive disorder*, *bipolar disorder*, and *post-traumatic stress disorder* arrived only recently. They are terms that were coined and promoted by psychiatrists and others in order to name what mental health clinicians are attempting to treat. When we apply these terms to our experience, this does more than simply *name* our experience. These labels also *shape* and *construct* our experience and our understanding of ourselves. They teach us to interpret human suffering and challenge through the language of mental illness, and to seek remedy through mental health care.

Mental health care has always named a complex, shifting, and often fragmented collection of practices, institutions, and practitioners addressing mental health needs in the population. These *structures* of mental health care require the *language* of mental health care for their legitimacy and their function. The language of mental health care—particularly the language of psychiatric diagnosis—gives form to mental health practices and institutions, and these practices and institutions likewise promote and legitimize the power of mental health language.

In this book, I critically examine some common practices and ways of speaking within the world of modern mental health care and propose how Christians might faithfully engage this world. I am a psychiatrist who for two decades has worked in the US Department of Veterans Affairs health care system and who has served as a resident and now a psychiatry faculty

14. K. M. Scott et al., "Post-traumatic Stress Disorder Associated with Sexual Assault among Women in the WHO World Mental Health Surveys," *Psychological Medicine* 48 (2018): 155–67.

15. Jessica J. Fulton et al., "The Prevalence of Posttraumatic Stress Disorder in Operation Enduring Freedom/Operation Iraqi Freedom (OEF/OIF) Veterans: A Meta-analysis," *Journal of Anxiety Disorders* 31 (2015): 98–107.

member at a large academic medical center.[16] Though Ann is not my patient, I have had the privilege of walking alongside hundreds of patients navigating similarly challenging mental health problems, many with elements in their story that resonate strongly with Ann's. As a psychiatrist, I am also a core participant in the mental health care system. My institution considers me a "mental health provider."

In addition, I am a Christian who is trained in theological ethics and now teaches at a Christian divinity school. As a Christian psychiatrist, I recognize that it is a privilege to work with those who seek my care. I feel a deep sense of calling and responsibility to care well for them, practicing psychiatry with excellence and integrity. (I know that many of my colleagues who are not Christian believe and feel the same way.)

But as a Christian, I see problems with mental health care as it is practiced in the United States and in many industrialized nations. It is not because psychiatry is somehow intrinsically anti-Christian, though it is true that some prominent early psychiatrists and psychologists like Sigmund Freud and John Broadus Watson sharply criticized Christianity, and that psychiatrists are still least likely of all physicians to identify as religious or as Christian.[17] In my experience, mental health clinicians these days see value in religious practice and belief and often are people of faith themselves. The problem is rather that psychiatry, the most person-focused and holistic of medical specialties, is all too often remarkably *im*personal. Patients come to us with deep and inchoate wounds, confusing experiences, and longings that they sometimes cannot name. We then virtually dissect and classify them, not into organs and tissues as a surgeon might, but into categories of symptoms that can be organized into diagnoses to which particular interventions can be applied. Patients come to us with suffering and with complex stories, and we are trained to see them as clusters of symptoms. On bad days, my work feels mechanical, like I am part of a big industrial process that fixes broken machines.

This would probably bother me even if I were not a Christian. I know that it bothers many of my colleagues. But it bothers me as a Christian because in the perspective of Christian faith, humans are not machines and should never

---

16. It is important to note that all of the views and opinions expressed in this book are my own and do not represent the views of the Durham VA Medical Center, the US Department of Veterans Affairs, or the Department of Psychiatry and Behavioral Sciences of Duke University Medical Center.

17. Farr A. Curlin et al., "The Relationship between Psychiatry and Religion among U.S. Physicians," *Psychiatric Services* 58 (2007): 1193–98.

be treated as machines. Humans are good, beloved creatures of God, bearing God's image, created for union with God.

In this book, I argue that important segments of modern mental health care, and especially my own field of psychiatry, operate according to what I call the machine metaphor. The machine metaphor, with roots going back at least to the 1600s, has deeply shaped the history of medicine, psychiatry, and psychology. The metaphor reflects a working assumption that the body and often the mind can be understood as machines. As machines, they can break down, giving rise to unwanted or disvalued experiences and behaviors that are labeled as symptoms. These symptoms indicate the presence of an underlying mental disorder, a dysfunction in the mind-body machine. Those with symptoms of such dysfunction are expected to seek the care of experts—mental health clinicians—who can observe the symptoms, infer the presence of one or more underlying disorders, and apply relevant interventions to ameliorate the symptoms. Treatments—whether physical technologies like pharmaceuticals or verbal technologies like structured forms of psychotherapy—are considered successful if they reduce symptoms in a reasonably reliable way across a population of people with the same disorder. Like all technologies, these interventions can be bought and sold.

The machine metaphor has sparked the development of remarkable and even life-saving mental health treatments, yet it leaves many longing for something more. In this book, I draw on the work of Saint Thomas Aquinas, the thirteenth-century philosopher, theologian, teacher, priest, and Dominican friar, to argue that the machine metaphor needs to be replaced with the Christian image of the human being as a wayfarer who journeys from God to God—always seeking, always loving, always on the way. In this image, mental health clinicians and those who seek care would ask not, "What is broken that needs fixing?" but rather "What is needed, right now, for the journey?" Humans are not machines in need of technological repair. We are wayfarers who need and deserve to be attended, nurtured, guided, and loved as we find our way forward together.[18]

18. In this work, I draw on and am indebted to authors and researchers who have modeled thick Christian theological consideration of personhood as it relates to mental health problems and mental health care. I have learned from first person memoirs such as David Finnegan-Hosey, *Christ on the Psych Ward* (New York: Church Publishing, 2018); Kathryn Greene-McCreight, *Darkness Is My Only Companion: A Christian Response to Mental Illness* (Grand Rapids: Brazos, 2015); and Monica Coleman, *Bipolar Faith: A Black Woman's Journey with Depression and Faith* (Minneapolis: Fortress, 2016). I look to the models of broader theological considerations of mental health in works such as John Swinton, *Resurrecting the*

This book is motivated by my own love for and deep dissatisfaction with the work of psychiatry, my corner of the mental health world. On one hand, the work of psychiatry braces me with the profoundness of its object, the human person. As a psychiatrist I attend and accompany people through the heights and depths of their lives. People tell me stories of joy, pain, triumph, and heartache that they might not disclose to anyone else. And yet the work of psychiatry frequently fails to match the dignity of those whom it seeks to serve.

I believe the approach outlined in this book can go a long way toward rendering psychiatry not only more healing but more meaningful both for clinicians and for those who seek our care. These principles have helped to sustain my own joy. But complex barriers get in the way: the requirement to see patients in isolation, as individuals; the mistaken assumption that one can speak intelligibly of mental health without a shared framework of understanding what human life is for; the presumption that negative emotions should be brought under technological control and that patients alone determine how and when this is to happen; the commoditization of care in quantifiable, remunerable units; the systemic treatment of adverse outcomes such as attempted or completed suicide as either clinician-specific practice failures or system engineering failures, rather than as tragedies to be lamented; and on and on.

In place of these dysfunctional symptoms of the machine metaphor, I have been captured by a vision of the human as a beloved, relational wayfarer—not

Person: Friendship and the Care of People with Mental Health Problems (Nashville: Abingdon, 2000); John Swinton, *Dementia: Living in the Memories of God* (Grand Rapids: Eerdmans, 2012); Swinton, *Finding Jesus in the Storm: The Spiritual Lives of Christians with Mental Health Challenges* (Grand Rapids: Eerdmans, 2020); Eric Johnson, *Foundations for Soul Care: A Christian Psychology Proposal* (Downers Grove, IL: InterVarsity Press, 2007); Marcia Webb, *Toward a Theology of Psychological Disorder* (Eugene, OR: Cascade, 2017); Jessica Coblentz, *Dust in the Blood: A Theology of Life with Depression* (Collegeville, MN: Liturgical Press, 2022); and Matthew LaPine, *The Logic of the Body: Retrieving Theological Psychology* (Bellingham, WA: Lexham, 2020). For work on Aquinas's account of psychology, I draw on Robert Edward Brennan's classic *Thomistic Psychology: A Philosophic Analysis of the Nature of Man* (New York: Macmillan, 1941), as well as more recent work, such as that which has been generated through the collaborations of the Institute for the Psychological Sciences of Divine Mercy University, including Romanus Cessario, Craig Steven Titus, and Paul C. Vitz, eds., *Philosophical Virtues and Psychological Strengths: Building the Bridge* (Manchester, NH: Sophia Institute Press, 2013); Benedict M. Ashley, *Healing for Freedom: A Christian Perspective on Personhood and Psychotherapy* (Arlington, VA: Institute for the Psychological Sciences Press, 2013); and Paul C. Vitz, William J. Nordling, and Craig Steven Titus, eds., *A Catholic Christian Meta-model of the Human Person: Integration of Psychology and Mental Health Practice* (Sterling, VA: Divine Mercy University Press, 2020).

a mechanism but a creature, not a sufferer of symptoms but a bearer of stories, not a consumer or a service user but, in the best sense, a patient, one who reclines into a secure and trusting relationship with a healer. This change of vision makes all the difference in how we understand and respond to mental health challenges.

The Practices and Institutions of Modern Mental Health Care

First, some background. How did the complex, shifting, and often fragmented collection of practices, institutions, and practitioners we call mental health care come to be? Though a detailed history lies beyond the scope of this book, several trends that have characterized mental health care over the past half century deserve attention.

Historical Trends

First, since the 1950s, the site of treatment for serious mental illness has moved away from psychiatric hospitals (especially large state institutions) toward community care, which in practice names a fragmented network of outpatient clinics, case management services, group homes, and other small institutions. In 1955, there were 558,239 inpatients in public psychiatric hospitals in the United States. By 1994, that number had dropped to 71,619, even as the US population grew 58 percent (a more than 95 percent reduction per capita).[19] The United States had approximately 170,000 inpatient hospital beds in 2014, roughly 77 percent fewer per capita than in 1970.[20] These changes were driven in part by the availability of antipsychotic medication starting with the introduction of chlorpromazine (Thorazine) in France in 1952 and in the United States in 1954, in part by commitments to reform state institutions that had become overcrowded and dehumanizing, and in part by forward-looking government programs such as the Community Mental Health Act

19. E. Fuller Torrey, *Out of the Shadows: Confronting America's Mental Illness Crisis* (New York: Wiley & Sons, 1997), 207, available in excerpted form at "Deinstitutionalization: A Psychiatric Titanic,'" *Frontline*, https://www.pbs.org/wgbh/pages/frontline/shows/asylums/special/excerpt.html.

20. "Trend in Psychiatric Inpatient Capacity, United States and Each State, 1970 to 2014," National Association of State Mental Health Program Directors, August 2017, https://www.nri-inc.org/media/1319/tac-paper-10-psychiatric-inpatient-capacity-final-09-05-2017.pdf.

of 1963 designed to fund and to grow community care. But the changes also were facilitated by states' desire to curtail their budgets allocated to mental health, and funding for outpatient mental health services did not keep pace with reductions in inpatient beds. As a result, people with serious mental illness often either lack mental health care entirely or are faced with under-staffed and overstretched mental health agencies that cannot meet their needs. One especially and frequently noted by-product of the closure of inpatient mental health beds is that people living with serious mental illness are at risk of chronic homelessness—more than 50 percent of unhoused people live with a chronic psychotic disorder, mood disorder, or substance use disorder—and of incarceration.[21] Currently, the largest inpatient institutions in the United States providing treatment for people with serious mental illness are the Cook County Jail in Chicago, the Los Angeles County Jail, and Rikers Island Jail in New York City.[22]

The second major trend is that since the Second World War, outpatient mental health services have expanded rapidly. In part, they have expanded to absorb the shift away from inpatient care, but they have also expanded in response to rising demand for mental health services from those who never would have been admitted to psychiatric institutions. Even in the first half of the twentieth century, psychiatrists and psychoanalysts practicing in the tradition of Freud were seeing patients in outpatient practices. But after the war, these were joined by a wide range of other practitioners in marketing and offering mental health services, including clinical psychologists (who emerged to meet the psychological needs of Second World War veterans in the late 1940s),[23] mental health social workers, pastoral counselors, licensed professional counselors, and others.

Third, as demand for mental health services has grown and as general health care expenditures have increased dramatically in recent decades, mental health care has become increasingly regulated by business models and structured by the demands of third-party payers in the United States and by government health systems in the United States and in other industrialized nations. Employer-sponsored health insurance plans in the United States, which formed during the Second World War as a way to incentivize domestic workers

---

21. Adriana Foster, James Gable, and John Buckley, "Homelessness in Schizophrenia," *Psychiatric Clinics of North America* 35 (2012): 717–34.

22. Alisa Roth, *Insane: America's Criminal Treatment of Mental Illness* (New York: Basic Books, 2018).

23. Ludy T. Benjamin, "A History of Clinical Psychology as a Profession in America (and a Glimpse of Its Future)," *Annual Review of Clinical Psychology* 1 (2005): 1–30.

in an era of wartime pay freezes but became a dominant way of funding health care in the postwar era,[24] slowly began covering outpatient psychiatric services.[25] Medicare and Medicaid, beginning in 1965, became important sources of funding for mental health care for the elderly and poor and for people living with disabilities. In the 1970s and 1980s, insurance plans and government funders began placing additional requirements and limits on mental health services, often limiting psychotherapy sessions, identifying preferred formularies for medications, and requiring preapproval by a company official for payment for any mental health services. Mental health services were often disproportionately limited and carved out of standard insurance policies, because until the Mental Health Parity and Addiction Equity Act of 2008 and the Patient Protection and Affordable Care Act of 2010, there was no meaningful, enforceable requirement for insurance companies to fund mental health care at a level consistent with funding for other kinds of medical services (mental health parity).[26]

Fourth, in recent decades and notably since the 1970s, mental health care has been dominated by medical models of care, with a focus on individuals. It is true that mental health care has always, by definition, been framed to some degree in medical concepts and language. It is also true that dominant models of mental illness in the United States and Europe in the late nineteenth and early twentieth centuries (Sigmund Freud's psychoanalytic ideas notwithstanding) were biological, often focused on somatic treatments such as insulin coma therapy and electroshock therapy. As we will explore in chapter 1, even Freud was a neurologist by training who worked for a time at the famed Salpetrière Hospital in Paris under the eminent neurologist Jean-Marie Charcot, and who wrote an early mechanistic work titled *Project for a Scientific Psychology*.[27] But it was also the case that the large asylums that came to dominate early twentieth-century care for persons with serious mental illness were

24. Aaron E. Carroll, "The Real Reason the U.S. Has Employer-Sponsored Health Insurance," *New York Times*, September 5, 2017, https://www.nytimes.com/2017/09/05/upshot/the-real-reason-the-us-has-employer-sponsored-health-insurance.html.

25. M. S. Ridgely and H. H. Goldman, "Mental Health Insurance," *Handbook on Mental Health Policy in the United States*, ed. D. A. Rochefort (Westport, CT: Greenwood, 1989), 341–62.

26. "The Mental Health Parity and Addiction Equity Act (MHPAEA)," Centers for Medicare and Medicaid Services, https://www.cms.gov/CCIIO/Programs-and-Initiatives/Other-Insurance-Protections/mhpaea_factsheet.

27. Sigmund Freud, "Project for a Scientific Psychology," in *The Standard Edition of the Complete Psychological Works of Sigmund Freud*, vol. 1, *Pre-Psychoanalytic Publications and Unpublished Drafts (1886–1899)* (London: Hogarth, 1966).

more than sites of medical intervention. In a time of large inpatient populations and long lengths of stay, they were centers of community, providers of
housing and shelter, and opportunities for meaningful work. Patients in these
institutions might see their attending psychiatrist once every few weeks—not
unlike the frequency of visits in outpatient settings today. In the early years of
deinstitutionalization, there were strong voices that the community, not the
clinic, was the appropriate incubator of mental health, and a tradition of social
psychiatry emphasized the role of communities in causing and also in curing
mental health problems.[28] Though community-oriented and group-oriented
approaches to mental health still exist and thrive in some contexts, modern
mental health care is now framed primarily in individualistic and medicalized
ways, with group therapy and community interventions understood as treatments *for individuals* and as adjuncts to whatever individualized treatments
a patient is prescribed. In part, this is related to the tremendous growth of
prescriptions of psychiatric medications over the last decades and extensive
marketing and promotion by the pharmaceutical industry not only of medications but also of the medical conditions for which they are prescribed. But
it also relates to conscious decisions by leaders in American psychiatry to
position psychiatry as a medical discipline that steers clear of political and
social critique,[29] and to the increasing alignment of mental health funding
with broader structures of health care reimbursement. Social psychiatry, as
it existed within American psychiatry in the 1960s, has now virtually disap-
peared.[30] People who seek mental health treatment nowadays mostly do so as
individuals, for conditions that they have, and for which individually tailored
treatment is prescribed and administered.

Mental Health Care Today

More than ever, modern mental health care is a complex and fragmented collection of practices, institutions, and practitioners, with high degrees of vari-
ability in geographic distribution, accessibility, and practices. For those who
can access them, there is an ever-expanding array of treatment options for all

---

28. Dan Blazer, *The Age of Melancholy: "Major Depression" and Its Social Origins* (New
York: Routledge, 2005), 59-76.
29. Hannah Decker, *The Making of DSM-III®: A Diagnostic Manual's Conquest of American Psychiatry* (New York: Oxford University Press, 2013).
30. Blazer, *Age of Melancholy*, 77-93.

forms of mental health conditions. Modes and practices of psychotherapy become ever more diverse as new practices are developed and tailored. Freudian psychoanalysis, always diverse and internally contentious, has given rise to newer analytic treatments such as mentalization-based treatment for borderline personality disorder and accelerated experiential dynamic psychotherapy (AEDP).[31] Traditional behavior therapy and cognitive behavioral therapy (CBT) is now complemented by a wide array of psychotherapy systems such as acceptance and commitment therapy (ACT) and mindfulness-based cognitive therapy (MBCT) that draw on cognitive-behavioral principles and often merge these principles with different philosophical or psychological systems. Many newer approaches target specific diagnostic categories, such as dialectical behavior therapy (DBT) for borderline personality disorder and cognitive processing therapy (CPT) for PTSD. Some newer modes of psychotherapy, such as DBT, feature group components in addition to individual therapy. Others are entirely group based, such as interpersonal group therapy (IPT-G). Psychotherapy is administered by a wide array of clinicians, including clinical psychologists (PhD or PsyD), therapists who are social workers, substance use counselors, marriage and family therapists, licensed counselors, psychiatrists, and pastoral counselors.

Medications also are used widely for the treatment of mental health problems. In the 2013 Medical Expenditure Panel Survey, 16.7 percent of American adults (including 11.9 percent of men and 21.2 percent of women) reported that they had filled a prescription for a medication used to treat anxiety, insomnia, bipolar disorder, or psychosis in the previous year.[32] Antidepressants, which in practice are used to treat a wide range of depression, anxiety, insomnia, and emotional lability, were the most commonly prescribed class of medication among US adults age 40-59 in 2016-2017; 15.4 percent of adults in this age range endorsed having been prescribed antidepressants in the previous thirty days.[33] Approximately 15-20 percent of adults in the United States and United Kingdom take a prescription medication to prevent or to alter unwanted ex-

31. On treatment for borderline personality disorder, see Peter Fonagy et al., *Affect Regulation, Mentalization, and the Development of the Self* (New York: Other, 2002), and for AEDP, see Diana Fosha, *The Transforming Power of Affect: A Model for Accelerated Change* (New York: Basic Books, 2000).

32. Thomas J. Moore and Donald R. Mattison, "Adult Utilization of Psychiatric Drugs and Differences by Sex, Age, and Race," *JAMA Internal Medicine* 177 (2017): 274-75.

33. Craig M. Hales et al., "Prescription Drug Use among Adults Aged 40-79 in the United States and Canada (NCHS Data Brief, no. 347)," Centers for Disease Control and Prevention (Hyattsville, MD: National Center for Health Statistics, 2019), https://www.cdc.gov

perience and behavior. Although psychiatrists, mental health nurse practitioners (NPs), and mental health physician assistants (PAs) have specialized training in the use of psychiatric medications and routinely prescribe them, most antidepressant and antianxiety medications in the United States are prescribed not by psychiatrists but by primary care clinicians, who prescribed nearly 75 percent of antidepressants in the early 2000s.[34]

Access to these treatment options varies widely by geography and socioeconomic status. A 2014 study of office-based American physicians found that only 43.1 percent of psychiatrists surveyed in 2009–2010 accepted Medicaid, only 54.8 percent accepted Medicare, and only 55.3 percent accepted any private noncapitated insurance plans, including employer-sponsored private plans. Effectively, many psychiatrists require patients either to be wealthy enough to pay the psychiatrist's fees out of pocket or resourceful enough to submit their expenses to their insurance companies for partial out-of-network reimbursement.[35] Similarly, those who seek psychotherapy must either pay therapists out of pocket or submit to the limits of their insurance plans regulating numbers of sessions and rates of payment. Many parts of the United States, particularly rural areas, have very few mental health practitioners. Even in highly resourced urban areas, demand for mental health services often exceeds supply, forcing people in psychological distress to search extensively for what they need.

In practice, American mental health care is less a rational system than a confusing consumer market, marked by all of the inequalities and complications of modern market economies. Some people seeking mental health services develop meaningful therapeutic relationships and benefit from high-quality treatments. Some engage in frustrating, lengthy searches for the right clinical care, navigating many procedural, geographic, and financial hurdles in the process. Some find themselves shunted from more resource-intensive therapies (e.g., weekly individual psychotherapy with a clinician) to less resource-intensive therapies (e.g., antidepressant medication prescribed by a primary care physician). And many others find themselves unable to access mental health services at all.

/nchs/products/databriefs/db347.htm#:~:text=Nearly%207%20in%2010%20adults,and%2018.8%25%20in%20Canada).

34. Ramin Mojtabai and Mark Olfson, "National Patterns in Antidepressant Treatment by Psychiatrists and General Medical Providers: Results from the National Comorbidity Survey Replication," *Journal of Clinical Psychiatry* 69 (2008): 1064–74.

35. Tara F. Bishop et al., "Acceptance of Insurance by Psychiatrists and the Implications for Access to Mental Health Care," *JAMA Psychiatry* 71 (2014): 176–81.

From Machines to Wayfarers, with Aquinas as Guide

In chapter 1 of this book, I present a historical and conceptual account of the machine metaphor in modern mental health care. The machine metaphor is characterized by the logic of the mechanization of the body, the mechanization of the mind, the standardization of diagnosis, and the industrialization of care. The metaphor is perpetuated by five presumptions that are at times therapeutically and practically helpful but that have serious negative consequences in the long run: individualism and internalism, self-symptom dualism, self-body dualism, technicism, and commodification. In the remaining chapters of the book, I draw on Scripture, philosophy, psychology, and (sometimes closely and sometimes more loosely) on the thought of Thomas Aquinas to inform a different vision of mental health care, focused not on the machine metaphor but on the image of the human as wayfarer.

Why Aquinas? What does a thirteenth-century medieval friar and theologian who lived and wrote before the rise of modern science have to offer to contemporary conversations about mental health care? I have chosen Thomas Aquinas as a central conversation partner in the latter chapters of this book not only because he captured my imagination at a critical period of my own study but also because his work embodies the kind of interdisciplinary intersections of theology, philosophy, psychology, and natural science that are critical for making sense of the practices and concepts of modern mental health care. Born around 1225 as the youngest son in a wealthy southern Italian family, Aquinas was designated by custom and tradition to serve the church, likely as a Benedictine monk at the nearby abbey of Monte Cassino. At the recently founded University of Naples, he was exposed not only to Christian thought but also to Greek and Roman philosophical, scientific, and medical ideas that had been interpreted and developed not only in Latin Christian Europe but also in Islamic centers of learning in Persia, Baghdad, Cairo, North Africa, and Spain. Entering adulthood, he shocked his family by pledging himself to a newly founded and countercultural order of itinerant, mendicant friars, the Order of Preachers, founded by the Spanish priest Dominic in the early 1200s and known to us as the Dominican Order. Bound to the Dominican commitments to study, preaching, teaching, and itineracy, and focused on cities rather than on rural monasteries, Aquinas continued his education at the universities of Paris and Cologne, where he studied under the Dominican philosopher, naturalist, physician, and theologian Saint Albert the Great (Albertus Magnus, who lived ca. 1200–1280). Completing the grueling medieval process of theological education in his early thirties, Aquinas was named a *magister in sacra pagina* (master of biblical sciences, or what we would now call a master of theology) in 1256, and spent most of the remainder of his brief life assigned by his Dominican superiors to teach and to study at the universities of Paris, Orvieto, and Naples (see figure 1).[36]

In just over two decades, from his late twenties until his death in his late forties, Aquinas wrote and dictated a massive body of scholarship. He produced numerous commentaries on books of Scripture, commentaries on the works of Aristotle and Boethius, philosophical treatises that were prompted by active disputes in his time, and three major overviews of Christian thought. The first is an extended commentary on the *Sentences* of Peter Lombard (ca. 1252–1254), the standard theological textbook of his time. The second is the *Summa contra Gentiles* (ca. 1258–1265), loosely translated as a "summary [of philosophy and theology] to oppose the pagans," which begins with systematic philosophical argument and ends with an exposition of revealed Christian doctrine and may have been intended to equip Dominican friars for mission work. The third, widely considered the most developed expression of Aquinas's mature thought, is the unfinished *Summa theologiae* (ca. 1265–1274), loosely translated as "summary of theology" and intended as an introductory textbook for advanced students of theology.[37]

Though I occasionally draw on Aquinas's other writings, including prayers and hymns attributed to him, the *Summa theologiae* (or *Summa* for short) is

---

36. Jean-Pierre Torrell, *Saint Thomas Aquinas*, vol. 1, *The Person and His Work*, rev. ed., trans. Robert Royal (Washington, DC: Catholic University of America Press, 2005); Torrell, *Aquinas' Summa: Background, Structure, and Reception*, trans. Benedict M. Guevin (Washington, DC: Catholic University of America Press, 2005).

37. Thomas Aquinas, *Summa theologiae*, part 1, prologue (*STh* Ia *proem.*). Hereafter, the title will be abbreviated as *STh*, followed by customary citations. All quotations from the *Summa theologiae*, unless otherwise noted, are from the 1911 translation Saint Thomas Aquinas, *Summa Theologica*, 5 vols., trans. Fathers of the English Dominican Province (New York: Benziger, 1948; repr., Notre Dame: Christian Classics, 1981). I generally refer to the 1911 translation rather than to the more recent Blackfriars translation (Saint Thomas Aquinas, *Summa Theologiae*, 61 vols. [Cambridge: Cambridge University Press, 1964; repr., Cambridge, Cambridge University Press, 2006]) due to ease of access and because of the internal consistency of translation in the 1911 edition compared to the Blackfriars translation. While Thomas states that the *Summa* was written for the instruction of "beginners" (*incipientes*), it is likely that this refers to advanced Dominican learners who already had broad exposure in Aristotelian logic and the study of Scripture. See Reinhard Hütter, *Bound for Beatitude: A Thomistic Study in Eschatology and Ethics* (Washington, DC: Catholic University of America Press, 2019), 113.

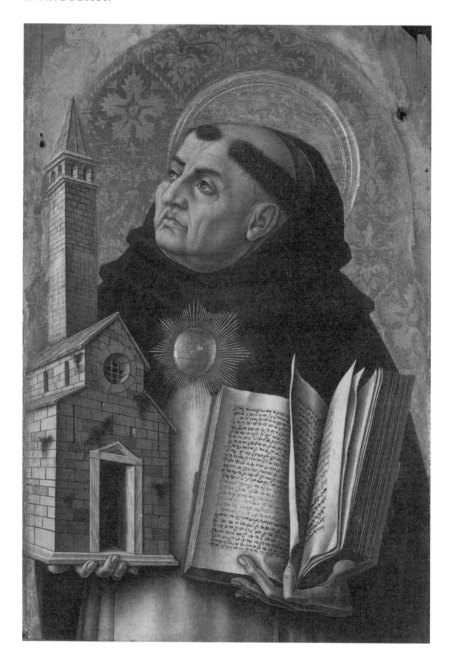

Figure 1. Carlo Crivelli, *Saint Thomas Aquinas*, 1476, National Gallery, London

the primary source for the argument of this book. The *Summa*, which was left unfinished at the time of Aquinas's death, is comprised of 512 questions that are divided into 2,669 articles, each of which poses a philosophical or theological question, considers various alternatives, and argues for an answer along with responses to the various alternatives. In the *Summa*, Aquinas paints a magisterial picture of God as the source and end of creation (see table 1). In the First Part, he speaks of God and the procession of creatures, including human beings, from God. In the Second Part, he speaks of human beings as wayfarers (*viatores*) on the way to God, first by a systematic exposition of human psychology, the virtues, and the work of sin, law, and grace, and then by a detailed description of the various embodied dispositions to action (virtues and vices) that enable or impede the wayfarer's journey. In the unfinished Third Part, he speaks of Christ as the way to God, and the sacraments as God's way of channeling grace to us. If the multivolume *Summa* were to be condensed to five sentences, it might be as follows: Like all creatures, human beings are from God. Unique among all creatures, human beings are equipped to know God, to love God, and to order our lives in God. We find our deepest fulfillment in union with God. We are wayfarers on the way. Jesus Christ, mediated through the sacraments, *is* the way.

I am drawn to Thomas as a source for this book because, as a premodern thinker who wrote before the dawn of modern mechanistic science, he displays in his thought a vision of human beings not as machines but as creatures, image-bearers, knowers, lovers, and wayfarers. His Aristotelian account of the relation of body and soul stands in stark contrast both to the mind-body dualism of Descartes and to modern forms of materialism that reduce mind and soul to body and matter. He offers a vision of human flourishing that is rooted in union with God marked by agency and freedom. He persistently draws readers to Scripture and to Jesus as the exemplar of what it means to live fully as human beings.[38] He offers a practical, life-giving, and detailed account of habits and virtues as helps for the journey, embodied dispositions to know and to do what brings happiness and freedom. And his thought and life are marked by a stance of wonder.[39] Aquinas's biographer Reginald of Piperno wrote shortly after his death that near the end of his life, Aquinas had some

---

38. Nicholas Healy, *Thomas Aquinas: Theologian of the Christian Life* (Burlington, VT: Ashgate, 2003).

39. In his *Commentary on the Sentences*, Aquinas writes that "the last end of this *doctrina* is the contemplation of the primary truth in the heavenly homeland." *In I Sent.* Pro., a. 3 sol. 1 and *ad1*; quoted in Jean-Pierre Torrell, *Saint Thomas Aquinas*, vol. 2, *Spiritual Master*, trans. Robert Royal (Washington, DC: Catholic University of America Press, 2003), 17.

sort of vision and remarked to his companions, "I cannot write any longer. All that I have written is but straw compared to what I have seen." He did not write much after that. His prodigious scholarly life, so full of words, ended in silence and wonder.[40]

Table 1. *Structure of Thomas Aquinas's* Summa theologiae

Part	Themes	Content
Ia (First Part, *Prima pars*)	Nature of sacred doctrine, God, creation, human nature, "God and creation"	Nature of sacred doctrine (q. 1) God's existence (q. 2) God's attributes and nature (qq. 3–43) God's work in creation (qq. 44–74) God's creation of human beings (qq. 75–102) Divine government (qq. 103–119)
IIa (Second Part, *Secunda pars*)	The rational creature (human) as a wayfarer returning to God	IaIIae (First Part of the Second Part, *Prima secundae partis*) Happiness (qq. 1–5) Human action and agency (qq. 6–21) The passions (qq. 23–48) Habits and virtues (qq. 49–70) Vice and sin (qq. 71–89) Law and grace (qq. 90–114) IIaIIae (Second Part of the Second Part, *Secunda secundae partis*) Faith (qq. 1–16) Hope (qq. 17–22) Charity (qq. 23–46) Prudence (qq. 47–56) Justice (qq. 57–122) Courage (qq. 123–140) Temperance (qq. 141–170) Particular vocations (qq. 171–189)

40. Denys Turner, *Thomas Aquinas: A Portrait* (New Haven: Yale University Press, 2013), 40–46; Josef Pieper, *The Silence of St. Thomas: Three Essays*, 3rd ed. (South Bend: Saint Augustine's, 1999); Torrell, *Saint Thomas Aquinas*, 1:289–93.

Part	Themes	Content
IIIa (Third Part, *Tertia pars*)	Christ, the way to God	Christ's nature (qq. 1–26) Christ's life (qq. 27–59) Sacraments (qq. 60–90 [unfinished]).

This book describes a vision of Christian engagement with mental health care with Aquinas as a guide.[41] In chapters 2 and 3, I argue that while Christian faith affirms that as creatures of dust we are bodies, it also affirms that we are always bodies in relation. We love, grow, and find ourselves in our relationships with God, with others, and with nonhuman creatures. This leads to a fundamentally biosocial and ecological account of being human. Mental health problems happen in the body but cannot be reduced to the body alone.

In chapters 4 and 5, I engage the complex manifestations of shame and stigma that hang like a cloud over many people with mental health challenges and also over many clinicians, and I argue that Christian faith offers powerful resources for engaging shame—most prominently in the central affirmation that before all else, we are known and loved by God. We are never alone, never left to generate the meaning of our lives. Further, Scripture teaches that humans are made in God's image and invited, by grace, to participate in the life of Jesus.

In chapters 6 through 8, I describe how Aquinas's vision of the human journey to God matters for engaging mental health care. In chapter 6, I compare modern conceptions of mental health with Aquinas's vision of *beatitudo*, often translated "happiness" or "flourishing" but more fruitfully understood as

41. Though not a guide in every way, Aquinas also embraced many views characteristic of his thirteenth-century culture that few of even the most committed Thomists would now defend. He held that while women are created in the image of God (chapter 5), men are more inclined to the use of reason than women (*STh* Ia q. 92 a. 1; q. 93 a. 4). He held that heretics deserved not only to be excommunicated but to be put to death because of their threat to the faithful (*STh* IIaIIae q. 11 a. 3). Aquinas is a theologian of the undivided (pre-Reformation) western church and an authority within the western Christian tradition. In the encyclical *Aeterni Patris* (1879), Pope Leo XIII recognized Aquinas as "master and prince" of the medieval theologians and recommended that Catholic teachers "do their best to instill the doctrine of Thomas Aquinas into the minds of their hearers; and let them clearly point out its solidity and excellence above all other teaching." But even for Catholic Christians, Aquinas must be read in the light of the ongoing teaching of the church.

"participation in blessing." Aquinas's concept of *beatitudo* shows how modern conceptions of mental health are too limited when compared with Aquinas's expansive vision of the soul's rest in God. In chapter 7, after discussing Aquinas's accounts of intellect and will, I describe contemporary debates about the nature of emotion and argue that for Aquinas, the emotions or passions are usually signs of love, helping us to understand whom or what we love and how to act in response. Even aversive emotions may need to be accepted and attended, prior to any attempt to eradicate or ameliorate them. In chapter 8, I turn to Aquinas's account of habit, virtue, and the gifts of the Spirit and argue that the virtues, aided by the gifts, are pathways to the forms of agency and freedom that are a central good of mental health care.

In chapter 9, I turn to the story of the man who lived in the tombs (Mark 5:1–20) and to Aquinas's account of two forms of life, the active life (*vita activa*) and the contemplative life (*vita contemplativa*), to argue that while control is a good of mental health care, it is not the highest good, and that the pursuit of control, if taken too far, can be self-defeating. What is ultimately needed is to move beyond the pursuit of control to the cultivation of wonder, which for Christians manifests itself in rest, Sabbath, play, worship, and praise.

In chapter 10, I consider Luke's account of the two grieving, weary disciples on the road to Emmaus who, unbeknownst to them, were accompanied by Jesus himself. These disciples recognized Jesus not in the information that he presented to them but in shared table fellowship and the blessing and breaking of bread. Healing is not a matter simply of *information* or technological *manipulation* but of communion. Against the machine metaphor, a Christian vision of mental health care is characterized by the movement from duality to unity, from individual to relational experience, from fixing to attending, and ultimately from the journey to a feast.

A Note on Language

There is no neutral or uncontested way to speak about experiences of psychological and emotional challenge and suffering. In this work, I refer to "mental disorder(s)" only when describing specific diagnostic categories or clinical settings, since this is the language of psychiatry and of its diagnostic guidebook, the *Diagnostic and Statistical Manual of Mental Disorders*. I sometimes use the term "mental illness" as a category of experience, recognizing that this language is embraced by some advocates and shunned by others. Most commonly, I speak of "mental health problems" and "mental health challenges."

When speaking of recipients of and seekers of mental health care, I use the words "patient" or "client" when referring to aspects of the therapist-client or doctor-patient relationship, but I most often speak of "people who seek mental health care." I refer to psychologists, psychiatrists, clinical social workers, professional counselors, pastoral counselors, and other professional caregivers as "mental health clinicians" or "mental health practitioners" but never "mental health providers."

CHAPTER 1

Modern Mental Health Care and the Machine Metaphor

Therapy as Technique

Wonderful are your works;
that I know very well.

—Psalm 139:14

A body, love insists, is neither a spirit nor a machine; it is not
a picture, a diagram, a chart, a graph, an anatomy; it is not
an explanation; it is not a law. It is precisely and uniquely
what it is. It belongs to the world of love, which is a world
of living creatures, natural orders and cycles, many small,
fragile lights in the dark.

—Wendell Berry, "Health Is Membership"[1]

It is eight o'clock on a Thursday morning, and as usual, I am about to begin
seeing outpatients in the Mental Health Clinic at the Durham VA Medical
Center, where I serve as a staff psychiatrist. The examination room, located
below ground level, is windowless, but I have done my best to humanize it,
adding bookshelves and some framed artwork to supplement the plexiglass-
enclosed impressionist prints that the hospital installed long ago. I sit in an
office chair with a monitor containing the electronic medical record close at
hand, looking at the small sofa and chair that my patients, and sometimes
their families, will occupy. Then I begin.

1. Wendell Berry, "Health Is Membership," in *Another Turn of the Crank* (Berkeley: Counterpoint, 1995), 86–109.

During the morning, I see seven to eight patients in thirty-minute slots—a luxury of time in an era where psychiatrists often spend ten to fifteen minutes with many of their patients for brief med checks. But the stories always exceed whatever time is allotted. Over the course of the morning I hear many stories, stories of pain, frustration, and sometimes of delight and triumph. I hear stories of grief and loss, of battle buddies who never returned from war, of children who died too soon from drug overdoses and motor vehicle accidents. I hear stories of sexual assault and intimate partner violence, sometimes told in detail. I hear stories of parents who drank too much and of childhood neighborhoods from which the rigors of military basic training were a welcome and dignifying relief. I hear stories of chronic pain, chronic loneliness, and hopelessness in the face of mounting chronic medical conditions. I hear stories of feeling anxious or depressed for no apparent reason at all. I hear stories of financial stress and reliance on disability income that requires the ongoing presence of symptoms. I hear stories of marriages and other intimate relationships: close and supportive relationships, loveless and hostile relationships in which a couple share a house but not a life, volatile relationships full of passion and anger. And I hear excited and hopeful stories: of relationships healed, of housing secured, of sobriety maintained, of community found, of spouses and children and grandchildren cherished.

With each of my patients, I listen as closely as I can to these stories, and we talk about them. Then, around the fifteen-minute mark of our thirty-minute visit, I turn to a mental checklist of things that I'm expected to document by the end of the appointment. I ask about thoughts of suicide, about substance use, about sleep and mood, about violence at home. Turning to the electronic medical record, I review the patient's electronic medication list, sometimes short and sometimes quite long, and ensure in a process called "medication reconciliation" that the list is accurate. I comply with clinical reminders and complete structured scales measuring symptoms and behavior. As required for coding and billing purposes, I assign a formal psychiatric diagnosis. More often than not, I discuss and prescribe medicines. All the time, I discuss other approaches to treatment, ranging from individual psychotherapy to group therapy to twelve-step groups to personal habits and practices. I make referrals when appropriate. I explore possibilities for expanding community ties and for cultivating meaningful and purposeful activity. I set a time for the patient to return, usually weeks or months in the future. Then I say goodbye and welcome my next patient.

I always feel tired at the end of a clinic session. The stories overwhelm. I cannot contain them, no matter how hard I try. I reflect on the deep privilege of being entrusted with those stories. I marvel that people trust me to walk alongside them, trust me with some of the deepest and most hidden shadows of their lives. But the stories are so complex, their pain and struggle so pervasive, that I cannot help but wonder, What am I doing? What is it for? And is it for the good?

"They're Turned into Mechanics"

For people who live with mental health problems, good mental health care can restore function and even prevent death. Somatic treatments such as electroconvulsive therapy (ECT) have helped countless people to recover from severe depression. Medications such as lithium have allowed people with bipolar disorder both to recover from and to avoid life-threatening mania and depression. Courses of individual psychotherapy have enabled people to recover from disabling depression, anxiety, and other mental health conditions, navigate relationships and other life challenges, and recover a sense of meaning and purpose. Interdisciplinary team models such as Assertive Community Treatment (ACT) have allowed people with serious mental illness to live independently and productively in community settings, decreasing the need for institutionalization.[2]

But all is not well in the world of mental health care. Too often those who seek mental health care experience it as inadequate and fragmented. Rather than being known and nurtured toward wholeness and healing, they find themselves being managed in ways that feel industrial and impersonal. This is especially the case in public mental health systems where people with complex and multidimensional mental health needs are treated in overburdened institutions with inadequate resources. A *New York Times* report described the difficulty that people with serious mental illness face in receiving care within New York City's public mental health institutions. Many find themselves in a "revolving door" of inpatient admissions, time in jail, and time on the streets.

2. Susan D. Phillips et al., "Moving Assertive Community Treatment into Standard Practice," *Psychiatric Services* 52 (2001): 772–79. See also "Assertive Community Treatment: The Evidence (DHHS Pub. No. SMA-08-4344)," Substance Abuse and Mental Health Services Administration (Rockville, MD: Center for Mental Health Services, Substance Abuse and Mental Health Services Administration, US Department of Health and Human Services, 2008), https://www.samhsa.gov/.

Psychologist Xavier Amador stated that "psychiatrists are no longer trained to look at someone's long-term needs. . . . They're turned into mechanics, dispensing psychopharmacology over a 72-hour period, or a one-week period, and then, 'My job is done.'"[3]

This perception of mental health care as industrial process shows up more subtly in sociologist Linda Blum's interviews with forty-eight socioeconomically and racially diverse mothers of children with "invisible disabilities" such as attention deficit/hyperactivity disorder (ADHD), learning disorders, and other mental disorders. For many of the mothers whom Blum interviewed, the "emphasis on brain power in an information- and innovation-based economy" meant that "taking extensive personal responsibility for the health of one's family also means vigilantly monitoring and maximizing children's brain development, working relentlessly to resolve or ameliorate innate flaws and imbalances."[4] This forced mothers to navigate complex and fragmented mental health care systems under pressure from school systems and others, and to accept medications when other forms of therapy were out of reach:

> Perhaps some years from now, new generations of parents will no longer confront the maze of private insurers and HMOs, barely able to decode the extent of their families' coverage let alone the array of emerging hyper-specialized fields. But for now we're left with the fact that pills are cheaper, more profitable, and a relatively quick fix compared to labor-intensive forms of one-on-one or family therapies, or to the multimodal approaches incorporating such practices with medications that have been found to be most effective.[5]

Blum argues that modern mental health care is often used to satisfy the demands and expectations of a modern neoliberal economic order that equates value with productivity and that places the burden on individuals to bear personal responsibility for their economic well-being.[6] She points out that while

3. Quoted in Andy Newman, Nate Schweber, and Chelsia Rose Marcius, "Decades Adrift in a Broken System, Then Charged in a Death on the Tracks," *New York Times*, February 5, 2022, https://www.nytimes.com/2022/02/05/nyregion/martial-simon-michelle-go.html.

4. Linda F. Blum, *Raising Generation Rx: Mothering Kids with Invisible Disabilities in an Age of Inequality* (New York: New York University Press, 2015), 34.

5. Blum, *Raising Generation Rx*, 31.

6. Blum defines neoliberalism as "the nation-state's corollary to New Economy entrepreneurialism [that] valorizes independence, small government, and the free market, while demanding that each citizen take 'personal responsibility' for all life outcomes, from wealth

the language of brain science helped to reduce mothers' sense of guilt and responsibility for the origin of their children's struggles, it paradoxically intensified "the neoliberal belief that the brain is an embodied object to be individually managed, manipulated, and optimized for improved productivity rather than the site of a potentially deep, self-reflective, unmanageable mind."[7]

The perception of mental health care as an industrial process aimed at helping individuals adapt to the demands of a market economy is not limited to public mental health systems or to situations where resources are scarce. Sociologist Joseph Davis interviewed eighty American adults who responded to an ad seeking those who "struggled with being sad, with being anxious in social situations, or with concentration and attention problems"—experiences that Davis calls "everyday suffering."[8] He found that around three quarters of his interviewees were engaged in some form of mental health care, and that they were less often seeking personal growth or deeper self-knowledge, and more often seeking to attain "viable selfhood" in a social and economic order that values efficiency, autonomy, productivity, and personal responsibility.[9] In their pursuit of viability, participants often were formed within a "neurobiological imaginary" that located the source of everyday psychological suffering in a physical malfunction of the body or brain—leading them not only to turn to medication as first-line treatment but also to describe mental

---

and poverty to health and illness"; *Raising Generation Rx*, 29. In this book, neoliberalism names, broadly, the economic and political theories and practices associated in Europe with the Austrian school of economics associated with Friedrich Hayek and Ludwig von Mises, in the United States by the Chicago school of economics associated with Milton Friedman and George Stigler, by numerous economic think tanks such as the American Enterprise Institute and the Heritage Foundation, and by the free-market economic and monetary policies that have been influential in the United States and United Kingdom at least since the elections of Margaret Thatcher in 1979 and Ronald Reagan in 1980. For a history of neoliberal thought that describes its internal complexity, see David Stedman Jones, *Masters of the Universe: Hayek, Friedman, and the Birth of Neoliberal Politics* (Princeton: Princeton University Press, 2014). Pastoral theologian Bruce Rogers-Vaughn describes neoliberalism as a social and economic system in which privatization, deregulation, and trust in the market has made competition and inequality core principles of our lives, and in which "every individual becomes an entrepreneur, managing and marketing the self as a personal enterprise and investment." See Bruce Rogers-Vaughn, *Caring for Souls in a Neoliberal Age* (New York: Palgrave Macmillan, 2016), 44.

7. Blum, *Raising Generation Rx*, 5. Blum is drawing from sociologist Victoria Pitts-Taylor's concept of the em-brained self.

8. Joseph E. Davis, *Chemically Imbalanced: Everyday Suffering, Medication, and Our Troubled Quest for Self-Mastery* (Chicago: University of Chicago Press, 2020), 4.

9. Davis, *Chemically Imbalanced*, 128–49.

health care as a matter of "fixing."[10] Many of Davis's interviewees did not find the industrial and mechanistic feel of mental health care to be a bad thing; they *wanted* this because they understood themselves as somehow broken and in need of repair.[11]

Adjusting Medicines, Managing Symptoms, Fixing Machines

Blum's and Davis's studies, along with the experiences of many clinicians and seekers of mental health care, suggest that prominent amid the diverse landscape of mental health care services is a tendency to approach mental health care as a matter of fixing something that is broken, or tuning something that is out of alignment. In my own experience as a psychiatrist, it is common for my colleagues and me to use the language of standardized processes and industry. Using a word rooted in the handling of horses and extended to the wielding of tools, we speak of "managing" a caseload of patients and helping patients to "manage" their symptoms.[12] We speak of "managing," "adjusting," and "tweaking" medications in order to bring particular symptoms or unwanted behaviors under "control." Within the Veterans Affairs health system, we refer to clinical interventions, including visits with clinicians, as "standard episodes of care." We assist patients with emotional and behavioral "self-regulation" and help them to "cope" with various "stressors."

This language points to the way that modern mental health care is influenced by what in this book I refer to as the machine metaphor. In its simplest form, the machine metaphor depicts the body and brain as a machine that, when broken, gives rise to mental health problems. As we will see, this metaphor of the body as machine is deeply woven into modern medicine and also into modern psychiatry and psychology. More broadly, however, the machine metaphor names the way that the imagination and practices of clinicians and patients alike are formed such that regardless of whether a particular mental health problem can be understood as a mechanical bodily dysfunction, the

---

10. Davis, *Chemically Imbalanced*, 129.

11. Davis notes that while certain forms of psychotherapy and counseling would push against this industrial model, psychotherapy itself can be just as mechanized as medication therapy: "as commonly practiced, psychotherapists can foster the very same regime of the self that I will be scrutinizing and can promote their own highly mechanistic view of suffering"; *Chemically Imbalanced*, 17.

12. *Online Etymology Dictionary*, s.v. "manage (v.)," https://www.etymonline.com/word /manage#etymonline_v_6769.

most fitting response is the application of standardized techniques and processes akin to those used in mechanical industries.

The machine metaphor displays itself in a way of speaking and thinking about mental health care (that is, a grammar and logic of mental health care) that, while not universal, will be recognizable to most clinicians and patients:

a. Mental health problems are characterized by unwanted or disvalued experiences and behaviors,
b. located in individuals,
c. operationally understood as constellations of symptoms and signs,
d. and often characterized as disorders of the brain or neural circuits,
e. that demand treatment by therapies (psychotherapies, pharmacotherapies, or somatic therapies) proven to be effective in reducing these symptoms.

In this chapter, after unpacking this grammar and logic, I will then briefly describe four historical roots of the machine metaphor and propose five powerful but problematic presumptions that correlate with the use of the machine metaphor in clinical practice.

Grammar and Logic of the Machine Metaphor

First, mental health problems are initially *recognized* as the presence of unwanted or disvalued experiences and behaviors. Most of the time, these experiences are unwanted, as when a college student struggles to complete a class because of severe anxiety, or when a successful executive recognizes that she needs help to cut down on her use of alcohol in order to function in different areas of her life. At other times, these experiences or behaviors are not unwanted but are *disvalued* by others, as when a person with bipolar mania who is on top of the world but doing dangerous things is brought to a psychiatric crisis center. Often the experiences and behaviors are both unwanted *and* disvalued.

These unwanted or disvalued experiences and behaviors are then understood to be located somehow within individuals. Most people who seek the services of a psychiatrist, therapist, or counselor do so as individuals. They say things—such as, "I am feeling very sad," or "my anxiety is horrible"—that locate the unwanted experience and behavior as somehow within themselves. Psychiatry's diagnostic guidebook, the *Diagnostic and Statistical Manual of Mental*

Disorders (*DSM*), contains operational definitions of diagnostic categories that overwhelmingly apply to individuals and specifies in its definition of "mental disorder" that mental disorders are signs of "dysfunction in the individual."[13]

Though there is nothing intrinsically medical or psychiatric about unwanted or disvalued experience and behavior as such, clinicians and patients assign this experience and behavior to the realm of the medical by labeling these experiences and behaviors as "symptoms" or "signs" of an underlying mental health condition. The *DSM* aids in this process by defining particular mental disorders as sets of symptoms and signs.[14] To have alcohol use disorder *just is* to display, in the words of *DSM-5-TR*, "a problematic pattern of alcohol use leading to clinically significant impairment or distress, as manifested by at least two" of eleven behaviors and experiences, such as drinking alcohol in larger amounts or over a longer period than intended and experiencing craving, or a strong desire or urge to use alcohol.[15] While various causal factors may lead to these problematic symptoms and signs, it is the presence of symptoms and signs that allows alcohol use disorder to be recognized and named as such.

The move to identify particular unwanted or disvalued experiences and behaviors as symptoms or signs that indicate particular mental disorders does not entail any particular account of what *causes* these unwanted experiences and behaviors.[16] But clinicians, research scientists, and pharmaceutical representatives all frequently speak about mental health problems as problems of the brain, of the body, or of neural circuits. As Davis's study makes clear, mental health advocacy communities and many care-seekers also speak about mental health problems in this way. The National Alliance on Mental Illness (NAMI), for example, affirms in its public policy platform that "in accordance with current scientific evidence, mental illness is *essentially biological in nature* sometimes triggered by environmental factors such as trauma, countering the

---

13. American Psychiatric Association, *Diagnostic and Statistical Manual of Mental Disorders*, 5th ed. rev. [*DSM-5-TR*] (Washington, DC: American Psychiatric Association, 2022),

14. The *DSM* is an iterative document that is now in its fifth major revision. The successive editions of the *DSM* are conventionally abbreviated as *DSM-I* (1952), *DSM-II* (1968), *DSM-III* (1980), *DSM-III-R* (1987), *DSM-IV* (1994), *DSM-IV-TR* (2000), *DSM-5* (2013), and most recently *DSM-5-TR* (2022). We will be engaging *DSM-III* (1980) in more detail below.

15. *DSM-5-TR*, 5.

15. *DSM-5-TR*, 553.

16. Indeed, the authors of the influential third edition of the *DSM* (*DSM-III*, published in 1980) made clear their intention that the *DSM* would be "atheoretical with respect to etiology." American Psychiatric Association, *Diagnostic and Statistical Manual of Mental Disorders*, 3rd ed. [*DSM-III*] (Washington, DC: American Psychiatric Association, 1980), 7.

myth that these conditions are failures of character and will. Mental illness affects behavior and behavior can affect mental illness, but mental illnesses are not behavioral."[17]

These ways of speaking and thinking build on one another. The designation of unwanted or disvalued experience and behavior as located in the individual and as symptoms that are often located in the brain specifies that the experience and behavior reflects a psychiatric disorder. This then gives moral legitimacy to the search for particular interventions that can remove or ameliorate the unwanted symptoms. As leaders within psychiatry and virulent critics of psychiatric power have recognized, naming experience and behavior as "mental illness" is a moral act because the labeled experience and behavior is then rendered the subject of mental health treatment.[18] Once one is labeled

17. "Public Policy Platform of the National Alliance on Mental Illness," National Alliance on Mental Illness, 12th ed., December 2016, https://www.nami.org/Advocacy/Policy -Platform. Quotation is from p. 3, italics mine.

18. This view was forcibly expressed by a diverse group of mid-twentieth-century clinicians and thinkers who are often described as members of an "antipsychiatry movement" because of their trenchant critiques of psychiatric power. The libertarian psychiatrist Thomas Szasz, for example, concerned about the way that psychiatry could underwrite the power of totalitarian governments as he had seen in his native Hungary after World War II, argued in his 1961 book *The Myth of Mental Illness* that experience and behavior labeled in his time as mental illness were actually "problems of living" that should not be pathologized. (Szasz left the door open for the machine metaphor, however, by arguing that behavior that results from a "physicochemical disorder of the body" would indeed be disease and properly treated by physicians.) See Thomas S. Szasz, *The Myth of Mental Illness: Foundations of a Theory of Personal Conduct*, rev. ed. (New York: Harper & Row, 1974), 36-37. Throughout his career, Szasz charged that the mental health disciplines inappropriately assume the medical model to describe conditions that are not valid medical disorders; that psychiatry uses this wrongly appropriated medical model to justify various forms of coercion, especially including involuntary commitment; and that psychiatric technology, particularly medication, is but one form of this coercion. See, for example, Thomas Szasz, "The Case against Psychiatric Coercion," *Independent Review* 1 (1997): 485-98; Szasz, "The Therapeutic State: The Tyranny of Pharmacracy," *Independent Review* 5 (2001): 485-521; Szasz, *Psychiatry: The Science of Lies* (Syracuse, NY: Syracuse University Press, 2008). Szasz's British contemporary R. D. Laing, well known in the 1960s counterculture, argued that psychiatric (and particularly psychoanalytic) jargon was a barrier, rather than an aid, in understanding patients, since it distances patients from their experience and implies that the psychiatrist can faithfully narrate "what is going on" in abstraction without careful attention to the *specificity* of a patient's self-narration of experience. See R. D. Laing, *The Divided Self* (New York: Pantheon Books, 1960), 18-21. Szasz and Laing were joined by a number of sociological thinkers, notably Erving Goffman and the more polemical Thomas Scheff, who were critical of the orga-

as "mentally ill," one can accept treatment or refuse treatment, but either way, "mental health care" wields power. As medical and mental health disciplines have turned increasingly to empirical analysis to determine treatments that are effective for specific conditions, therapies that are shown to be evidence based—that is, when tested empirically, ideally in placebo-controlled double-blind clinical trials, they result in statistically significant improvement in the symptoms and signs that constitute mental disorders—gain social prestige and power. Further, to the extent that one assumes that the unwanted or disvalued experience is caused by dysfunction in the brain or body, one is likely to prioritize treatments that are most clearly understood to operate biologically, such as medication.

Historical Roots of the Machine Metaphor

The machine metaphor is not just an image but rather a complex way of seeing, understanding, and acting in the world. As Joseph Davis has recognized, it is what philosopher Charles Taylor has called a "social imaginary," an account of "the ways in which [people] imagine their social existence, how they fit together with others, how things go on between them and their fellows, the expectations which are normally met, and the deeper normative notions and images which underlie these expectations."[19] As a social imaginary, it has complex cultural, scientific, and philosophical roots.[20] While it is beyond the

---

nization of psychiatric care and, in Scheff's case, argued that mental illness itself was social construction. See Erving Goffman, *Asylums: Essays on the Social Situations of Mental Patients and Other Inmates* (Piscataway, NJ: Aldine Transaction, 2007); Thomas J. Scheff, *Being Mentally Ill: A Sociological Theory*, 3rd ed. (Piscataway, NJ: Aldine Transaction, 1999). Though he was less connected to the clinical literature, Michel Foucault in *Folie et Deraison: Histoire de la Folie a L'age Classique* (published in English in abridged form as *Madness and Civilization*) argued that contemporary psychiatry continues the modern project of sequestering unreason from reason and that far from liberating the mentally ill, modern psychiatry shackles them with invisible chains. See Michel Foucault, *Madness and Civilization: A History of Insanity in the Age of Reason*, trans. Richard Howard (New York: Vintage Books, 1965).

19. Charles Taylor, *A Secular Age* (Cambridge: Belknap, 2007), 171.

20. Vladimir Glebkin argues that while classical writers typically used the Greek and Latin words for mechanism and machine only to describe human-crafted products and contrivances, writers in the medieval era employed these terms much more broadly to apply to the cosmos, the human body, and even the church. This broadening of the concept's range, Glebkin argues, may have set the stage for the increasing mechanization of world and body

scope of this book to provide a detailed account of these roots, it is clear that the machine metaphor builds on four conceptual developments—some centuries old and some quite recent—that are important for understanding modern medicine, psychiatry, and psychology: the mechanization of the body, the subsequent mechanization of the mind, the standardization of psychiatric diagnosis, and the industrialization of care.

The Mechanization of the Body

René Descartes (1596-1650), to whose work we will return below, is most often associated with his affirmation *cogito ergo sum*—"I think, therefore I am"—and by his insistence that "the mind by which I am what I am, is wholly distinct from the body."[21] Descartes is often dismissed by modern mental health researchers and clinicians as a dualist who denies the vital role of the body in determining experience. But in fact Descartes was deeply interested in the emerging medical sciences of his time. He devotes much of part 5 of the *Discourse on Method* (1637) to a rapt account of the physiology of the heart, which he adopted from William Harvey's recently published *De Motu Cordis* ("On the Motion of the Heart," 1628). He concludes that the human body is "a machine made by the hands of God, which is incomparably better arranged, and adequate to movements more admirable than is any machine of human invention."[22] While Descartes was not the first to describe the body as a machine,[23] he was a forceful early advocate of this view.[24]

---

in the early modern era. Glebkin, "A Socio-Cultural History of the Machine Metaphor," *Review of Cognitive Linguistics* 11 (2013): 145-62.

21. René Descartes, *Discourse on the Method of Rightly Conducting the Reason and Seeking Truth in the Sciences*, trans. John Veitch, in *The Rationalists* (New York: Anchor, 1960), 63. While *cogito ergo sum* was the Latin affirmation of Descartes in his *Meditations on First Philosophy*, his affirmation in the *Discourse on Method*, written in French, was *je pense, donc je suis*.

22. Descartes, *Discourse on Method* 5. Quotation is from *Rationalists*, 80.

23. Shakespeare's Hamlet referred to his body as a machine several decades before Descartes wrote, in perhaps the first use of this term in the English language. See William Shakespeare, *Hamlet*, act 2, scene 2; Daryl W. Palmer, "Hamlet's Northern Lineage: Masculinity, Climate, and Mechanician in Early Modern Britain," in *William Shakespeare's Hamlet*, ed. Harold Bloom (New York: Bloom's Literary Criticism, 2009), 26; Daniel Black, *Embodiment and Mechanisation: Reciprocal Understandings of Body and Machine from the Renaissance to the Present* (Burlington, VT: Ashgate, 2014), 8.

24. Stephen Gaukroger, *Descartes: An Intellectual Biography* (Oxford: Clarendon, 1995), 269-90. Gaukroger argues that Descartes's advocacy of mechanism was influenced by the

The Mechanization of the Mind

While Descartes enthusiastically affirmed that the body is a machine that can be understood as *res extensa* (extended substance), he was not ready to affirm that the human mind operates like a machine. (He did not extend the same exception to nonhuman animals, which he understood as soulless machines who are "destitute of reason" and in which "nature acts . . . according to the disposition of their organs.")[25] It was important to Descartes that the mind/soul (the *res cogitans*, thinking substance) is immaterial in part to *avoid* mechanization, for treating the mind as mechanism would then deny the soul's immortality and erode Christian moral teaching.[26]

Even in Descartes's own subsequent writing, however, the image of the body as machine began to encroach on what we would today understand as the life of the mind. While Descartes was keen to maintain a metaphysical dualism between mind and body, he expressly rejected the view that the soul inhabits and directs the body as a captain inhabits and directs a ship. It is rather "necessary for [the soul] to be joined and united more closely to the body, in order to have sensations and appetites similar to ours, and thus

---

work of mathematician, priest, and Minim friar Marin Mersenne (1588–1648), who was an intellectual peer of Descartes and for whom the affirmation of matter's inertness was a way to combat "renaissance naturalism," broadly understood as practices and ideas in which nature was understood to bear intrinsic powers that did not require reference to God, as well as mortalism, the doctrine that the soul is "not a separate substance but simply the 'organizing principle' of the body." Both naturalism and mortalism were threats to established religion and gave rise to what might now be called occult or nature-worship practices, and "Mersenne's solution is to cut them off at the root, by depriving them of the conception of nature on which they thrive" (149). It is ironic that a mechanistic theory intended by Mersenne and Descartes to safeguard the importance of God for the natural order paved the way for a mechanistic conception of nature in which God was even more rigorously banished.

25. Descartes, *Discourse on Method* 5. Quotation is from *Rationalists*, 82.

26. Descartes writes, "For after the error of those who deny the existence of God, an effort which I think I have already sufficiently refuted, there is none that is more powerful in leading feeble minds astray from the straight path of virtue than the supposition that the soul of brutes is of the same nature with our own, and consequently that after this life we have nothing to hope for or to fear, more than flies and ants; in place of which, when we know how far they differ we much better comprehend the reasons which establish that the soul is of a nature wholly independent of the body, and that consequently it is not liable to die with the latter; and, finally, because no other causes are observed capable of destroying it, we are naturally led thence to judge that it is immortal." See Descartes, *Discourse on Method* 5. Quotation is from *Rationalists*, 82.

constitute a real man."[27] He elaborated on this in his last major published work, *The Passions of the Soul* (1649), in which he maintained that emotions (feelings, passions) occur when the body transmits particular physical "animal spirits" to the brain, which are received by the immaterial soul through the medium of the pineal gland. The passions of the soul, Descartes holds, are "perceptions or sensations or excitations of the soul which are referred to it in particular and which are caused, maintained, and strengthened by some movement of the spirits."[28] While for Descartes the mind is not a machine, the contents of mental experience are in part the products of the machine-body.[29]

Notwithstanding Descartes's intentions, it did not take long for the machine metaphor to claim the territory of mental experience. In *Man a Machine*, first published in 1748, the French physician and philosopher Julien Offray de La Mettrie (1709-1751) argued that the mind is so dependent on and related to the body that both are subject to mechanistic description and explanation:

> But since all the faculties of the soul depend to such a degree on the proper organization of the brain and of the whole body, that apparently they are but this organization itself, the soul is clearly an enlightened machine. . . . The soul is therefore but an empty word, of which no one has any idea, and which an enlightened man should use only to signify the part in us that thinks. Given the least principle of motion, animated bodies will have all that is necessary for moving, feeling, thinking, repenting, or in a word for conducting themselves in the physical realm, and in the moral realm which depends upon it.[30]

"Let us then conclude boldly," La Mettrie stated in a direct challenge to Descartes's substance dualism, "that man is a machine, and that in the whole universe there is but a single substance differently modified."[31]

La Mettrie's views were consistent with a larger "mechanization of the world picture" that characterized much of seventeenth- and eighteenth-century Eu-

27. Descartes, *Discourse on Method* 5. Quotation is from *Rationalists*, 82.

28. Descartes, *Passions of the Soul* 27. See René Descartes, *The Passions of the Soul*, trans. Stephen H. Voss (Indianapolis: Hackett, 1989), 33-34.

29. Gary Hatfield, "The *Passions of the Soul* and Descartes' Machine Psychology," *Studies in History and Philosophy of Science* 38 (2007): 1-35.

30. Julien Offray de La Mettrie, *Man a Machine* (Chicago: Open Court, 1912), 57, available at https://www.gutenberg.org/files/52090/52090-h/52090-h.htm.

31. La Mettrie, *Man a Machine*, 80.

ropean scientific thought.[32] This tendency to a thoroughgoing materialism and mechanization of the mind was reinforced by rapid advances in the understanding of human anatomy and the new science of human physiology in the late eighteenth and early nineteenth centuries. Writing in the 1840s, French zoologist Henri Milne-Edwards captured the way that the machine metaphor operated in nineteenth-century science:

> Who, when reflecting upon these phenomena [of the movement of animals], and the actions we ourselves execute, does not experience the desire to scrutinize the interior of these complicated machines, to know by what agents, by what mechanism all these movements are executed; to examine the processes, by which all organized beings assimilate to their own substance the foreign substances by which they are nourished; and to inquire the uses of the different organs, of which the body is composed?[33]

This assumption that the body and mind could be understood mechanistically influenced the development of nineteenth- and early twentieth-century psychology and psychiatry. Nineteenth-century German researchers developed laboratories that successfully identified what are now considered to be foundational discoveries in neural science. For example, Herman von Helmholtz (1821–1894), rejecting the idea of an intrinsic vital principle of life and applying Newtonian physics to physiology, calculated the speed of conduction

32. For Charles Taylor, this "mechanization of the world picture" (a term associated with historian of science E. J. Dijksterhuis) emerges from the centuries-long rejection of intrinsic teleology, the belief that things have ends internal to their nature, within European thought. First, philosophical nominalists held that things do not have ends in themselves but are directed to their proper ends by God, who "relates to things as freely to be disposed of according to his autonomous purposes." But this means that humans must also relate to other creatures not according to intrinsic ends but according to the purposes that they are assigned by God. But it would not be long, Taylor argues, when God would mostly drop out of the picture in favor of "a new understanding of being, according to which, all intrinsic purpose having been expelled, final causation drops out, and efficient causation alone remains. There comes about what has been called 'the mechanization of the world picture.' And this in turn opens the way for a view of science in which a good test of the truth of a hypothesis is what it enables you to effect. . . . A radical shift has taken place. . . . The world is God's creature. Moreover, it is an ordered whole. But now the order is no longer normative, in the sense that the world exhibits the (more or less imperfect) instantiations of a system of normative patterns, on which we should model ourselves. Rather the world is a vast field of mutually affecting parts"; *A Secular Age*, 97–98.

33. Henri Milne-Edwards, *Outlines of Anatomy and Physiology* (Boston: Little & Brown, 1841), 1.

in sensory and motor nerves and offered experimental evidence for the view that color is encoded in the retina and optic nerve not by different kinds of energy but by color-specific receptors. Gustav Fechner (1801–1877) systematically explored the relationship between the force of stimuli and perceptions associated with them in a process that he named "psychophysics."[34] Wilhelm Wundt (1832–1920), whose establishment of a laboratory at the University of Leipzig in 1879 is often marked as the founding event of modern psychology, treated conscious mental processes as law-governed phenomena that like chemical processes could be experimentally modified, extending the machine metaphor to the contents of conscious experience. "As soon as the psyche is viewed as natural phenomenon," Wundt stated, "and psychology as a natural science, the experimental methods must also be capable of full application to this science."[35]

Reflecting his training as a neurologist, a young Sigmund Freud (1856–1939) wrote a highly speculative treatise that described human mental experience as the interaction of neuronal systems. Freud begins this 1895 treatise, untitled and unpublished in his lifetime but later published in English as *Project for a Scientific Psychology*, with the claim that "the intention of this project is to furnish us with a psychology which shall be a natural science: its aim, that is, is to represent psychical processes as quantitatively determined states of specifiable material particles and so to make them plain and void of contradictions."[36] While in subsequent early work, notably *The Interpretation*

34. Morton Hunt, *The Story of Psychology* (New York: Doubleday, 1993), 114–26.

35. Quoted in Hunt, *Story of Psychology*, 129. Of note, not all early psychologists shared the reductive view of Wundt and the physiologists. The American philosopher and psychologist William James, always suspicious of enclosed systems of thought whether religious or scientific, criticized "the automaton-theory" in his influential *Principles of Psychology* (1890). The theory that brain states cause mental states but that mental states do not cause each other or cause changes in the brain fails the test of "common-sense." "Psychology is a mere natural science, accepting certain terms uncritically in her data, and stopping short of metaphysical reconstruction. Like physics, she must be *naïve*, and if she finds that in her very peculiar field of study ideas *seem* to be causes, she had better continue to talk of them as such." See William James, *The Principles of Psychology* (Mineola, NY: Dover, 1950), 137.

36. Sigmund Freud, "Project for a Scientific Psychology," in *The Standard Edition of the Complete Psychological Works of Sigmund Freud*, vol. 1, *Pre-Psychoanalytic Publications and Unpublished Drafts (1886–1899)* (London: Hogarth, 1966), 355. More recently, contemporary psychoanalyst Mark Solms has called *Project for a Scientific Psychology* "the Rosetta Stone of neuropsychoanalysis" and has offered a revised version that seeks to bring Freud's model into conversation with the twenty-first-century brain sciences. See Mark Solms, "New Project for a Scientific Psychology: General Scheme," *Neuropsychoanalysis* 22 (2020):

of Dreams (1900), Freud abandoned a reductive neurophysiological model of mind in favor of what is often called his "topographical" model of conscious, preconscious, and unconscious mental systems, the influence of nineteenth-century neurology is still evident in his thinking.

The rise of behaviorism as a rejection of the introspective methods of Wundt, James, and other early psychologists was in some ways a methodological doubling-down on the metaphor of mind as a machine. In his seminal paper "Psychology as the Behaviorist Views It," the American behaviorist John Broadus Watson (1878–1958) argued that psychology is a "purely objective experimental branch of natural science. Its theoretical goal is the prediction and control of behavior. Introspection forms no essential part of its methods."[37] A benefit of this, Watson argued, is that "this suggested elimination of states of consciousness as proper objects of investigation in themselves will remove the barrier from psychology which exists between it and the other sciences. The findings of psychology become the functional correlates of structure and lend themselves to explanation in physico-chemical terms."[38]

Having influenced the development of psychoanalysis and behaviorism, the metaphor of mind/brain as machine is perhaps most evident in the writings of champions of a biological approach to psychiatry. The development of effective (that is, associated with symptom reduction) medications for schizophrenia, depression, anxiety, and other conditions in the 1950s through 1970s gave rise to a generation of medication-oriented psychiatrists who used mechanistic imagery about mental illness to describe and to justify their biological interventions.[39] In a popular work titled *From Sad to Glad*, psychiatrist and antidepressant pioneer Nathan Kline argued that while depression is related both to biochemical problems and to relational and social problems, the root problem is often mechanistic and biochemical:

1–2, 5–35, https://doi.org/10.1080/15294145.2020.1833361; also Solms, *The Hidden Spring: A Journey to the Source of Consciousness* (New York: Norton, 2021).

37. John Broadus Watson, "Psychology as the Behaviorist Views It," *Psychological Review* 20 (1913): 158.

38. Watson, "Psychology," 177.

39. Historian of science Evelyn Fox Keller comments that "one might argue that psychopharmaceuticals have been more effective in persuading people of their essentially mechanistic and physical-chemical nature than all of modern science put together." See Evelyn Fox Keller, "Whole Bodies, Whole Persons? Cultural Studies, Psychoanalysis, and Biology," in *Subjectivity: Ethnographic Investigations*, ed. João Biehl, Byron Good, and Arthur Kleinman (Berkeley: University of California Press, 2007), 357.

Why can one person handle stress and another not? There are, to be sure, many factors in personality development, but I am convinced that one critical element is biochemical. Among those who habitually blow up I suspect that a marginal, quite dithery brain chemistry is overwhelmed when stress situations introduce a flow of unmanageable pressures. And I am convinced that many suffer from a poorly organized biochemical system that simply functions only marginally even when external pressures are not a factor.

I have noted that we now have practical ways to correct some of these malfunctions. Simply stated, we accomplish it through drugs that adjust the biogenic amine levels up or down as the case may require.[40]

Perhaps the most influential popular champion of the view that mental illness is a matter of a broken brain and that the mind functions like a machine is Nancy Andreasen, a literature scholar who became a psychiatrist and prominent schizophrenia researcher, a prominent contributor to the third and fourth editions of the *DSM*, and later the editor of the flagship *American Journal of Psychiatry*. In *The Broken Brain: The Biological Revolution in Psychiatry*, Andreasen claimed that

psychiatry, like the prodigal son, has returned home to its place as a specialty within the field of medicine. It has become increasingly scientific and biological in its orientation. Psychiatry now recognizes that the serious mental illnesses are *diseases* in the same sense that cancer or high blood pressure are diseases. Mental illnesses are diseases that affect the brain, which is an organ of the body just as the heart or stomach is. People who suffer from mental illness suffer from a *sick or broken brain*, not from weak will, laziness, bad character, or bad upbringing.[41]

While most contemporary writers on mental illness avoid Andreasen's metaphor of the "broken brain" in favor of more polyfactorial approaches to

40. Nathan S. Kline, *From Sad to Glad: Kline on Depression*, rev. and updated ed. (New York: Ballantine Books, 1974), 88.

41. Nancy C. Andreasen, *The Broken Brain: The Biological Revolution in Psychiatry* (New York: Harper & Row, 1984), 8. Later she makes clear that her view of life is fundamentally materialist: "The brain is the source of everything we are. It is the source of everything that makes us human, humane, and unique. It is the source of our ability to speak, to write, to think, to create, to love, to laugh, to despair, and to hate" (83). As we will examine in chapter 2, Aquinas provides a way to acknowledge the brain's contribution to life without reducing life itself to the brain.

mental illness, the idea that psychiatry proves its worth as a medical specialty by being "scientific and biological" is deeply rooted in the culture of American psychiatry.[42] The image of the broken brain still guides the way that mental health research funding is allocated in the United States. Writing in the influential journal *Science* in 2015, two psychiatric leaders and architects of the National Institute of Mental Health B. R. A. I. N. Initiative write that all effective therapy, including targeted psychotherapy, is fundamentally a matter of tuning disordered brain circuits:

> As new diagnostics will likely be redefining "mental disorders" as "brain circuit disorders," new therapeutics will likely focus on tuning these circuits. What is the best way to tune a negative valence or social processing circuit? Medications might be useful, but recent attention has focused on devices that invasively (deep brain stimulation) or noninvasively (transcranial magnetic stimulation) alter brain circuit activity. Paradoxically, one of the most powerful and precise interventions to alter such activity may be targeted psychotherapy, such as cognitive behavioral therapy, which uses the brain's intrinsic plasticity to alter neural circuits and as a consequence, deleterious thoughts and behavior.[43]

The Standardization of Diagnosis

The tendency to view the human body and then the human mind through the image of the machine, and mental illness as a matter of a broken or dysfunctional machine, has both fostered and been reinforced by efforts to develop an efficient, standardized system of diagnosing mental illness. This standardization of diagnosis is a third feature of the machine metaphor of

42. Writing in 1998, psychiatrist and Nobel laureate Eric Kandel argued that "all mental processes, even the most complex psychological processes, derive from operations of the brain" and that "as a corollary, behavioral disorders that characterize psychiatric illness are disturbances of brain function, even in those cases where the causes of the disturbance are clearly environmental in origin." See Eric Kandel, "A New Intellectual Framework for Psychiatry," *American Journal of Psychiatry* 155 (1998): 460. Kandel argued that "the psychiatrists we are training today [in 1998] will need more than just a nodding familiarity with the biology of the brain. They will need the knowledge of an expert, a knowledge perhaps different from but fully comparable to that of a well-trained neurologist" (466).

43. Thomas R. Insel and Bruce N. Cuthbert, "Brain Disorders? Precisely: Precision Medicine Comes to Psychiatry," *Science* 348 (2015): 500.

mental health care. German psychiatrist Emil Kraepelin (1856–1926), who studied under Wilhelm Wundt and came to prominence as a psychiatrist at the University of Heidelberg, recognized that biological research in psychiatry would be fruitful only if psychiatric diseases could be described clearly and distinctly: "the principle requisite in the knowledge of mental diseases is an accurate definition of the separate disease processes."[44] Focusing on disease course and prognosis rather than on presumed cause, Kraepelin meticulously recorded the time course of symptoms and behavior of patients in Heidelberg's university clinic and published several editions of an influential textbook, *Ein Lehrbuch der Psychiatrie*, that distinguished distinct syndromes of mental illness, including for the first time contrasting *dementia praecox* (which, using Eugen Bleuler's language, is described today as schizophrenia) from manic-depressive psychosis (now described as bipolar disorder).

Kraepelin's method was so influential for twentieth-century American and European psychiatry that historian Edward Shorter argues that "it is Kraepelin, not Freud, who is the central figure in the history of psychiatry."[45] Specifically, Kraepelin's views profoundly affected the development of the *DSM*, which has emerged as the most influential system of naming and classifying mental health problems over the last half century, both in the United States and (through its influence on the World Health Organization's *International Classification of Diseases*, or ICD) in many other countries. By establishing norms for the language of mental disorder, the *DSM* has played an outsized role in the structures and practices of modern mental health care and the perpetuation of the machine metaphor.

First published as a slender volume in 1952 by the American Psychiatric Association (APA), the *DSM* replaced a series of coding manuals that had been used in the early twentieth century to classify inpatients in large psychiatric hospitals. These early manuals, published prior to the availability of antipsychotic drugs, focused on classifying severe and chronic psychoses and other neurodegenerative conditions (e.g., cerebral syphilis) that would today be treated by neurologists and infectious disease specialists.[46] But the first *DSM* (*DSM-I*) was published with outpatients in mind, in part to aid psychiatrists

44. Emil Kraepelin, *Clinical Psychiatry: A Text-Book for Students and Physicians*, trans. A. Ross Diefendorf (New York: Macmillan, 1912), 115.

45. Edward Shorter, *A History of Psychiatry: From the Era of the Asylum to the Age of Prozac* (New York: Wiley & Sons, 1997), 100.

46. National Committee for Mental Hygiene and Committee on Statistics, American Psychiatric Association, *Statistical Manual for the Use of Hospitals for Mental Diseases*, 10th ed. (Utica, NY: State Hospitals Press, 1942).

within the Veterans Administration to care for the many returning veterans who sought their services in the aftermath of the Second World War.[47] For the next two decades, *DSM-I* and its equally slender successor, *DSM-II* (1968), played a modest and mostly background role in guiding the way that mental disorders were classified and coded by psychiatrists.

In the 1960s and 1970s, however, to the dismay of many leaders of American psychiatry, critics of psychiatry increasingly challenged the legitimacy of psychiatric theory and practice. To name a few examples, in the influential journal *Science*, D. L. Rosenhan and his colleagues reported that twelve researchers without mental illness had faked their way into inpatient psychiatry units by reporting auditory hallucinations such as "thud" and "empty." Although these researchers posing as patients ceased reporting any symptoms after admission, they were nonetheless held on these units for an average of nineteen days (range seven to fifty-two days) and nearly all were discharged with diagnoses of schizophrenia or manic-depressive illness "in remission."[48] Journalist Susannah Calahan has recently sharply challenged the validity of Rosenhan's study, showing that the paper was at minimum improperly reported and very likely fraudulent, but this does not change the fact that it helped to shape public narratives about psychiatry in the 1970s.[49] Around the same time, a transatlantic study of psychiatric diagnosis in the United States and United Kingdom showed that patients in the United Kingdom who would be diagnosed with manic depression or personality disorder would often be diagnosed with schizophrenia in the United States, challenging the reliability of *DSM-II*'s diagnostic constructs.[50] Most prominently, early self-described "gay liberation" activists began to publicly challenge the inclusion of homosexuality in *DSM-II*'s list of disorders of sexual behavior, which resulted in the eventual deletion of homosexuality from *DSM-II* in 1973 and its replacement by the more limited but still pathologizing "ego-dystonic homosexuality."[51] All of these controversies, and more, led prominent American psychiatrists to conclude that psychiatry would lose its professional and public perception

47. Gerald N. Grob, "Origins of *DSM-I*: A Study in Appearance and Reality," *American Journal of Psychiatry* 148 (1991): 421–31.

48. D. L. Rosenhan, "On Being Sane in Insane Places," *Science* 179 (1973): 250–58.

49. Susannah Calahan, *The Great Pretender: The Undercover Mission That Changed Our Understanding of Madness* (New York: Grand Central, 2019).

50. R. E. Kendell et al., "Diagnostic Criteria of American and British Psychiatrists," *Archives of General Psychiatry* 25 (1971): 123–30.

51. Ronald Bayer, *Homosexuality and American Psychiatry: The Politics of Diagnosis* (Princeton: Princeton University Press, 1981).

as a legitimate medical specialty unless it developed a more secure scientific foundation for classifying mental disorders. In an extraordinarily complicated, personality-driven, and still-contested scientific and political process, psychiatrist Robert Spitzer led an overhaul and expansion of the *DSM* that resulted in the publication of the third edition the *DSM*, *DSM-III*, in 1980.[52]

DSM-III was influenced by a group of psychiatric researchers centered at Washington University in Saint Louis who argued, following the example of Kraepelin, that psychiatric diagnosis should avoid the speculative theories of psychoanalysis. Instead, they sought to ground diagnosis on observable syndromes that would be identified by criteria such as description of symptoms, laboratory studies, differentiation from other disorders, longitudinal follow-up study, and studies of how similar symptoms appear in family members.[53] *DSM-III* introduced for the first time a set of now-familiar diagnostic categories such as major depressive disorder, bipolar disorder, and post-traumatic stress disorder, together with lists of standard descriptive criteria.

In doing so, *DSM-III* transformed psychiatric diagnosis from a project that focused on narrative understanding of a person's life to a project focused on *symptoms*. The diagnoses of *DSM-III* and each of its subsequent editions have focused on description rather than cause: to have major depressive disorder *just is* to experience enough of the signs and symptoms of major depressive disorder to qualify for the diagnosis. (Under the current criteria for major depressive disorder, to be depressed is to meet five of nine criteria such as depressed mood, decreased energy, increased or decreased appetite, increased or decreased ability to sleep, excessive guilt, difficulty concentrating, and thoughts of suicide.) The scientific merits and clinical wisdom of this descriptive approach to psychiatric diagnosis, as we will consider later, are actively debated by clinicians, philosophers, and scientists. But *DSM-III* was a political coup for psychiatry's influence in the broader culture. Broad reaches of human experience—depressed mood, anxiety, inattention, difficulty complying with social norms—were placed into the criteria sets for *DSM-III* categories such as attention deficit disorder, major depression, generalized anxiety disorder, and conduct disorder. By virtue of this classification, people with these experiences could now be understood to have a major mental illness. Under the

52. Hannah Decker, *The Making of DSM-III*: *A Diagnostic Manual's Conquest of American Psychiatry* (New York: Oxford University Press, 2013); Allan V. Horwitz, *DSM: A History of Psychiatry's Bible* (Baltimore: Johns Hopkins University Press, 2021).

53. Eli Robins and Samuel B. Guze, "Establishment of Diagnostic Validity in Mental Illness: Its Application to Schizophrenia," *American Journal of Psychiatry* 106 (1970): 107–11.

broad category of "mental disorder," *DSM-III* included conditions that had always been understood as serious mental or neurologic illness (e.g., dementia, schizophrenia, bipolar mania, melancholic depression), conditions that were understood as rooted in personality and character (e.g., borderline personality disorder, histrionic personality disorder), conditions defined by problematic behaviors (e.g., alcohol abuse), and conditions that described unwanted and common areas of human experience, such as chronic depression and anxiety. All alike were rendered "mental disorders," which opened in a new way to psychiatric research and mental health treatment.[54]

DSM-III and its successors enabled unprecedented large-scale epidemiological study of mental disorders. Within a few years of its 1980 publication, numerous studies documented the prevalence of *DSM*-defined mental disorders in the United States and other populations.[55] It became possible to know with scientific precision, for example, that 1.3 percent of the US population meets criteria for bipolar disorder (according to the seminal Epidemiologic Catchment Area study)—because the *DSM* had for the first time specified what is meant by "bipolar disorder."[56]

54. Mitchell Wilson, "*DSM-III* and the Transformation of American Psychiatry: A History," *American Journal of Psychiatry* 150 (1993): 399–410. Writing in 1993, Mitchell argues that while *DSM-III* was not based on large-scale empirical studies, by presenting itself as a work of science the document shaped its social reception: "The project of descriptive psychiatry, officially established by DSM-III and continued by the development of DSM-III-R, has become much more than an expression of fashion. This is because the language of DSM-III is being applied in daily teaching and practice and necessarily takes on the look of something that, more and more, seems natural—not made by human hands. As with any professional discourse applied in teaching and clinical settings, reification of the discourse of descriptive psychiatry through daily use of DSM-III and DSM-III-R seems unavoidable. In addition, the ideological power of science cannot be underestimated as a contributing factor in the hegemony of the discourse of descriptive diagnosis in contemporary psychiatry. The seeming objectivity of science is science's own justification. The seeming objectivity of the project of descriptive psychiatry serves, rhetorically, as the most persuasive argument in its own behalf" (408). Wilson laments the way that *DSM-III* focused on the "superficial and publicly visible," rather than on "depth of mind," replaced "the unfolding of life over time" with a snapshot view of symptoms, and de-emphasized "personality and the ongoing development of character, unconscious conflict, transference, family dynamics, and social factors" (408).

55. These studies included the Epidemiological Catchment Area (ECA) Study, the National Comorbidity Study (NCS), and among Vietnam veterans, the National Vietnam Veteran Readjustment Study (NVVRS).

56. Myrna M. Weissman et al., "Affective Disorders," in *Psychiatric Disorders in America: The Epidemiologic Catchment Area Study*, ed. L. N. Robins and Darryl A. Regier (New York: Free Press, 1991), 53–80, cited in Ronald C. Kessler et al., "The Epidemiology of Major Depressive Disorder: Results from the National Comorbidity Survey Replication (NCS-R),"

The diagnostic categories of *DSM-III* quickly became the standard for psychiatric diagnosis not only in the United States but around much of the world, which shaped the way that mental illness is understood, researched, and treated globally. *DSM-III* gave language and form to the world of modern mental health care.

The Industrialization of Care

The standardization of diagnosis brought about by *DSM-III* stipulated that mental disorders *just are* syndromes of unwanted or disvalued experience and behavior. By specifying mental health problems as symptoms, *DSM-III* and its successors made it possible to conceive of mental health care as a standardized set of interventions in which particular technologies—whether talk therapies, medications, or somatic therapies such as electroconvulsive therapies—are implemented for specific disorders in ways that allow for systematic study. Mental health care became an industry with standard processes of product development, implementation, surveillance, and quality control. This began with newly standardized and scaled clinical research made possible by the clinical definitions of *DSM-III*. Because *DSM-III* defined a disorder known as major depressive disorder, epidemiologists could then investigate the prevalence of major depression in the US population and establish, for example, that 1.7 to 3.4 percent of Americans were depressed at any given time using *DSM-III* criteria.[57] Mood disorder researchers could then work to identify helpful treatments for depression, and so the diagnosis of major depressive disorder has shaped a generation's understanding of what forms of medication therapy and psychotherapy count as effective treatments for depression.[58] Be-

---

JAMA 289 (2003): 3095–3105. Of note, while the authors of *DSM-III* claimed that its categories were reliable (in that clinicians working in different places and contexts would be able to use the same language for the same presenting problems), the *DSM* made no claim that these diagnoses were *valid* (existing in nature); this was the task of researchers working in the wake of the *DSM* to prove. Robert L. Spitzer, Janet B. W. Williams, and Andrew E. Skodol, "*DSM-III*: The Major Achievements and an Overview," *American Journal of Psychiatry* 137 (1980): 151–64. More recently, however, in a critical examination of the *DSM-III* field trials, Stuart Kirk and Herb Kutchins have questioned whether even this claim to reliability is well founded. See Stuart A. Kirk and Herb Kutchins, *The Selling of DSM: The Rhetoric of Science in Psychiatry* (New York: Aldine de Gruyter, 1992).

57. Weissman et al., "Affective Disorders."

58. "VA/DOD Clinical Practice Guideline for the Management of Posttraumatic Stress Disorder and Acute Stress Disorder," The Management of Posttraumatic Stress

cause *DSM-III* defined a disorder known as PTSD, trauma researchers could then work to identify those suffering from PTSD so defined as well as helpful treatments for this condition. So the diagnosis of PTSD has shaped a generation's understanding of what forms of medication therapy and psychotherapy count as effective treatments for PTSD.[59]

In addition to its formative and structuring effect on mental health research, *DSM-III* and its successive revisions also shaped practices of coding and billing within mental health services. By ensuring that the international standard for medical coding and billing, the World Health Organization's *International Classification of Diseases and Related Health Problems* (*ICD*), was aligned with the *DSM* for the vast majority of conditions, the architects of *DSM-III* secured for the *DSM* both clinical and economic authority. After *DSM-III*, insurance companies, government programs such as Medicare and Medicaid, and other third-party payers required clinicians to diagnose patients with one or more *DSM/ICD* mental disorders in order to receive payment for their work. This cemented the *DSM* as the central organizing diagnostic framework of mental health care and forced clinicians to use its categories, notwithstanding reservations clinicians may have had about the framework.

By shaping how we think about and speak of mental illness, how research in mental health is conducted, and how clinicians are recognized and reimbursed for their work, the *DSM* has profoundly shaped mental health care practices and systems in the United States and in other countries. The *DSM*'s categories became the perfect medium for the rise of managed care within mental health, as funding conditions could be tied to particular diagnoses and in some cases approved only for care that is "evidence based" for these diagnoses.

Problematic Presumptions of the Machine Metaphor

Enabled by imaging the body and then the mind as a machine, reinforced by the standardization of psychiatric diagnosis, and brought to practical fulfillment in systems that understand mental health care as a kind of standardized industry, the machine metaphor exerts a powerful influence in modern mental health care. Having described the content of the machine metaphor

---

Disorder Work Group, 2017, https://www.healthquality.va.gov/guidelines/MH/ptsd/VADoDPTSDCPGFinal012418.pdf.

59. "VA/DOD Clinical Practice Guideline."

and having suggested some of its historical and professional sources, I now turn to five problematic presumptions of the machine metaphor that are all challenged by the Christian approach to mental health and mental illness that I will offer in subsequent chapters.

Individualism and Internalism

First, modern mental health care is structured by the dual presumptions of *individualism and internalism*, the idea that mental health problems are essentially located within (internal to) individual persons. The latest version of the *DSM* published in 2022, *DSM-5-TR*, makes this presumption explicit in its definition of "mental disorder":

> A mental disorder is a syndrome characterized by clinically significant disturbance in an *individual's* cognition, emotion regulation, or behavior that reflects a *dysfunction in the psychological, biological, or developmental processes underlying mental functioning.* Mental disorders are usually associated with significant distress or disability in social, occupational, or other important activities. An expectable or culturally approved response to a common stressor or loss, such as the death of a loved one, is not a mental disorder. Socially deviant behavior (e.g., political, religious, or sexual) and conflicts that are primarily between the individual and society are not mental disorders unless the deviance or conflict results from a *dysfunction in the individual*, as described above.[60]

This definition emerges in part from a desire not to pathologize experience and behavior that is rooted in social deviancy or protest, but also from the belief that treatment should focus on the experience and behaviors of *individuals*.[61] Even treatments that do not focus on individuals alone, such as couples therapy and family therapy, are typically used as adjuncts to the mental health care of individuals. They are started because a problem (treated as)

60. *DSM-5-TR*, 14, italics mine. Although there is little evidence that the definition of mental disorder in *DSM-5-TR* and prior editions have had any significant influence over which disorder categories are included in the volume, nevertheless they display how the architects of the *DSM* understand the conditions that psychiatrists treat.

61. Warren A. Kinghorn, "The Biopolitics of Defining 'Mental Disorder,'" in *Making the DSM-5: Concepts and Controversies*, ed. Joel Paris and James Phillips (New York: Springer, 2013), 47–61.

internal to an individual requires broader intervention (e.g., parent training therapy for a behaviorally dysregulated child). While most mental health clinicians and researchers readily affirm that mental disorders may be caused, exacerbated, or perpetuated by factors outside of an individual (e.g., delayed healing from PTSD due to an ongoing abusive relationship), these "social determinants of mental health" are often framed as risk factors for individually focused pathology.[62]

It is not surprising that mental health care characteristically focuses on the individual. The experience of mental illness is often deeply personal and, in many ways, unsharable. The emptiness of major depression, for instance, can be described to, but not fully understood by, persons other than the sufferer. As such, therapeutic relationships understandably focus on the individual's experience and behavior in a confidential context.

Locating mental illness inside individuals, though, can obscure the social and political contexts in which people live and that contribute to mental health problems. This is displayed in a pharmaceutical advertisement for the "minor tranquilizer" Serax (oxazepam), which appeared in the *Journal of the American Medical Association* in 1967 (see figure 2).[63] While the advertisement is dated, its themes remain relevant today.

In the advertisement, a young white woman (pharmaceutical advertisements for depression and anxiety medications often picture young white women) is sitting anxiously behind what appear, on first glance, to be prison bars. On closer inspection, however, the bars are the handles of various household cleaning tools: mops, a broom, and so on, while an iron and sponges sit before her, and a child's tricycle behind her. The advertisement reads as follows:

> You can't set her free. But you can help her feel less anxious.
>
> You know this woman. She's anxious, tense, irritable. She's felt this way for months.
>
> Beset by the seemingly insurmountable problems of raising a young family, and confined to the home most of the time, her symptoms reflect

62. Michael T. Compton and Ruth S. Shim, eds., *The Social Determinants of Mental Health* (Washington, DC: American Psychiatric Publishing, 2015).

63. I am indebted to a blog post by the journalist and writer Katherine Sharpe for introducing me to these advertisements. See Katherine Sharpe, "Bad Mothers and Single Women: A Look Back at Antidepressant Advertisements," *Huffington Post*, June 11, 2012, http://www.huffingtonpost.com/katherine-sharpe/antidepressant-advertising_b_1586830.html.

a sense of inadequacy and isolation. Your reassurance and guidance may have helped some, but not enough.

Serax (oxazepam) cannot change her environment, of course. But it can help relieve anxiety, tension, agitation, and irritability, thus strengthening her ability to cope with day to day problems.

This advertisement displays the problems of the individualistic and internalist presumptions of the machine metaphor. The "symptoms" of the woman "reflect a sense of inadequacy and isolation" that is related to the "seemingly insurmountable problems" of parenting young children and being confined to the home. Contemporary readers of this ad are likely to have a number of questions about her relational and social world. Why is she "confined to the home"? What kind of relationship does she have, if any, with a spouse or partner? How is she connected to others in her family and community, including a religious community, and how might social connection help to reduce her sense of isolation? What vocational dreams or aspirations has she had, or does she have, and what is preventing them from being fulfilled? But the advertisement does not entertain any of these questions: the physician's "reassurance and guidance" is presumed to be ineffective, and the physician is therefore encouraged not to ask deeper and more probing questions, or to work to empower her agency, but rather to reduce her internal "symptoms" through prescribing a short-acting anxiety medication.

We will consider the problems of individualism and internalism in more detail in chapters 2 and 3, but the advertisement points to two problems. First, individualism within mental health care reflects individualism and social disconnection within modern culture that perpetuates many of the experiences and behaviors that mental health care is intended to treat. Social support and close interpersonal relationships, for example, are often associated with lower rates of depression.[64] If treatment for depression simply reproduces individualism, then it may perpetuate the problem it is meant to solve.

There is no good reason to frame mental health problems primarily as problems of individuals that happen to affect the individual's social and communal context. Mental health problems might be framed just as well—if not more profitably—as problems of communities and cultures that somehow

64. Geneviève Gariépy, Helena Honkaniemi, and Amelie Quésnel-Vallée, "Social Support and Protection from Depression: Systematic Review of Current Findings in Western Countries," *British Journal of Psychiatry* 209 (2016): 284-93; Linda K. George et al., "Social Support and the Outcome of Major Depression," *British Journal of Psychiatry* 154 (1989): 478-85.

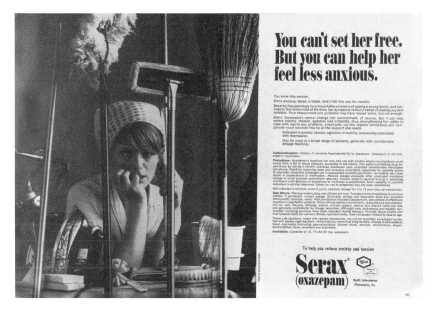

Figure 2. Advertisement in *Journal of the American Medical Association* 200, no. 8 (1967): 206

affect that community's individual members. In this social view of mental health, some individuals might be more vulnerable to effects of the community's disease, just as some children living in poverty are more vulnerable to developing asthma from tobacco smoke, vehicle exhaust, and cockroach dander. But the fact that only some children suffer does not make asthma a problem of those children alone. It is a community problem that is displayed in some of that community's children.

The second problem with the individualism and internalism exemplified by the advertisement above is that these link illness and diagnosis to identity. If my mental health problem is mine alone, belonging in a deep way to me and resting within me, I naturally wonder whether my mental health problem defines me. Maybe I simply *am* a depressive, or a borderline, or a bipolar/manic-depressive, or a schizophrenic, or an alcoholic. To some people, such as proponents of Mad identity,[65] linking diagnosis to identity frees and em-

65. Mohammed Abouelleil Rashed, *Madness and the Demand for Recognition: A Philosophical Inquiry into Identity and Mental Health Activism* (New York: Oxford University Press, 2019).

powers. But many others seek ways to distance their unwanted experience and behavior from their identity—and to do so they often turn to the presumptions of self-symptom dualism and self-body dualism.

Self-Symptom Dualism

Most mental health clinicians and advocates are keen to emphasize that mental disorders are not what a person *is* but rather something that a person *has*. *DSM-IV* stipulated this distinction as a basic rule for diagnostic language:

> A common misconception is that a classification of mental disorders classifies people, when actually what are being classified are disorders that people have. For this reason, the text of DSM-IV . . . avoids the use of expressions as "a schizophrenic" or "an alcoholic" and instead uses the more accurate, but admittedly more cumbersome, "an individual with Schizophrenia" or "an individual with Alcohol Dependence."[66]

Note the clear distinction between one's self (who one is) and one's symptoms and experiences (which one has). Just as I can *have* or *suffer from* influenza, so I can *have* or *suffer from* anxiety. My symptoms are external to my self.

The dynamics of this self-symptom dualism are displayed in another, more recent pharmaceutical advertisement (published in the *American Journal of Psychiatry* [2004]; see figure 3) for a commonly prescribed anxiolytic/ antidepressant medication. On the left panel of the advertisement, another young white woman is pictured alone and in front of a crooked window. Below are three statements that she is presumably saying to herself: "My sadness just won't go away." "I don't have the energy to go out with friends." "My constant worry is affecting my job." The physician reader is encouraged to "see depression." Presented with a stylized interpretation of selected research findings, the physician is then encouraged to "see the data." Then, on the right panel, the same woman is pictured again, this time surrounded by others, laughing and arm-wrestling. The physician is encouraged to "see a difference"—presumably the difference the antidepressant has made in reducing depression's symptoms.

66. American Psychiatric Association, *Diagnostic and Statistical Manual of Mental Disorders*, 4th ed. [*DSM-IV*] (Washington, DC: American Psychiatric Association, 1994), xxii.

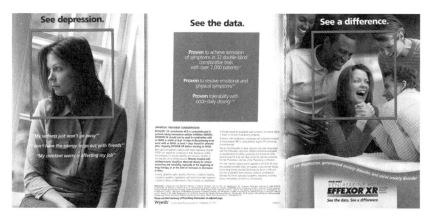

Figure 3. Advertisement that appeared in the *American Journal of Psychiatry* (July 2004): A41–A43

This advertisement shows how psychiatric diagnosis can become a way of *seeing* experience and behavior as separate from the self. Many find this way of seeing appealing because it avoids much of the shame and stigma that accompanies the association of illness with identity. It also encourages a hopeful orientation toward recovery: if I *have* depression, or bipolar disorder, or anxiety, then I can eventually *not have* these things, and still remain myself. Most of all, this way of seeing allows clinicians and patients to join forces against a common enemy: the symptoms and experiences that a person has and wants to be rid of. Mental health care becomes a collaborative fight against these externalized symptoms and behaviors.

Externalizing symptoms from the self can be helpful, but it also can mislead. First, there is a danger that the symptoms still continue to dominate people's self-understanding or the way that others perceive them, or both. The woman in the advertisement above is known to us not by her given name but only as "depression." If others see her only as depression and if she sees herself only as depression, then diagnosis has become identity, and self and symptoms are still fused. As we will explore in more detail in chapters 4 and 5, the way to ensure that illness does not define identity is not to externalize symptoms but to establish that human identity is rooted in our nature as creatures who are loved and known by God, created in the image of God, and invited to participate in God's life, regardless of the presence of any symptoms.

Second, however, there is an inverse danger that externalizing symptoms from the self might enforce too stark a separation. It is not always possible for me to identify a self apart from the experience and behavior that constitutes my self at any given point of my life. People who live for years or decades with mental illness may not find it easy to extract these experiences and behaviors from who they are; nor would all wish to do this. To live with anxiety, or depression, or schizophrenia, is in many cases to learn to inhabit one's world in particular ways that cannot be disentangled from those experiences—and to find in them blessings as well as challenges.

Self-Body Dualism

It is possible to understand mechanistic mental health care simply by reference to symptoms, without any attempt to describe what is causing the symptoms. But more often self-symptom dualism—splitting symptoms apart from the self—goes hand in hand with some version of René Descartes's self-*body* dualism. In self-body dualism, not only are *symptoms* separable from the self, but it is the *body* or *brain*, or both, that produces these symptoms—not the self, much less the social context. As a result, in self-body dualism, the very *body* is separate from and alien to the self. When mental illness is attributed to the body as a way of externalizing mental illness from the self, then modern mental health care tacitly embraces Descartes's mind-body dualism.

To be sure, few psychiatrists or other modern mental health clinicians would endorse Cartesian dualism. Most would reject Descartes's philosophical substance dualism, the theory that the human *res cogitans*, or thinking substance, is a substance distinct from the human *res extensa*, the extended material body. Most psychiatrists, after all, believe that mental illness is not a matter only of the mind. Mental illness is embodied.

Yet there is more than one way to be a Cartesian. Descartes lived and wrote at a time when early modern science was beginning to supplant the Aristotelian physics and metaphysics that had dominated European thought for the previous fifteen hundred years, and he affirmed what became known as substance dualism for more practical as well as speculative reasons. The *Discourse on Method* (1637), in which Descartes first articulated his theory of mind and affirmed famously, "I think, therefore I am," is a comparatively brief prologue to his three-volume work on optics, geometry, and meteors. For Descartes, the *Discourse* was a methodological primer on how to go about scientific progress. He wanted to open the natural world, including the world of the body, to scientific investigation but to do so without allowing the new science—the investigation of matter as space and extension—to subsume human life itself.

By positing that what makes us essentially human is our capacity for thought, and by further positing that this capacity for thought is "entirely distinct from the body," Descartes permitted science to investigate and manipulate the body in a way that left the human "essential self" unscathed. He was one of the first major thinkers to argue for the metaphor of the body as machine. The machine metaphor, rather than his mind-body dualism, constitutes Descartes's primary legacy for the world of medicine and mental health care.

When modern mental health clinicians and advocacy groups seek to decrease shame and stigma associated with mental illness by framing mental disorders as "brain disorders," they are engaging in Descartes's essential project. This form of dualism attempts to separate the body, posited as the bearer of disorder, from the essential self, posited as the self that is afflicted by the brain disorder. This dualism does not claim (nor did Descartes) that the mind is independent of the body, but it does abstract the self from the body in a way that makes the body safe for medical research, experimentation, and manipulation.

As with self-symptom dualism, self-body dualism can be a way to emphasize that mental illness does not determine one's identity. If mental illness is a problem of the brain, then mental illness is something that one *has* rather than something that one *is*. Empirical studies support this way of seeing: in two meta-analyses of studies of stigma and biological explanations for mental disorders, psychologists Nick Haslam, Erlend Kvaale, and William Gottdiener found that people who adopted "biogenetic explanations" for their own mental illness blamed themselves less and were viewed by others as less to blame for their illness.[67] Ann, whose story we encountered in the introduction to this book, affirms that biological accounts of mental health challenges can be helpful:

> I like to have things make sense and to recognize and accept that as human beings, we have chemistry. With some, chemistry makes you . . . want to talk to everybody and run for Congress or whatever. Someone else, you're sitting back and observing and not jumping right in. The whole extrovert,

67. Erlend P. Kvaale, Nick Haslam, and William H. Gottdiener, "The 'Side Effects' of Medicalization: A Meta-analytic Review of How Biogenetic Explanations Affect Stigma," *Clinical Psychology Review* 33 (2013): 782–94; Erlend P. Kvaale, William H. Gottdiener, and Nick Haslam, "Biogenetic Explanations and Stigma: A Meta-analytic Review of Associations among Laypeople," *Social Science and Medicine* 96 (2013): 95–103. Tanya Luhrmann comments more bluntly that "biology is the great moral loophole of our age." See Tanya Luhrmann, *Of Two Minds: The Growing Disorder in American Psychiatry* (New York: Knopf, 2000), 8.

introvert thing I think is all rooted in this, the fact that we are biological and chemical, and human beings. In so many ways, we're not the same. In some other ways, we are the same. I go, "Okay. Yeah. Good." Then I can accept who I am. I think that's been helpful. Because I think for years, I just thought, "There's something wrong with me. I can't be like that. I can't be more this or more that. There's just something wrong with me."[68]

But like self-symptom dualism, self-body dualism comes at a cost. First, we lack sufficient evidence to reduce any major mental disorder to a biochemical or bodily state of affairs.[69] A systematic umbrella review of studies documenting the association between the neurotransmitter serotonin and depression, for example, found "no consistent evidence of there being an association between serotonin and depression, and no support for the hypothesis that depression is caused by lowered serotonin activity or concentrations."[70] Second, self-body dualism can undermine patients' agency and increase stigma. The same meta-analyses that recorded lower self-blame and attribution of responsibility with biogenetic explanations also found that people with mental illness who accept biogenetic explanations are more pessimistic about their own chances for recovery, and more likely to be avoided by others. Third, because the problem is now outside the self, self-body dualism separates people from their own experience and makes them dependent on clinicians both to interpret experience and to find ways to change it.[71] Fourth, self-body dualism legitimizes biological interventions and especially psychiatric medication as first-line treatments for mental illness even when this is not clearly based in evidence. Insofar as mental illness is conceived as a brain disorder, then medications or other somatic treatments that directly target the brain (such as electroconvulsive therapy, ECT, or repetitive transcranial magnetic stimulation [rTMS]) appear the obvious choice for therapy. Research in other contexts, however, does not support the superiority of medication over psychotherapy as a first-line treatment for

68. Personal interview, June 3, 2022.

69. There are arguably exceptions to this, such as major neurocognitive disorder with Lewy bodies, but these are exceptions rather than the rule among *DSM* diagnostic categories.

70. Joanna Moncrieff et al., "The Serotonin Theory of Depression: A Systematic Umbrella Review of the Evidence," *Molecular Psychiatry* 28 (2023): 3243–56.

71. Nick Crossley, "Prozac Nation and the Biochemical Self: A Critique," in *Debating Biology: Sociological Reflections on Health, Medicine, and Society*, ed. Simon J. Williams, Lynda Birke, and Gillian A. Bendelow (New York: Routledge, 2003), 245–58.

mental disorders, though there are good reasons to prioritize medications in some cases and with some manifestations of mental disorder (e.g., active psychosis and acute bipolar mania). For example, in a sweeping practice guideline of the treatment of PTSD, the US Department of Defense and Department of Veterans Affairs clearly recommends short-term trauma-focused psychotherapy, rather than medication, as a first-line treatment for PTSD.[72]

Technicism

Individualism, self-symptom dualism, and self-body dualism lead directly to the problematic presumption of *technicism*, in which mental health interventions are wielded as instruments or tools to achieve prespecified ends, and progress in mental health care is marked by the development of more precise and sophisticated tools. Mental health care becomes a form of technology, a manifestation of the classical concept of *technē*, described by Joseph Dunne as a way of practicing in which (a) the end or goal is specified in advance of the application of method or technology, (b) the focus is on the best method or technology by which to attain the prespecified end, and (c) the successful application of the method or technology does not directly depend on the moral character of the practitioner.[73] Mental health care—whether in the form of psychotherapy, pharmacotherapy, or somatic treatments—becomes a technology that is applied to and used by individuals (individualism) to alleviate symptoms and signs (self-symptom dualism), often by targeting specific changes in the body (self-body dualism). The autonomous patient becomes the user or consumer of this technology, as well as the object of its action.

Technological models are so deeply ingrained within modern mental health care that it is hard for many clinicians, patients, and advocates to see them as a problem. The entire enterprise of evidence-based medicine and evidence-based psychotherapy displays the logic of *technē*: "evidence-based" or "effective" treatments are standardized treatments, designed to effect particular prespecified outcomes, that in principle can be applied by any clinician with requisite technical training and experience. Medications provide the paradigmatic examples of technology.

72. "VA/DoD Clinical Practice Guideline."
73. Joseph Dunne, *Back to the Rough Ground: "Phronesis" and "Techne" in Modern Philosophy and in Aristotle* (Notre Dame: University of Notre Dame Press, 1993).

In modern life, no one can avoid technology, and technology is often quite helpful. If I need to travel from North Carolina to California, I am grateful that aviation technology allows me to do so quickly and safely (if not always comfortably). If my appendix becomes inflamed, I am grateful that skilled practitioners can employ surgical instruments and techniques to remove my appendix with only minor risk of complications, thereby allowing me to resume my life with little interruption. If I become severely depressed, I am grateful that medication, psychotherapy, and treatments like electroconvulsive therapy (ECT) and repetitive transcranial magnetic stimulation (rTMS) can help me to recover.

But it is important to recognize the costs of technicism along with its benefits. First, when mental health care is understood as technique and mental health practitioners operate as technicians, this can leave patients feeling like experimental subjects. Commenting on her own experience of working with a psychiatrist to take antidepressant medication, Ann says,

> There wasn't a whole lot of talk [about medication]. There was an agreement between us that we'll try these things. If it doesn't work, we'll try something else. We did that for a year or two. Then, I just got tired of it. . . . I got tired of the laborious process. . . . It's just a hit and miss. I think none of us know anything about this. It's trial and error.[74]

Ann's comment is a vivid illustration that, as Martin Heidegger made clear, when humans take up with technology, we do not simply use technology. We are changed in the process; we begin to interpret the world through the capabilities and limitations of our technological power. Just as for a person with a hammer, everything looks like a nail, so also for a clinician with a prescription pad, all unwanted experience and behavior can begin to look like symptoms. For a psychotherapist trained in cognitive-behavioral therapy, the same experience and behavior can look like the product of cognitive distortions. For someone struggling with unwanted experience and behavior, the ubiquitous presence of mental health technologies shapes the character of that experience and behavior. For worse or for better, what might have been sadness becomes major depression, what was habitual drunkenness becomes substance use disorder, each named to fit particular mental health interventions. Though this technological framing of experience can lead to practically powerful results, it also can lead those struggling with un-

---

74. Personal interview, June 3, 2022.

wanted experience and behavior to find their identities increasingly labeled and subsumed by health care.[75]

A second cost of technicism is that it diverts our attention toward the sophistication of our instruments—our new medications, our manual-driven models of psychotherapy, our electroconvulsive therapy and transcranial magnetic stimulation therapy machines—and away from the ends or goals for which these instruments are deployed. Ends or goals remain: all mental health care is administered for some reason, with some end in mind. But technicism tends to reduce these ends to what the technology itself can intelligibly make happen, rather than asking how a mental health intervention is contributing to one's ability to live well. Ask a psychiatrist who prescribes antianxiety medication what the goal of his or her prescribing is for an anxious patient, and he or she likely will respond, "to help the patient to be less anxious"—where "anxiety" is understood as a symptom, or as a constellation of symptoms set forth in the *DSM* or in a standard rating scale like the Hamilton Anxiety Scale (HAM-A). This end seems straightforwardly worthy—until we remember that the *DSM* constructs for anxiety disorders were developed in large part to facilitate the development of antianxiety psychotherapies, medications, and other treatments. Sometimes pharmaceutical companies have sponsored expensive public awareness campaigns about specific disorders in order to sell a medication approved for that disorder, marketing a drug by marketing the disorder that it is intended to treat.[76] Saying that an anxiety medication works because it reduces symptoms of anxiety, while self-referentially true, is a lot like saying that earplugs work because they reduce the amplitude of sound waves that reach the eardrum from the external world. It is good to have earplugs when you need them. But it is also good to ask, "Is this a situation in which blocking my ability to receive sound waves is good for me?" The answer to that question is not dependent on whether the earplugs consistently work. In the same way, anxiety-reducing medication may work for anxiety, but this obscures the broader question of whether blunting the experience of anxiety is in the best interest of the person as a whole. To answer that question, one must consider a broader set of ends that technology alone cannot specify. But

---

75. For development of these themes within the context of Chistian ethics, see Jeffrey P. Bishop, "Of Minds and Brains and Cocreation: Psychopharmaceuticals and Modern Technological Imaginaries," *Christian Bioethics* 24 (2018): 224–45; Bishop, "Technics and Liturgics," *Christian Bioethics* 26 (2020): 12–30; Brian C. Brock, *Christian Ethics in a Technological Age* (Grand Rapids: Eerdmans, 2010).

76. Carl Elliott, *Better Than Well: American Medicine Meets the American Dream* (New York: Norton, 2003), 54–76.

who is empowered to determine these ends? This leads us to commodification, the fifth problematic presumption of modern mental health care.

Commodification

Who decides what mental health care is for? Mental health clinicians like to think that we do not decide for patients what is good for them—that instead we look to patients to guide their own use of mental health care services. We call this disposition by different names—patient autonomy, patient self-determination, patients' rights to set their own recovery goals. Even the concept of shared decision making, which acknowledges that clinicians have a role in shaping patient decisions, focuses on the right of a patient to determine the course of his or her care.[77]

Though modern mental health care places a high value on patient autonomy, it does so within limits. Involuntary commitment laws give mental health clinicians not only the right but the legal obligation to force particular forms of mental health care (e.g., hospitalization) on people who appear imminently dangerous to themselves or to others as a result of mental illness. Clinicians sometimes decline to provide mental health technologies even when patients demand them (e.g., controlled substances for patients who have been overusing or diverting them). These exceptions notwithstanding, however, modern mental health care is increasingly framed in the language of market exchange. As a psychiatrist, I am called a mental health "provider." Mental health care is a service (or, in some cases, a material good) that is "provided" to patients (often called "consumers") in some form of monetary exchange. Mental health care becomes a commodity: goods and services rendered in exchange for money.[78]

As with the other presumptions named in this section, commodifying mental health care brings benefits. It helps to establish boundaries: if patients treat me as a vendor, they retain power as customers. If they do not like what I provide, they can (and do) vote with their feet and go elsewhere. If I treat patients as customers or consumers, then I am less likely to treat them as friends or family members. Clear professional boundaries can foster safe intimacy in clinical re-

---

77. Glyn Elwyn et al., "Shared Decision Making: A Model for Clinical Practice," *Journal of General Internal Medicine* 27 (2012): 1361–67.

78. Farr Curlin and Christopher Tollefsen refer to this as the "Provider of Services Model," pervasive in contemporary health care, in contrast to their preferred "Way of Medicine." See Farr Curlin and Christopher Tollefsen, *The Way of Medicine: Ethics and the Healing Profession* (Notre Dame: University of Notre Dame Press, 2021).

lationships. Some patients will share their deepest concerns with me precisely because my relationship with them is professional and not personal.

But when commodification becomes the central way of organizing support for people living with mental health problems, it distorts the clinician-patient relationship and obscures therapeutic approaches that are truly healing. To begin, when health care (including mental health care) becomes a product for market exchange as it is in the United States, then it can be accessed only by those who can pay for it, either from their own resources or with the aid of third-party payers or beneficiary programs like the Veterans Health Administration. Those who cannot pay go without mental health care entirely, find themselves shunted to resource-strained public agencies, or end up in emergency departments or (most tragically) jails and prisons.

Framing mental health care as a commodity for market consumption also shapes and limits our imagination for what counts as mental health care and what is privileged within mental health care systems. Care becomes a unit of trade, fixed with a price. This privileges any aspect of care that can be commodified: bottles of medications, office visits with clinicians, sessions of rTMS therapy, days in inpatient mental health units, and so on. Clinicians learn to prioritize these commodified units, since these lead to reimbursement, income, and status. Interventions that cannot be easily commodified—exercise, participating in community organizations, healthy eating—lose visibility. Aspects of care that escape commodification—such as the quality of a therapist's relationship with a patient—often fade from view entirely, visible only in the crude proxies of patient satisfaction ratings and dropout rates.[79]

Finally, commodifying mental health care suppresses the question of what mental health care is for. It offloads the task of discerning the end of mental health care to the impersonal structures of the market economy, which treat the end of mental health care as whatever those who consume and purchase

---

79. Jennifer Radden critiques the model of the mental health practitioner as "technical/technological expert" by pointing out its presumptions that "(1) the consumer acts with full agency, and (2) enjoys rough social equality with the expert, with whom (3) purposes and understandings are also shared; that the relationship is (4) governed by a contract nullified when either party violates its terms, and finally (5) incidental to the effectiveness of the transaction beyond the maintenance of basic 'contractual' trust" (267). But given the disparities of power between mental health clinicians and patients, particularly in times of crisis, none of these presumptions are valid. For Radden, this points to the need to prioritize the virtues in the formation and education of mental health clinicians. See Jennifer Radden, "Thinking about the Repair Manual: Technique and Technology in Psychiatry," in *Philosophical Perspectives on Technology and Psychiatry*, ed. James Phillips (New York: Oxford University Press, 2009), 263–78.

it say it is. Consumer demand establishes the goal of mental health care. But consumer demand is shaped by other forces that have their own ends. Particular forms of mental health care, such as medication prescription, are marketed and promoted by those who stand to profit from them: medications are for the shareholders of pharmaceutical companies as well as for patients. Payment for mental health care is justified by the promise of avoiding more significant expenses to third-party payors.[80] Mental health care systems support high-paying jobs within local economies. Mental health care becomes "for" a lot of things: the alleviation of patient suffering, yes, but also the satisfaction of consumer demand, the profitability of those who sell mental health services, the sustenance of the economy's health care sector, and the formation of people for economic productivity. These ends might, or might not, align with what is good for the person living with mental illness.

Rethinking Mental Health Care: The Need for a Different Approach

It is good that modern mental health care exists. As a psychiatrist, I am humbled that people will entrust themselves at some of the most painful and vulnerable times of their lives to the care of mental health clinicians. I celebrate when someone experiences healing and recovery related to that care. I am humbled also by the deep wisdom that many of my colleagues display after years of attending people who are suffering. As someone who has both received and offered mental health care, I am grateful.

But mental health care in the United States is broken, and the standard solutions for this brokenness—more research, more funding, more psychiatrists and clinicians, better third-party payment—may help but will not heal. To begin to heal the brokenness of mental health care we must answer three questions. *Who* is mental health care for? *What* is mental health care for? And following on these, *how* is modern mental health care to be engaged?

Who Is Mental Health Care For?

When asked, "Who is mental health care for?" the obvious answer is, "Well, of course, it is for the patient." And indeed all mental health care can in some

---

80. "Issue Brief: Parity," Mental Health America, https://www.mhanational.org/issues/issue-brief-parity.

way be narrated as *for* the patients who receive it. But a closer look reveals that mental health care is not *only* for patients: it is for many other things besides. These other things need to be named and evaluated. Sometimes mental health care is for not only the patient but also the health and safety of others, as when patients are involuntarily committed to psychiatric units due to clinicians' concern that they will harm others. Sometimes mental health care is for not only the patient but also the well-being of an institution, as when universities expand student mental health services and launch wellness initiatives to decrease their risk of student suicide, sexual assault, and other adverse mental health outcomes. Sometimes mental health care is for not only the patient but also the efficient functioning of a social collective, as when children deemed disruptive within classrooms are diagnosed and medicated for attention deficit/hyperactivity disorder.

As I will argue in the following chapters, mental health care cannot be for the patient alone, because human beings do not live in isolation, and the flourishing of one cannot be isolated from the community to which one belongs. Mental health care will always, in some way, be *for* persons as we live together in community. The key question, then, is not how to make mental health care serve only the patient but rather how mental health care can be genuinely for the patient as he or she lives in community, without sacrificing the good of the former to the latter. But this requires a nonindividualistic account of personhood and a noncommodified account of mental health care.

What Is Mental Health Care For?

To engage mental health care with integrity, one needs some account, however tacit, of what mental health care is for. Unfortunately, many clinicians and mental health leaders have no ready answer to this question. None of the most straightforward answers satisfy. Some may say that mental health care is for mental health, but that only raises the questions, "What is mental health?" and the corollary question, "Who has the authority to decide what mental health entails for a particular patient?" Others may say that mental health care is for the relief of suffering, or for the attainment of happiness, or for the cultivation of autonomy, or for maximization of economic productivity and meaningful work—all judgments about the nature of mental health, and all contestable. Others, seeking to alleviate clinicians of the moral burden of adjudicating the meaning of mental health, may respond that mental health care should be for whatever the patient wants it to be for. But beyond the fact

that this approach reinforces the individualism, technicism, and commodification of mental health care already discussed, it also contradicts practices
that mental health clinicians believe are well justified. Mental health clinicians routinely say no to requests for interventions the clinician judges to be
unhelpful or unsafe—such as prescriptions of opioids and benzodiazepines to
patients who are drinking high amounts of alcohol. In other cases, clinicians
are prohibited by law or professional rules from offering some interventions,
such as prescription of lethal doses of barbiturates for terminally ill patients
or offering therapy intended to change a patient's sexual orientation, even if
patients request them. In practice, mental health care is usually guided by the
preferences of the patient, but this fact does not settle the question of what
ends are legitimate for mental health care to pursue. We need a better moral
and philosophical account of the nature of mental health and, following this,
the goals of mental health care.

How Is Mental Health Care to Be Engaged?

This third question is the central practical question of this book, but it follows
directly from the first two and cannot be answered without them. Only when
we have at least provisionally answered the questions of *who* mental health
care is for and *what* mental health care is for can we begin to address the question of how to engage particular mental health care practices.

These three questions, the first two directly informing the third, will guide
the remainder of this book.

CHAPTER 2

From Duality to Unity

We Are Creatures of Earth Formed for Relationship and Love

> My frame was not hidden from you,
> when I was being made in secret,
>   intricately woven in the depths of the earth.
> Your eyes beheld my unformed substance.
> In your book were written
>   all the days that were formed for me,
>   when none of them as yet existed.

—Psalm 139:15–16

You are not enough. You are not valued. You are not loved. You are alone. People who live with mental illness find these messages all too present. Many of my patients who live with chronic depression, anxiety, PTSD, substance use, and other mental health problems have experienced rejection from communities, fracturing of relationships, and the loss of goals and dreams. Rarely have patients sought my help simply because of an isolated bothersome symptom, such as difficulty sleeping or panic attacks, when everything else in life is going well. Much more commonly the symptoms with which people present are the tip of the iceberg, the visible evidence of a host of deeper questions and concerns about relationships, vocation, identity, and worth. Any Christian engagement with mental health care, then, must start from the right place— not focused primarily on symptoms and how they might best be ameliorated technologically but focused on who we are as human beings before one another and before God.

In the previous chapter, I argued that modern mental health care displays the influence of the machine metaphor. The machine metaphor depicts our bodies as complex machines that when broken in particular ways can give rise to mental illness. This image of the body as machine is influenced by René Descartes's self-body dualism—the belief that I, as a self, can stand apart from and in judgment of my machine-body. It is also associated with the closely related self-symptom dualism, in which I envision *my symptoms* as things that are separate from me, things I *have*. These dualisms lead us to imagine mental health care as technology that can be commodified, bought and sold in a market economy.

Each of the chapters that follow will show how this mechanistic image of the body and of mental health care contradicts a Christian understanding of the human person and undermines a Christian approach to mental health care. The machine metaphor leads to an image of humans as mechanisms from which consciousness somehow emerges, who grasp for control in a universe in which we are alone. But Christian faith affirms something quite different: that humans are multidimensional beings who are loved by God, who are summoned on a journey, who find our fulfillment in wonder, love, and praise. This chapter and chapters 3, 4, and 5 focus on *who humans are* and on the irreducibly relational character of human life, affirming that we are creatures of earth formed for relationship and love (chapter 2) who become who we are in relationship with others and with the world around us (chapter 3), and then that far from being alone in the universe, we are known and loved by God and invited to be held in the life of Jesus (chapters 4–5). Chapters 6–9 then focus on *where humans are going*, affirming that we are wayfarers on a journey (chapters 6–8) and that we are called not to control but to wonder, love, praise, and sabbath rest (chapter 9).

Creatures of Earth

Christian engagement with mental health must begin with the earthiness of our bodies. We are dust. But there is more: we are dust that has been formed by God to be fit for relationship. We find ourselves not only in the dust of our bodies but in fabrics of relationship with others, with the world around us, and with God.

Genesis 2 teaches that "the LORD God formed man [*adam*] from the dust of the ground [*adamah*], and breathed into his nostrils the breath of life, and the man became a living being [*nephesh*]. And the LORD God planted a garden in Eden, in the east; and there he put the man whom he had formed" (Gen. 2:7–8). Dust from dust, *adam* from *adamah*: the first human was intimately connected to soil, to plants, to other animals, and eventually to another human, "bone of my bones, and flesh of my flesh" (Gen. 2:23). It was as body, as dust, as flesh and bone, that the first humans lived as creatures before God. Of note, the enlivening breath or spirit (*ruah*) imparted by God did not constitute humans as disembodied souls that could exist in completeness apart from the body. The first humans existed in body-soul unity. As Wendell Berry writes,

> My mind, like most people's, has been deeply influenced by dualism, and I can see how dualistic minds deal with this verse. They conclude that the formula for man-making is: man = body + soul. But that conclusion cannot be derived, except by violence, from Genesis 2:7, which is not dualistic. The formula given in Genesis is not man = body + soul; the formula there is soul = dust + breath. According to this verse, God did not make a body and put a soul into it, like a letter into an envelope. He formed man of dust; by breathing his breath into it, he made the dust live. Insofar as it lived, it was a soul. The dust, formed as man and made to live, did not *embody* a soul; it *became* a soul. "Soul" here refers to the whole creature. Humanity is thus presented to us, in Adam, not as a creature of two discrete parts temporarily glued together but as a single mystery.[1]

The creation accounts in the Psalms and in Hebrew wisdom literature consistently celebrate the dust-nature of human life. Our nature as dust reminds us of our radical vulnerability and dependency on God. Sometimes this dust-nature leads to affirmation and assurance:

> As a father has compassion for his children,
>> so the LORD has compassion for those who fear him.
> For he knows how we were made;
>> He remembers that we are dust. (Ps. 103:13–14)

At other times, our dust-nature terrifies and confuses:

> Your hands fashioned and made me;
>> and now you turn and destroy me.
> Remember that you fashioned me like clay;
>> and will you turn me to dust again?

---

1. Wendell Berry, "Christianity and the Survival of Creation," in *Sex, Economy, Freedom, and Community: Eight Essays* (New York: Pantheon, 1992), 106.

> Did you not pour me out like milk
>> and curdle me like cheese?
> You clothed me with skin and flesh,
>> and knit me together with bones and sinews.
> You have granted me life and steadfast love,
>> and your care has preserved my spirit. (Job 10:8–12)

But always, our dust-nature reminds us that we never live except as connected with the soil, the environment, and the world of living beings. We are created *from* the ground, we live *on* the ground, and we are profoundly affected by the ground conditions in which we live. The health of our bodies—including our mental health—is deeply connected to what we eat, what we breathe, and where we live. Chronically exposed to environmental toxins, we become polluted and diseased. Sleep-deprived and information-overloaded in a world of artificial light that extracts and distances us from natural rhythms of night and day, we grow weary, inattentive, and anxious.[2] Again, Wendell Berry:

> Our bodies are involved in the world. Their needs and desires and pleasures are physical. Our bodies hunger and thirst, yearn toward other bodies, grow tired and seek rest, rise up rested, eager to exert themselves. All these desires may be satisfied with honor to the body and its maker, but only if much else besides the individual body is brought into consideration. We have long known that individual desires must not be made the standard of their own satisfaction. We must consider the body's manifold connections to other bodies and to the world. The body, "fearfully and wonderfully made," is ultimately mysterious both in itself and in its dependences.[3]

The biblical teaching that human bodies are dust means that there is no essential conflict between Christian faith, properly understood, and biological observations showing a connection between the body and mental illness. Because we are dust, because we live as bodies, we can hardly be surprised that bodily states of affairs show up in our lived experience and behavior. When our bodies are fighting infection and we develop a fever, we feel depleted and

2. Gabriel Natan Pires et al., "Effects of Acute Sleep Deprivation on State Anxiety Levels: A Systematic Review and Meta-analysis," *Sleep Medicine* 24 (2016): 109–18.

3. Wendell Berry, "Health Is Membership," in *Another Turn of the Crank* (Berkeley: Counterpoint, 1995), 86–109.

exhausted. When we have slept poorly, we feel inattentive, impulsive, and emotional. When we drink a cup of strong coffee, we feel more alert, and when we drink three, perhaps fidgety and irritable. When multiple small strokes kill millions of brain cells, we experience trouble with memory and cognitive function. When biological researchers show connections between the body and mental illness, Christian faith responds: yes, we are dust.

Configured Dust: The Need for a Multidimensional View of Human Beings

But that we are dust does not imply that our mental health problems can be understood simply by reference to the body or brain. After all, *all* human experience and behavior occurs in the brain and body—not just the forms of experience and behavior that come to be labeled "mental illness." The love that lovers feel for each other, or that a parent feels for a small child, happens in the brain and body. When a concert pianist plays Rachmaninoff's Piano Concerto no. 3 to a rapt audience, the playing happens in her brain and body, and the listening and enjoyment happen in the audience members' brains and bodies. My typing of these words is happening in my brain and body. But no one would say that the bodily location of parental or romantic love, performing or appreciating great music, or writing a book is an adequate explanation of these things. It only names their material conditions.

The machine metaphor and Christian teaching agree that human beings are dust—or, at least, that understanding humans, and the way that humans suffer, requires paying close attention to the biological material of the human body. Unlike Christian teaching, however, the machine metaphor assumes that human beings are *only* dust, and that any meaning of the body is assigned to it by the self who occupies that body or by others. In the machine metaphor, bodies just *are*, and it is the task of the self or others to understand how they are to be used.

Thomas Aquinas had a very different view of the body. He shares the view that human bodies are dust. As those composed of the mud of the earth (*de limo terrae*), humans share this earthiness with all other embodied creatures (*STh* IaIIae q. 91 a. 1 *resp.*). But the statement that we are dust, while true, doesn't explain very much. Just as knowing that a car is composed of various plastics, fabrics, and metals is useful but insufficient for understanding the car, so also knowing that a human body is composed of fat, water, proteins, and so on is useful but insufficient for understanding human beings. Understanding why requires that we unpack how Thomas Aquinas understands the concept of substance.

Substance, for Aquinas, has a precise meaning, drawn from Aristotle, that is not reflected in our contemporary language (especially the contemporary mental health language of "substance use"). For Aquinas, a substance is at root an existing thing, considered as simply as possible apart from any incidental and nonessential characteristics (these incidental and nonessential characteristics are called accidents). While Aquinas holds that some substances, like the angels, are immaterial, he primarily understands substance as material things—creatures, that is, of dust. Substances like rocks, plants, animals, and humans are natural, in that that they are not formed by craft or industrial process and manifest a self-determining directive course of action. By contrast, marble statues, violins, and toasters are artifacts.[4] None of these, however, can be understood in full simply by reference to their matter. Rather, Aquinas holds that to understand the nature of something, one needs to consider four dimensions that make that thing what it is. Aquinas describes these as *causes*, though they are more expansive than the way that we think of causes in our time. They are better understood as determining factors in making a thing what it is. Because each of these causes names a particular dimension according to which a thing can be understood, I will refer to this as Aquinas's four-dimensional approach.

What are these four determining factors, or causes? First, things have a *material* cause, which is the matter of which a thing is composed. The material cause or dimension of my body is the dust of which my body is made: water, amino acids, fat, carbohydrates, and so on.[5] For Aquinas, matter is important because it is the foundation of individuality. When I am standing in a grocery store aisle and looking for a particular brand of cereal, no others (to their dismay and annoyance) can occupy the precise spot where I am standing,

---

4. Robert Edward Brennan, *Thomistic Psychology: A Philosophic Analysis of the Nature of Man* (New York: Macmillan, 1941), 32–33; Jason Eberl, *The Nature of Human Persons: Metaphysics and Bioethics* (Notre Dame: University of Notre Dame Press, 2020), 152–53; Edward Feser, "Nature versus Art," *Edward Feser* (blog), April 30, 2011, http://edwardfeser .blogspot.com/2011/04/nature-versus-art.html.

5. Aquinas, *De Principiis Naturae*, chap. 1, secs. 2–4, 6, from Joseph Bobik, *Aquinas on Matter and Form and the Elements: A Translation and Interpretation of the* De Principiis Naturae *and the* De Mixtione Elementorum *of St. Thomas Aquinas* (Notre Dame: University of Notre Dame Press, 1998). We will soon see that even these chemical components are formed matter. For Aquinas, matter is the potentiality to receive form, but matter without form (prime matter) is not a substance (because it has no form) and does not exist in nature.

because I am there. They would have to use their own bodies to displace mine. The matter of my body is the site of my life, anchoring me to a specific time and place, and the site of my growth and change as a person over time.[6]

At the same time, however, very little of who we are can be known by examining the matter of our bodies. Much more interesting to clinicians and scientists, including neuroscientists, is how the matter of our bodies is *configured* to make complex cells, tissues, organs, and organ systems, and how those systems work together to sustain the body's life. Aquinas referred to this configuration, or form, as the second determining factor that makes a thing what it is. A true substance is never matter alone or form alone; it is always "configured matter," the union of matter and form.[7] Aquinas would affirm, in fact, that there is no actual existent matter that has not been configured, or shaped, in some way. Even the molecules of my body are formed into molecules, and the same is true for the atoms and subatomic particles that comprise them.

For Aquinas, a thing's form is what makes it what it is. Matter specifies *that* a thing is, and *where* and *when* it is, but it is matter's configuration or form that specifies *what* it is. The same molecules of carbon, oxygen, calcium, iron, and so on can be configured into the body of a warthog or into the body of a human being. The matter is the same, but the form, and therefore the thing itself, is different. The same principle applies to different individuals of the same species. Any two humans—Elizabeth and Mehul, for instance—share a common substantial form, that of humanness. But they are different because the matter of their bodies individuates them into two people, one of whom is named Elizabeth and the other of whom is named Mehul. Furthermore, the bodies and minds of Elizabeth and Mehul are configured differently in innumerable ways—height, weight, skin complexion and tone, temperament, even gender.[8] These additional configurations—characteristics that distinguish people from one another but that don't alter their common humanity—are what Aquinas calls "accidental forms." (For Aquinas, as stated above, accidents are not mishaps or unfortunate occurrences but rather simply happenings, nonessential and incidental things that happen to or occur in a substance without changing its nature.) Elizabeth is a unique individual because the dust of her body is

6. *STh* Ia q. 50 a. 1 *resp.*; Eberl, *Nature of Human Persons*, 31–34.

7. Eleonore Stump, "Non-Cartesian Substance Dualism and Materialism without Reductionism," *Faith and Philosophy* 1995 (12): 505–31; Stump, *Aquinas* (New York: Routledge, 2003), 200–206.

8. William Newton, "Why Aquinas's Metaphysics of Gender Is Fundamentally Correct: A Response to John Finley," *Linacre Quarterly* 87 (2020):198–205.

configured in particular ways—with the substantial form of humanness and with the many accidental forms that make her uniquely who she is. Aquinas refers to the form of any living human—the particular configuration of matter that marks that matter as alive—as one's soul (*STh* IaIIae q. 75 a. 5).

Matter and form, then—what Aquinas would call "material cause" and "formal cause"—are the two essential ingredients of substances and necessary for understanding them. But Aquinas held that there are two other dimensions that are essential for understanding substances, which he referred to as "efficient cause" and "final cause."

"Efficient cause" names what in ordinary language is often described simply as "cause." It is the power or process—the agent—that has led to the substance's specific form or configuration. For nonnatural entities—artifacts—it is often easy to identify an efficient cause.[9] The efficient cause of a violin is the luthier, who works with specialized tools that enable her to bend and shape various kinds of wood into a violin. For natural substances like oak trees and humans, specifying efficient causation is more complex and is a central project of biological science. In the case of a human being, for example, one's parents are efficient causes, having initiated a new, unique life through (in most cases) the act of sexual union. The natural, immanent processes of embryological and postnatal development—what Aquinas understood as the powers of the soul—are also efficient causes.[10] External factors, as varied as viruses, diet, and relationships, are also efficient causes that shape the configuration of our bodies in particular ways. As humans grow, make choices, and act on them, our choices and actions are efficient causes of our further development and change. We become, as Aquinas says, "intelligent beings endowed with free will and self-movement," capable of acting causally on ourselves (*STh* IaIIae *proem.*).[11]

---

9. There is debate among scholars of Aquinas, reflecting some ambiguity in Aquinas's own writing, about whether artifacts are substances—that is, whether things produced by art, such as a violin, are united by substantial form (making the thing a substance) or by accidental forms. If the latter, then a violin is not a substance proper but an artifact composed of integral parts, such as wood and catgut, which are themselves proper substances. To avoid this debate, I use the term "entities" for artifacts. See Michael Rota, "Substance and Artifact in Thomas Aquinas," *History of Philosophy Quarterly* 21 (2004): 241-59; Anna Marmodoro and Ben Page, "Aquinas on Forms, Substances and Artifacts," *Vivarium* 54 (2016): 1-21.

10. Benedict Ashley, *The Way toward Wisdom: An Interdisciplinary and Intercultural Introduction to Metaphysics* (Notre Dame: University of Notre Dame Press, 2006), 112.

11. More precisely, one's parents are efficient causes of one's essential humanness, in that they made it possible for a unique human being to exist. Causes related to prenatal or postnatal environment, development, and so on are efficient causes of accidental, not essential, forms.

For Aquinas, efficient causation is important, but it is not enough only to ask how something came to be. It is also important to understand what a thing is tending toward, or where it is going, which Aquinas describes as its *final cause*. The final cause of a thing is the end or goal toward which it tends, the realization of which allows the thing to be most fully what it is. As is the case with efficient cause, it is easiest to identify final cause in the case of artifacts. The final cause of a toaster is toasting bread. The final cause of a violin is the production of a particular range and tenor of beautiful sound. Understanding what a toaster or violin is *for* is central for understanding what these things are.

Identifying the final cause of natural substances becomes more difficult in proportion to the complexity of the natural thing. The final cause of a rock is, well, to be a rock—to occupy space with a certain mass and density and, presupposing a gravitational field, to fall to the ground when dropped. The final cause of a daffodil is to sprout, to flower, and to reproduce. Aquinas holds that unlike rocks, living organisms are equipped with intrinsic tendencies to actualize their own fulfillment. Understanding these intrinsic tendencies is crucial for understanding the living organism.[12]

But what is the final cause of humans, the goal toward which humans naturally tend in order to realize our fulfillment? Aquinas calls this *beatitudo*, often translated as "happiness" or "flourishing." I will sometimes refer to *beatitudo* in these ways, but I will argue that the term is best rendered as "participation in blessing." We will explore *beatitudo* much more in chapters 6 and 9, but stated briefly, Aquinas holds that like all living creatures, humans *just are* the kind of beings who act toward what we consciously or unconsciously believe will lead to our fulfillment (*STh* IaIIae q. 1 aa. 1, 6, 7). We do not wake up one day, say at age fifteen, and think, "Hey, now that I've lived in this body for fifteen years, I will now set life goals and begin to act according to my values in ways that will meet my needs and make me happy." We *already* do this, from the moment of conception and long before we are able to reflect consciously on our experience. We are always beings who act toward ends that

---

12. Benedict Ashley argues that the concept of final causation "is commonly rejected in modern science, yet it is a concept absolutely necessary to the explanatory power of scientific thought," because it names the expected and stable effects that result from the movement of efficient causes. When my dog Burley jumps with excitement at the sound of dry food landing in his bowl, the cumulative result of the multiple efficient causes at work in that situation, from the stimulus of the food to the multiple movements in Burley's brain and gut, can be understood by saying that Burley is hungry and is drawn to satisfy his own need for nutrition. See Ashley, *Way toward Wisdom*, 82.

we discern to be good for us. Even our most mundane choices about what we do each day—my deciding to write this book, or your deciding to read it, or my son's decision to brush his teeth—are in some way connected to a deeper desire for our fulfillment. For Aquinas, consideration of goals or ends (final cause) is deeply important because it is impossible to understand human beings unless we seek to understand not just from where we have come but where we are trying to go.

Centering Persons, Not Diagnoses

What does all of this have to do with understanding mental health and mental illness? Why are Aquinas's accounts of substance and of the four dimensions (or causes) important for understanding humans?

Listening to Aquinas will lead us to center *persons* rather than disorders or diagnoses as the focus of mental health care. Under the influence of the machine metaphor, it is all too easy to speak about mental health in ways that sideline or even erase the people who are seeking and receiving mental health care. Clinicians may speak about diagnosing depression, treating bipolar disorder, or preventing suicide. They may say, more specifically, that "clozapine is the only drug with proven efficacy in schizophrenia that does not respond to other antipsychotics."[13] But for Aquinas, no pattern of experience and behavior, including those patterns of experience and behavior that we would now call mental illness, is a substance. "Mental illness" is rather a *label* that is broadly used to categorize these particular patterns. These patterns at best reflect *configurations* of body and mind that affect but do not efface or replace the identity of the person. Just as height, weight, and skin color are accidental forms—that is, occurrences or happenings—that affect someone without changing their essential humanness, so also any particular manifestation of experience and behavior that is labeled "mental illness" is at best an accidental form. My illness can never be my identity. And as a psychiatrist, I do not treat "depression." I treat Elizabeth and Mehul, unique persons who, for a time, are experiencing what psychiatrists have come to call depression.[14]

13. R. J. Flanagan et al., "Clozapine in the Treatment of Refractory Schizophrenia: A Practical Guide for Healthcare Professionals," *British Medical Bulletin* 135 (2020): 73–89.

14. Aquinas's account of accidental forms provides a way to affirm that mental illness does not define identity, yet without slipping into the externalization of self-symptom dualism (see chapter 1). As accidental form, my experience shapes me and is a dimension of who I am but does not define my essence.

"Person" (*persona*) is an important concept for Aquinas, just as it was for his medieval theological contemporaries. In part related to the complex debates in Christian theology about what it means for the Father, Son, and Holy Spirit to exist as three persons in one nature, the concept of person shifted in the early centuries of the church from denoting particular social roles or legal designations (for example, a role in a stage play) to denoting particular, existing individuals capable of action and self-communication. A person, that is, is not the role that an actor may assume, but the actor herself. Following the influential definition of the sixth-century philosopher Boethius, Aquinas defined "person" as "a subsistent individual of a rational nature" and as "individual substance of a rational nature."[15] As individual substances of a rational nature, persons are knowing and loving *subjects* capable of some degree of self-awareness and of directing their own action. To be a person, that is, is to be "someone," not "something."[16] W. Norris Clarke furthermore argues that to be a human person is to be an embodied spirit who is not only capable of directing one's own action (self-possession and self-determination) but also grows and forms through relationship with others (self-communication and receptivity) and is drawn ultimately toward God as the "One Center and Source of the whole universe" (self-transcendence).[17]

We will explore throughout this chapter and this book what it means for the person to be embodied, rational, capable of directing action, relational, and drawn to God, especially when mental health problems or disability make it harder to feel or to realize these attributes. Suffice it to say, for now, that one does not cease to be a person, or become somehow less of a person, if these characteristics are not evident. That status is given by God in creation, regardless of capacity (see chapter 5). But it makes all the difference for clinicians to regard our patients as *persons* rather than as collections of symptoms.

Aquinas's affirmation of personal existence, along with his account of substance and the four causes, also makes clear that human experience and behavior can never be understood only by a reductive focus on the body and

---

15. *STh* Ia q. 29 a. 3 *resp.*; q. 29 a. 4 *resp.* Aquinas clarifies that because "person" is "what is most perfect in all nature," it can be attributed to God, though "in a more excellent way," by analogy. The divine persons are properly not individual substances but rather subsistent relations. See also Thomas Joseph White, *The Trinity: On the Nature and Mystery of the One God* (Washington, DC: Catholic University of America Press, 2022), 448–49.

16. Robert Spaemann, *Persons: The Difference between "Someone" and "Something,"* trans. Oliver O'Donovan (New York: Oxford University Press, 2006), 16–33; *STh* Ia q. 29 a. 1.

17. W. Norris Clarke, SJ, *Person and Being: The Aquinas Lecture, 1993* (Milwaukee: Marquette University Press, 1993).

brain. In order to understand what is happening with any substance (including a person), one must consider all four causal dimensions: material cause, formal cause, efficient cause, and final cause—or, for shorthand, *matter, form, agent*, and *end* (*De Principiis Naturae*, chap. 3, secs. 15-17). To understand Mehul, one must consider the location and elemental composition of Mehul's body (matter), the way that his body is configured (form), the multidimensional factors that have led to that configuration (agent), and the purposes or goals toward which he is tending, either consciously or unconsciously (end). If I neglect any one of these dimensions, I've left out something essential, and I won't really understand Mehul.

If this four-dimensional approach applies to understanding a person, it surely applies to understanding how a person develops, lives with, and responds to mental health problems. Most clinicians and neuroscientists understand the value of attending to material and formal cause: Of what matter is this body composed, and how is it configured? They also are comfortable with attention to efficient cause: What powers or processes led this matter to be configured in this particular way? But Aquinas encourages us to attend also to final cause: How is this person able to move toward the goals that help them to realize their potential? Aquinas's embrace of final causation (or teleology, the study of a being's *telos* or end) challenges modern reductionism, because it suggests that we can't really understand a thing unless we understand the end toward which it is directed, either by its natural properties (as with inanimate objects), by natural properties and instinct (as with animals), or by natural properties, instinct, and free will (as with human beings). The question of whether a person is moving toward ends or goals that are life-giving is not a neurochemical question but a moral question. Answering it requires a frame of judgment that is as broad as human life and culture itself. It is to ask, How does this bodily configuration relate to the well-lived life for this person? It requires attending not only to neurons and brain circuits but also to a person's life narrative, culture, hopes, fears, dreams, and goals. All of these are essential for understanding the context of a person who is experiencing mental health challenges.[18]

18. In debates about the ethics of psychiatric diagnosis, this is known as the *caseness* problem: When does a particular constellation of experience and behavior become a *case* of mental disorder? While some philosophers such as Christopher Boorse have attempted to define disease or disorder in naturalistic ways, for instance as deviation from species-typical functioning, most philosophers, social scientists, and clinicians who have engaged this question conclude that the definition of caseness requires judgments of value—judgments, for example, about whether the person or others are harmed. See John Sadler,

Dust Formed for Relationship

While Aquinas affirms that humans are creatures of dust, his four-dimensional approach to understanding substances forces questions that push against biological reductionism and the machine metaphor. If we apply Aquinas's teaching to our understanding of mental health challenges, we must consider not only the matter of the body (material cause) but how that body is configured (formal cause), what has led to that configuration (efficient cause), and how the configuration affects the person's pursuit of ends that will lead to flourishing (final cause). But so far, we have not explored *how* humans, as creatures of dust, are formed. What does Christian faith teach about our created nature?

Christian faith teaches that God has configured the dust of our bodies to be capable of relationship with others, with ourselves, and with God. As Reinhard Hütter, following Aquinas, has put it, we are "dust bound for heaven."[19] Humans are unique among creatures not because we are something other than dust but because God has equipped us, starting with our created nature and perfected through God's grace, to participate and to share in God's life. We are creatures of dust who by God's breath have been fitted to know and to respond to God. We do this not as disembodied minds temporarily trapped in physical bodies but as ensouled dust being drawn to God.[20]

Values and Psychiatric Diagnosis (New York: Oxford University Press, 2005); K. W. M. Fulford, "'What Is (Mental) Disease?': An Open Letter to Christopher Boorse," *Journal of Medical Ethics* 27 (2001): 80–85; Fulford, "Facts/Values: Ten Principles of Values-Based Medicine," in *The Philosophy of Psychiatry: A Companion*, ed. Jennifer Radden (New York: Oxford University Press, 2004), 205–34; Christopher Boorse, "On the Distinction between Disease and Illness," *Philosophy and Public Affairs* 5 (1975): 49–68; Boorse, "Wright on Functions," *Philosophical Review* 85 (1976): 70–86; Boorse, "What a Theory of Mental Health Should Be," *Journal of the Theory of Social Behavior* 6 (1976): 61–84; Boorse, "Health as a Theoretical Concept," *Philosophy of Science* 44 (1977): 542–73. It is important to attend to a person's life narrative, culture, hopes, fears, dreams, and goals even when people lack the capacity to articulate this in language, as with profound intellectual disability or advanced neurocognitive disorders. In that case, clinicians must be attuned to other forms of communication and to the way that these things are known and articulated within a person's family and community.

19. Reinhard Hütter, *Dust Bound for Heaven: Explorations in the Theology of Thomas Aquinas* (Grand Rapids: Eerdmans, 2012).

20. Aquinas holds that God grants humans an intellectual or rational faculty of the soul that does not depend on the body for its function (though our everyday experience of thinking, which generally involves sensation and emotion, does depend on the body). But this is not a disembodied soul; the rational soul is still the form of the body (*STh* Ia q. 76 a. 1).

As creatures of dust, we are not meant to be alone. The creation account of Genesis 2 reports that the first man was created alone and that God said, "It is not good that the man should be alone; I will make him a helper as his partner" (Gen. 2:18). God created the other animals, but "for the man there was not found a helper as his partner" (2:20). God then created the first woman "out of man," and the man responds to her with delight, recognizing her as "bone of my bones and flesh of my flesh" (2:23). The text then comments that "therefore a man leaves his father and his mother and clings to his wife, and they become one flesh. And the man and his wife were both naked, and were not ashamed" (2:24-25).

No human since Adam has had to wait for a special creation of God to find communion and relationship. Communion and relationship precede us and surround us from the earliest stages of embryonic development. We form in intimate relationship, and we are born—naked and not ashamed—in relationship with our mothers. After birth, we continue to depend on the nurture and care of others, toward whom we are drawn. As Wendell Berry states above, we are creatures who "yearn toward other bodies." Relationship is not an optional add-on to human existence. It is a basic necessity for our growth and security as creatures of dust.[21] As Dave, the husband of Ann whose story we encountered in the introduction, frames it, "The communityness of our life is vital. . . . The community has been the context where I have been encouraged, instructed, guided to see myself in the narrative, to see myself as part of the story."[22]

Christian theology affirms that relationship is not unique to humans or to creatures. Relationship lies in the heart of the triune God. God is not a static, staid, solitary overlord of human affairs. Rather, as Aquinas affirmed, God is *actus purus*, pure act, eternal and unimpaired dynamism (*STh* Ia q. 2 a. 3; q. 9 a. 1). The three persons of the Trinity are in eternal and real relation with

---

See Adam Wood, *Thomas Aquinas on the Immateriality of the Human Intellect* (Washington, DC: Catholic University of America Press, 2020).

21. That is not to say that all humans experience or navigate relationships in the same way. Dixon Kinser has persuasively argued that when a "personal relationship with Jesus" and close relationships with others at church are used as markers of faithfulness, this marginalizes people on the autism spectrum. It is not that people on the autism or neurodiversity spectrum do not need or even long for relationship. But they do have different ways of seeking and expressing that relational need. See D. Dixon Kinser, "Reimagining Relationship: What Autism Reveals about What It Means to Relate to God," DMin thesis, Duke University, 2021.

22. Personal interview, June 3, 2022.

each other (*STh* Ia q. 28).[23] Furthermore, the triune God's activity is first and foremost love, which is to say, an activity that reaches forth in relationship. Love characterizes the way that the three persons of the Trinity—Father, Son, Holy Spirit—relate to each other in the joyful dance of the triune life (*STh* Ia q. 28). And this relational love *in* God extends *from* God to give being and life to all of God's creatures (*STh* Ia q. 20 a. 2).[24] As we will explore in chapter 5, God's creating is an act of love, in which God says, "It is good that you exist; it is good that you are in this world!"[25]

The affirmation that God loves God's creatures means that no material substance—whether a rock, a molecule, a tree, or a human being—is isolated. The most foundational thing about us—the fact that we *are*, that we exist—is a continual gift of the triune God. "In [Christ]," Colossians affirms, "all things hold together" (1:16). Aquinas affirmed that every creature bears the trace of the Trinity (*STh* Ia 1. 45 a. 7).[26] Relationship is built into the heart of being itself. There is no being without being-in-relation.[27]

For Aquinas, created beings are able to reciprocate and to act in relationship according to the complexity and limits of their bodies. This for Aquinas is a continuum that progresses from inanimate objects, which are least capable of reciprocal relationship, to humans, who are most capable in accord with our natural capacities. Rocks cannot move themselves and cannot respond to their surroundings. But plants can stretch their stems and unfurl their leaves in the direction of life-giving sunlight and extend their roots deep into the ground in search of water and nutrients. Animals, endowed not just with the capacity for nutrition, growth, and reproduction but also with the capacities for sensation, perception, appraisal of threat, and desire-pursuit, can act according to love that is appropriate to their natures. In many cases, animals can

23. White, *The Trinity*, 297–305, 448–49.

24. Aquinas clarifies that while humans love things because of their goodness, or honor what is good within them and wish them greater good, God *imparts* goodness in virtue of God's love for them; White, *The Trinity*, 337–39.

25. Josef Pieper, *Faith, Hope, Love* (San Francisco: Ignatius, 1997), 164.

26. Aquinas follows Augustine in arguing that insofar as things subsist, they show the Father, the "principle from no principle"; insofar as things have form and species, they represent the Word "as the form of the thing made by art is from the conception of the craftsman"; insofar as things have relation of order, they represent the Holy Spirit "inasmuch as He is love, because the order of the effect to something else is from the will of the Creator." Creatures that possess both intellect and will bear not only a trace of the Trinity but also the image of the Trinity, as we will explore further in chapter 5.

27. W. Norris Clarke, *Explorations in Metaphysics: Being–God–Person* (Notre Dame: University of Notre Dame Press, 1994), 102–22.

develop complex social systems of nurture, care, protection, and reciprocity that approximate the way that humans love and care for each other and from which humans can meaningfully learn (*STh* Ia q. 72; q. 96 a. 1).[28] But only humans, in Aquinas's view, have the created and graced capacity to live as friends of each other and of God (*STh* Ia q. 20 a. 3 *ad3*; q. 93). It is the specific way that God has configured us.

Dust Formed for Love

Friendship, for Aquinas, presupposes love. For Aquinas the concept of love covers a lot of ground. It is most basically the inclination that follows the apprehension that someone or something is good for us or good in general. Love fosters the will's desire to attain the good that is loved. Because love orients and fuels desire, love is the psychological root of what animals (including humans) desire and what we do. All experience or behavior that relates to action, Aquinas argues, presupposes love as its root and origin,

> for nobody desires anything nor rejoices in anything, except as a good that is loved: nor is anything an object of hate except as opposed to the object of love. Similarly, it is clear that sorrow, and other things like to it, must be referred to love as their first principle. Hence, in whomsoever there is will and appetite, there must also be love: since if the first is wanting, all that follows is also wanting. (*STh* Ia q. 20 a. 1 *resp.*)

Aquinas uses a range of Latin words for love. The most inclusive term is *amor*, which we might call ordinary love because of its omnipresence in human and animal life, directing all emotion and action.[29] Somewhat more specific is *dilectio*, a term that is not easily rendered in modern English but that for Aquinas names love that follows from a prior choice of reason. We might therefore call *dilectio* directed love—expressed, for example, when someone loves exercising, or going to church, or eating beets, having already decided that these activities are good for her. Even more specific is *caritas*, charity,

28. See Alasdair MacIntyre, *Dependent Rational Animals: Why Human Beings Need the Virtues* (Chicago: Open Court, 2001); Norman Wirzba, *This Sacred Life: Humanity's Place in a Wounded World* (New York: Cambridge University Press, 2021), 63–89.

29. Aquinas affirms that God also loves with the love of *amor*, though unlike humans only in the manner of will and not in the manner of bodily passion. *STh* Ia q. 20 a. 1 *ad1*.

which is love that not only follows reason but is directed toward something that one holds very dear.[30] While Aquinas allows in principle that *caritas* might be directed toward others without reference to God, in practice he describes *caritas* as the love of God by which God grants us the capacity to love God for God's sake and to be friends of God and, in God, of each other. I will therefore refer to *caritas* as extraordinary love, because it is possible only through a special act of God. We will consider ordinary love, *amor*, in this chapter, and then consider *caritas* more fully in chapter 8.

Ordinary love (*amor*) is inclination that follows the apprehension that something or someone is good for us, or good in general.[31] It is a kind of connection. Love gives birth to desire, by which we seek to be with or to attain what is loved, but love precedes desire. In love, we are already connected to what we perceive to be good. Aquinas describes ordinary love as *complacentia boni*, "complacency in good" (*STh* IaIIae q. 26 a. 1 *resp.*). He distinguishes between two kinds of ordinary love. First is gratification-love, by which the good is loved for the sake of another or for oneself, as when I love a cheeseburger so that my hunger might be satisfied. Second is friendship-love, by which what is good is loved for his or her own sake (*STh* IaIIae q. 26 a. 4). Gratification-love helps us to get what we need to care well for ourselves and for others. But friendship-love unites us with others in an intimate union that Aquinas calls "mutual indwelling": "every love makes the beloved to be in the lover, and vice versa" (*STh* IaIIae q. 28 a. 2 *sed contra*). Aquinas's description of lovers' mutual indwelling is profoundly intimate: "The lover is not satisfied with a superficial apprehension of the beloved, but strives to gain an intimate knowledge of everything related to the beloved, so as to enter into their interior self" (*STh* IaIIae q. 28 a. 2 *resp.*).[32] When we love another as friend (or lover), they become so united to us as to become part of who we are, and vice versa:

30. *STh* IaIIae q. 26 a. 3; Daniel Joseph Gordon, *The Passion of Love in the* Summa Theologiae *of Thomas Aquinas* (Washington, DC: Catholic University of America Press, 2023), 70–87.

31. Aquinas calls love the "first inclination of the appetite towards the possession of good" (*STh* IaIIae q. 36 a. 2 *resp.*); see also Nicholas Lombardo, *The Logic of Desire: Aquinas on Emotion* (Washington, DC: Catholic University of America Press, 2011), 58–59. Daniel Joseph Gordon helpfully states that "love is the adaptation of the lover to the beloved. It is a change that takes place in the lover on account of and in response to the beloved" (Gordon, *The Passion of Love*, 68).

32. The last phrase is modified for better fit with modern English language use. It is important to note that this mutual indwelling always respects and preserves the dignity and integrity of each human person.

in the love of friendship, the lover is in the beloved, inasmuch as he reckons what is good or evil to his friend, as being so to himself; and his friend's will as his own, so that it seems as though he felt the good or suffered the evil in the person in his friend. . . . Consequently, in so far as he reckons what affects his friend as affecting himself, the lover seems to be in the beloved, as though he were become one with him; but in so far as, on the other hand, he wills and acts for his friend's sake as for his own sake, looking on his friend as identified with himself, thus the beloved is in the lover. (*STh* IaIIae q. 28 a. 2 *resp.*)

Love draws us outside of ourselves, into another. Our lives are shaped by our loves. As embodied creatures, we are profoundly open to the world around us, to other humans, and even to God. We are naturally drawn to mutually indwelling friendship with others. Love draws others into us, making them part of who we are, just as we become part of those who love us. The intimacy and vulnerability of this mutual indwelling will vary according to the kind of relationship that is enjoyed. The mutual indwelling that my wife and I enjoy is—and should be—deeper, more intimate, and more vulnerable than the mutual indwelling that I experience with my students, with colleagues, with superiors, with other friends, and even with other members of my family. But insofar as I am drawn to all of these people as good in some way, they are a part of me, making me who I am. We are creatures of earth formed for relationship and love.

CHAPTER 3

From Inside Out to Outside In

We Find Our Selves in Relationship, Community, and Culture

> O LORD, you have searched me and known me.
> You know when I sit down and when I rise up;
>   you discern my thoughts from far away.
> You search out my path and my lying down,
>   and are acquainted with all my ways.
>
> —*Psalm 139:1–3*

When Ann tries to make sense of why her family members have struggled with depression and other mental health challenges, she finds herself thinking not only of the individuals but of their relationships to others in their community. We always find ourselves in community, and communities always shape our experiences. At the same time, people within the same community will often respond differently to their context. Ann's three sisters were all affected by her mother's illness, but each in a different way. Ann ascribes this to their unique positions in the family system and to their different "wiring." She notes, "how we deal with [communal or family stress] is going to be different depending on that wiring."[1] But early and formative relationships also matter:

> It's not weird that [when] my sisters and I get together, fifty years after my mother has died, . . . we still talk about her every time we get together. It's just a testimony to family being that impactful community. It matters. You have to look at it. If you have mental health issues, you have to look at those things. You can't just isolate the body, the machine, over here and feed it

1. Personal interview, June 3, 2022.

some antidepressants and expect it to go back [to a stressful family system]. Because even on medication, you still have to deal with that.[2]

Ann is grappling with a question at the center of any mental health care encounter: where do mental health challenges come from? Do they emerge from inside of a person's body or personality to then show up on the outside, affecting that person's relationships, community, and culture? This inside-out view is implied when mental health clinicians, and especially psychiatrists, frame mental health problems as constellations of symptoms and signs that reflect disorders of the brain or neural circuits. Or is it sometimes the other way around? Do mental health problems sometimes result from problems outside a person—problems in relationships, communities, and cultures—that then show up on the inside of a person's body, brain, and personality?

In this chapter, I argue that both the inside-out view and the outside-in view are valid ways of understanding mental health problems.[3] The inside-out view, however, dominates modern mental health care, overshadowing other ways of thinking. But Aquinas's vision of humans as creatures of earth who grow and who love in relationship calls us out of simplistic inside-out thinking to a contextual, ecological, biosocial view of mental health problems.

The Machine Metaphor and an Inside-Out View of Mental Health Problems

Modern mental health care is dominated by the idea that mental health challenges emerge from *within* individuals. As discussed in chapter 1, *DSM-5-TR* defines mental disorder as "a syndrome characterized by clinically significant disturbance in an individual's cognition, emotion regulation, or behavior that reflects a dysfunction in the psychological, biological, or developmental processes underlying mental functioning."[4] *DSM-5-TR* does not take this in-

2. Personal interview, June 3, 2022.
3. This use of the terms "inside-out" and "outside-in" is related to but different from its use by Sadler, who uses these terms to distinguish between diagnosis that objectifies a patient through categories and diagnosis that emerges within an effective therapeutic alliance. See John Sadler, *Values and Psychiatric Diagnosis* (New York: Oxford University Press, 2005), 144–46.
4. American Psychiatric Association. *Diagnostic and Statistical Manual of Mental Disorders*, 5th ed. rev. [*DSM-5-TR*] (Washington, DC: American Psychiatric Association, 2022), 14. *DSM-5-TR* goes on to stipulate that a mental health diagnosis should have clinical utility but need not be identified with the need for treatment. Furthermore, evidence used to clas-

dividualist and internalist stance because neuroscience research has shown that mental disorders can be explained by internal factors without regard to external factors (it has not). Nor does it do so because psychiatric researchers have characterized "psychological, biological, or developmental processes underlying mental functioning" to such an extent that one can pinpoint areas of dysfunction in these processes where they exist (they have not).[5] Rather, mental disorders are said to reflect "dysfunction in the individual" because saying this fits our culture's expectations for medical conditions. If the thought, emotion, and behavior classified as "mental disorder" were only "an expectable or culturally approved response to a common stressor or loss, such as the death of a loved one," "socially deviant behavior (e.g., political, religious, or sexual)," or due to "conflicts that are primarily between the individual and society," then we could accuse psychiatrists of miscategorizing ordinary problems of living as medical conditions to bolster their own power.[6] But if this experience and behavior reflects "dysfunction in the individual," then psychiatrists and psychologists speak with the authority of medical expertise.[7]

The *DSM* reflects mental health clinicians' and the broader public's assumptions about mental illness as much as it shapes those assumptions, and both clinicians and the public assume that mental illness starts *inside* an individual and then shows up *outside* through the individual's communication and behavior. This assumption runs all through mental health care.

---

sify particular mental disorders includes "antecedent validators (similar genetic markers, family traits, temperament, and environmental exposure), concurrent validators (similar neural substrates, biomarkers, emotional and cognitive processing, and symptom similarity), and predictive validators (similar clinical course and treatment response)"—though the document makes clear that the search for "incontrovertible etiological or pathophysiological mechanisms" that will "fully validate specific disorders or disorder spectra" are still lacking.

5. Anne Harrington, *Mind Fixers: Psychiatry's Troubled Search for the Biology of Mental Illness* (New York: Norton, 2019); Andrew Scull, *Desperate Remedies: Psychiatry's Turbulent Quest to Cure Mental Illness* (Cambridge: Belknap, 2022).

6. *DSM-5-TR*, 14. This was the charge of Thomas Szasz, described in chapter 1, in *The Myth of Mental Illness: Foundations for a Theory of Personal Conduct* (New York: Harper & Row, 1974). By arguing that "physicochemical disorder[s] of the body" (34) are the proper domain of medicine, Szasz can be read as a champion of a truly biological psychiatry, one focused on the body and its dysfunction and therefore of the machine metaphor.

7. Warren Kinghorn, "The Biopolitics of Defining Mental Disorder," in *Making the DSM-5: Concepts and Controversies*, ed. Joel Paris and James Phillips (New York: Springer, 2013), 47–61. Of course, in this case, the fox is placed in charge of the coop: clinicians with incentive to apply diagnoses are the ones who make the decisions regarding whether, in any given situation, a particular example of socially deviant behavior might reflect "dysfunction in the individual."

In this inside-out view, mental illness begins when the brain breaks down or at least loses some of its normal function, thereby giving rise to the subjective experience of mental disorder and its characteristic associated behaviors. Relational stress and environmental stressors such as poor nutrition, unemployment, poor housing, and pollution matter primarily as risk factors that precipitate and perpetuate brain dysfunction.

The inside-out model of mental disorder brings corollary approaches to mental health research and mental health care. Because mental disorders stem from dysfunction in brain circuits, research focuses on identifying the particular biological dysfunction (e.g., dysfunction of a brain circuit) associated with a particular manifestation of mental illness. Such research prioritizes basic science, the psychology laboratory, and the imaging suite, seeking to trace out the dysfunctional operations of brain circuits that correspond to particular mental health problems. In this model, the most successful mental health treatments are those that prevent, correct, or eliminate these underlying biological dysfunctions. Failing that, successful treatments would blunt the harmful effects of the dysfunctions, such as by reducing symptoms or by enhancing other brain circuits, as when stimulants are used for adjunctive treatment of major depression.

Philosophical (and Christian) Roots of the Inside-Out Model

To be fair, neither biological psychiatry nor the machine metaphor originated the idea that humans have a subjective inside and that psychological suffering might result from what is inside. The idea predates psychiatry and is rooted deeply in Christian thought. It relies on a view of the self as a site of what philosopher Charles Taylor refers to as inwardness. In this view, Taylor writes, "the opposition 'inside-outside' plays an important role. . . . We think of our thoughts, ideas, or feelings as being 'within' us, while the objects in the world which these mental states bear on are 'without.'"[8]

That we have interior selves seems obvious to most Westerners today, but Taylor argues that this view of the self was historically and culturally constructed. It was not always present even in western literature. Taylor argues that in the epics of Homer, for example, there is no word that can unproblematically be translated as "mind" or even as "soul" in the sense of a "unique

8. Charles Taylor, *Sources of the Self: The Making of the Modern Identity* (Cambridge: Harvard University Press, 1989), 111.

locus where all our different thoughts and feelings occur" (Taylor, 118). The rise of inwardness, he argues, can be seen in the work of four thinkers who foundationally shaped Western thought.

Plato began the process, in Taylor's account, by describing the virtuous person as one in whom the rational faculty (*to logistikon*) rules thought and action, which brings order to the soul. This account of the soul "requires some conception of the mind as a unitary space" (Taylor, 119; see Plato, *Republic* 4). But in an important way, Plato's account of the soul resisted the language of "inside" and "outside," because the source of reason was not inside the soul but rather in the world of unchangeable, eternal forms: "to be ruled by reason means to have one's life shaped by a pre-existent rational order which one knows and loves." This Platonic vision of reason as in some sense outside a person was continued with modification in the writings of Aristotle and the Stoics. For Plato, Aristotle, and the Stoics, the soul functions not to establish an interior self but to rightly integrate goals and desires, conforming them to a preexistent rational order (Taylor, 124).

For Taylor, Saint Augustine of Hippo (365–430) is a key figure in the development of an inward self. Augustine adopts Plato's theories of the Good and the eternal forms and modifies them to fit the demands of Scripture and Christian theology: all creation participates in God, derives being and goodness from God, and comes to perfection in God. To flourish is to have one's love (not just, as in Plato, one's attention) rightly ordered to God (Taylor, 128). But God is not simply "out there" as an object of contemplation. God is also

> the basic support and underlying principle of our knowing activity. God is not just what we long to see, but what powers the eye which sees. So the light of God is not just "out there," illuminating the order of being, as it is for Plato; it is also an "inner" light. It is the light "which lighteth every man that cometh into the world" (John 1:9). (Taylor, 129)

It is in the "radically reflexive" site of our first-person experience that we encounter God's presence to us. The way to find God, for Augustine, was therefore to look inward.[9] Taylor comments that "it is hardly an exaggeration to say that it was Augustine who introduced the concept of radical reflexivity and bequeathed it to the Western tradition of thought" (Taylor,

---

9. Taylor quotes Augustine, "*Noli foras ire, in teipsum redi; in interiore homine habitat veritas* (Do not go outward, return, within yourself. In the inward man dwells truth)"; Taylor, *Sources of the Self*, 129.

131). In contrast to what followed after, however, for Augustine this interior experience pointed outside of itself to God: "by going inward, I am drawn upward" (Taylor, 134).

René Descartes, to whom I attributed (chapter 1) the self-body dualism that is so problematic within modern mental health care, continued this Augustinian emphasis on radical reflexivity, searching for truth in his first-person experience. But whereas for Augustine the most important moral sources are outside of us—in God and in the ideas of God—for Descartes those moral sources are within us (Taylor, 143). Descartes, unlike Augustine, lived in a time when early modern scientific thinkers such as Francis Bacon and Galileo were describing a world that was increasingly understood mechanistically, with reference to efficient and material but not to formal and final causes. In this mechanistic world, knowing could not be a matter of participating in eternal forms or ideas outside of the self. Rather, it had to be a matter of the mind correctly representing external reality in mental experience. Even the notion of an idea was changed from something existing out there, in the world of forms or in God, to something inside the mind. Taylor argues, "the order of ideas ceases to be something we *find* and becomes something we *build*" (Taylor, 144).

The mind comes to be understood expressly by its abstraction from the body. Whereas for Plato and Augustine the mind came to fulness through participating or being absorbed into the immutable, eternal forms (or God), for Descartes the mind finds itself by objectifying and controlling the body (Taylor, 146). The mechanistic universe of matter, including the matter of the body, is not for Descartes a "medium of thought or meaning"; it is rather "expressively dead" (Taylor, 148). Meaning, insofar as it exists, must be built by the mind through rational control. The move toward the self-contained, autonomous self is well underway. For Descartes even the priority of the self with relation to God is reversed from his predecessors. Whereas for Augustine the turn inward, to oneself, is a way to find God and to discover one's radical dependence on God, for Descartes God matters primarily as the one whose existence guarantees the certainty of Descartes's own knowledge (Taylor, 157).

Taylor locates a further critical step in the development of modern inwardness in the philosophy of John Locke (1632-1704). In *An Enquiry concerning Human Understanding*, Locke agreed with Descartes that the world outside the mind is expressively dead, void of intrinsic moral meaning. But whereas Descartes held to the view that some ideas—such as red or sweet—exist in the mind prior to experience, Locke understood the mind as a passive space, a clean slate or *tabula rasa*, in which sense impressions are received and conjoined. The reason, far from projecting its own innate concepts onto these sense impressions, rather is tasked with ordering them rightly, to correspond to the world outside the mind. In doing so, Taylor argues, Locke reifies the mind as a space of continuous self-remaking. The self or "I" is not constituted by participating in external reality, or even by its ideas received from the senses, but rather by the power to stand back from all experience as a "punctual" self, fixing things as objects without being extended in or among them (Taylor, 49, 171-72). This extensionless self resides in consciousness, and the self is continuous only if consciousness is continuous over time. The punctual self disengages from and objectifies everything in its experience, from its own ideas to the world of people and society, so as to control them. Modern disengagement "calls us to a separation from ourselves through self-objectification" (Taylor, 175).

Descartes and Locke did not single-handedly construct this modern account of the self. They were building on, embedded within, and responding to broader economic, religious, and social contexts—including the rise of early modern science, the rise of colonialism, and the Protestant reformation. Their theories both emerged from and contributed to these broader cultural contexts. But though those engaged in modern mental health care may never have studied the thought of Descartes or Locke, the self that these philosophers describe is familiar. That self, sometimes equated with mind, is found in conscious experience and awareness that is somehow influenced by the body.[10] The body, including the brain, though foundational for the self's experience, is also a thing external to the self. One can intelligibly say, "My brain is playing tricks on me." The mind, by means of the brain and the nervous system, develops ideas corresponding to things and events in the external world. Things and events in the external world, such as the loss of a job or the chronic threat of intimate partner violence, can trigger painful and unwanted thoughts and feelings, and these thoughts and feelings can be labeled "mental illness" if they lead to marked distress or functional impairment. But these thoughts and feelings remain inside the person. Psychiatric and psychological treatments seek to understand where inside the person these problematic thoughts and feelings are located and to find ways of controlling them—using whatever technology suits that purpose.

---

10. In different ways, psychological theorists and scientists since Freud have mostly agreed that Descartes was wrong in equating mind with consciousness, as they have held that important mental functions relevant for emotion and behavior occur prior to or outside of conscious experience.

Problems with the Inside-Out View

The inside-out view of mental health problems sets the context for the *DSM* and most attempts to label and diagnose mental disorders, as well as for a great deal of modern mental health care. But when it is the sole narrative for mental health care, this view is inadequate and misleading in several ways.

First, research based on the inside-out view has had limited success clarifying the causes of mental illness or developing preventive or curative interventions. Though research into the biological roots of mental illness has produced vast data on thousands of phenomena,[11] biological psychiatry has so far failed to describe causal biological pathways for most forms of major mental illness.[12] Genome-wide association studies of genetic risk factors for major depression, for example, have identified more than eighty genetic variants that are associated with increased risk of depression, most located in genes associated with the brain's frontal cortex, though the mechanisms by which these genes contribute to depression remains unclear.[13] Some widely publicized findings have not been consistently replicated in follow-up research.[14] While the amply funded Research Domain Criteria (RDoC) project of the US National Institute of Mental Health (NIMH) may eventually identify at least some of these causal mechanisms, it has not yet done so.[15] Thomas Insel, who as the director of

11. Brain science accounts for the vast majority of US National Institute of Mental Health (NIMH) research investments. NIMH allocated $847 million for basic and brain science research in fiscal year 2021, compared to $185 million for mental health services and intervention research. These numbers reflect extramural research (grants to other institutions, like universities) only and do not include $547 million in translational research, much of which is also focused on the brain sciences. See "FY 2022 Budget—Congressional Justification," National Institute of Mental Health, https://www.nimh.nih.gov/about/budget/fy-2022-budget-congressional-justification.

12. Harrington, *Mind Fixers*; Scull, *Desperate Remedies*.

13. David M. Howard et al., "Genome-Wide Meta-analysis of Depression Identifies 102 Independent Variants and Highlights the Importance of the Prefrontal Brain Regions," *Nature Neuroscience* 22 (2019): 343–52.

14. An example is the report of a particular genetic variant associated with a protein that transports the neurotransmitter serotonin across the membrane of brain cells with the risk of developing major depression in response to stress. See Avshalom Caspi et al., "Influence of Life Stress on Depression: Moderation by a Polymorphism in the 5-HTT Gene," *Science* 301 (2003): 386–89; R. C. Culverhouse et al., "Collaborative Meta-analysis Finds No Evidence of a Strong Interaction between Stress and 5-HTTLPR Genotype Contributing to the Development of Depression," *Molecular Psychiatry* 23 (2018): 133–42.

15. Bruce N. Cuthbert, "Research Domain Criteria: Toward Future Psychiatric Nosologies," *Dialogues in Clinical Neuroscience* 17 (2015): 89–97; Thomas Insel and Bruce Cuthbert,

NIMH from 2002 to 2015 focused research funding on biological paradigms, startled many in a 2017 interview when he stated,

> I spent 13 years at NIMH really pushing on the neuroscience and genetics of mental disorders, and when I look back on that I realize that while I think I succeeded at getting lots of really cool papers published by cool scientists at fairly large costs—I think $20 billion—I don't think we moved the needle in reducing suicide, reducing hospitalizations, improving recovery for the tens of millions of people who have mental illness.[16]

Insel subsequently has argued that while "mental illnesses are fundamentally brain disorders with a biology that involves the same kind of cellular and molecular changes found in other medical illnesses," the most urgent needs related to therapy are broader social and structural interventions: access to mental health care, social connection, housing support, income and employment support, and so on.[17] He states, "I have come to think of mental illness as a medical problem that requires a social solution,"[18] adding that he learned from a "very wise clinician working on Los Angeles's skid row" that recovery from mental illness was all about "the three P's"—not "Prozac, Paxil, Prolixin," or even "psychotherapy, psychoeducation, psychoanalysis," but rather "people, place, and purpose."[19]

"Research Domain Criteria (RDoC): Toward a New Classification Framework for Research on Mental Disorders," *American Journal of Psychiatry* 167 (2010): 748–50.

16. Adam Rogers, "Star Neuroscientist Tom Insel Leaves the Google-Spawned Verily for . . . a Startup?," *Wired*, May 11, 2017, https://www.wired.com/2017/05/star-neuroscientist -tom-insel-leaves-google-spawned-verily-startup.

17. Thomas Insel, *Healing: Our Path from Mental Illness to Mental Health* (New York: Penguin Books, 2022), 17.

18. Insel, *Healing*, 167.

19. Insel, *Healing*, 160. It is notable, despite this admission, that Insel never concedes any misjudgment in focusing NIMH research funding on basic science: "I have no regrets about NIMH funding for genomics and neuroscience" (xxvi). He simply wants a broader approach to treatment that includes social interventions in addition to biomedical interventions. In this, I believe that his view is still too limited. He never calls into question his own professional, epistemic, and moral authority as a biological psychiatrist, or the usefulness of medical models for describing psychological suffering. In this, he remains firmly fixed in what I am calling the inside-out view. In contrast to Insel's view that "mental illness is a medical problem that requires a social solution" (167), it's my position that mental health challenges are often social and medical problems that require social and medical solutions, with prudential judgment necessary for understanding what narrative and what solutions are most fitting and appropriate.

The second problem with the inside-out view is that philosophers have successfully challenged the idea of an inner, private self that is distinct from the world of relationships. Ludwig Wittgenstein (1889-1951), in a series of philosophical aphorisms, challenged the idea that anyone could use language in a way that is private, accessible to the self and not to others. Language, Wittgenstein argues, is formulated and negotiated within particular social forms of life and is otherwise meaningless. Even to say "I am having a sensation" presumes that the words "having" and "sensation" are commonly understood.[20] The impossibility of a private language calls into question the possibility of truly private experience, as any attempt to understand or to express this experience, even silently and privately, will inevitably draw on words, concepts, and utterances derived from their use within a community.

Taylor echoes Wittgenstein's critique, countering the Cartesian-Lockean "punctual self" with his own argument that "one is only a self among other selves." Taylor adds,

> My self-definition is understood as an answer to the question Who I am. And this question finds its original sense in the interchange of speakers. I define who I am by defining where I speak from, in the family tree, in social space, in the geography of social statuses and functions, in my intimate relations to the ones I love, and also crucially in the space of moral and spiritual orientation within which my most defining relations are lived out.[21]

A self exists, Taylor argues, only in "webs of interlocution."[22]

By the time Wittgenstein wrote, the privacy of the self already had been challenged by thinkers in the American pragmatist tradition, particularly the University of Chicago social behaviorist George Herbert Mead (1863-1931). Mead held that minds and selves were "essentially social products" that arose from the world of social interaction and not from either the brain or from "a substantive soul endowed with the self of the individual at birth."[23] Social interaction gives rise to socially significant gestures and symbols that

20. Ludwig Wittgenstein, *Philosophical Investigations*, trans. G. E. M. Anscombe (Malden, MA: Blackwell, 2001), 79 (§261).

21. Taylor, *Sources of the Self*, 35.

22. Taylor, *Sources of the Self*, 36. As Alasdair MacIntyre puts it even more succinctly, "I can be said truly to know who and what I am, only because there are others who can be said to know who and what I am." See Alasdair MacIntyre, *Dependent Rational Animals: Why Human Beings Need the Virtues* (Chicago: Open Court, 1999), 95.

23. George Herbert Mead, *Mind, Self, and Society: From the Standpoint of a Social Behav-*

carry meaning both for the one making the gesture and for those to whom the gesture is directed, and mind is the internalization of these "significant symbols" (42–51). Mead argues that "mind arises through communication by a conversation of gestures in a social process or context of experience—not communication through mind" (50). For Mead, consciousness—the experience of subjectivity that has been so difficult to explain for modern neurobiology—is foundationally a social process. Consciousness is "functional, not substantive," and is located not in the brain but "in the objective world . . . it belongs to, or is a characteristic of, the environment in which we find ourselves" (112). The brain is, at best, the site of "the physiological process whereby we lose and regain consciousness: a process which is somewhat analogous to that of pulling down and raising a window shade" (112). The body, Mead argues, "is not a self, as such; it becomes a self only when it has developed a mind within the context of social experience" (50).

Mead, Wittgenstein, and Taylor are but the tip of a large iceberg of contemporary philosophers, social theorists, and psychologists who have criticized the Cartesian-Lockean self as the site of private, first-person experience that is related only distantly to the external world. Important critiques have been offered by phenomenologists such as Edmund Husserl and Maurice Merleau-Ponty and by post-structuralist thinkers such as Jacques Derrida and Judith Butler. Within the world of mental health care, as we will examine further below, the Cartesian-Lockean self also has been qualified or undercut by psychoanalytic object relations theory, by attachment theory, and by modern neuroscientific work on self-development.

The Cartesian-Lockean self and the inside-out model of mental illness that correlates with it present not simply an intellectual puzzle but a moral and practical problem that stands in the way of mental health care that honors humans as wayfarers rather than reducing them to mechanisms. When it is the only narrative guiding mental health care, the model harms in at least five ways.

Stigmatization of the private. First, by teaching that mental health problems are private experiences that occur in the secluded space of an individual's mind or self, this model feeds shame and stigma. It teaches the one who is struggling that the cause is a problem inside of them. The outside world may contribute various stressors, but the fundamental problem is a deficit in the individual's response to such stress. This emphasis often triggers worry about negative judgments from others and leads those who are suffering to retreat

---

iorist, ed. Charles W. Morris (Chicago: University of Chicago Press, 1962), 1. Subsequent page references are given in parentheses in the text.

into an isolating cocoon of shame. Meanwhile, those surrounding the one who is struggling have a reason to mark them as ill and respond with pity, avoidance, or scorn—all defining marks of stigma.

Objectifying focus on the body. Second, the inside-out model objectifies the body as the causal site of mental illness. If mental illness resides inside me, then its location must be the mind or the body. If I experience psychological suffering not only as unwanted but also as an intruder, alien to me, then I naturally attribute such suffering to the body, which I can easily—even if mistakenly—imagine as something other than my inmost self. But as I stand apart from my body and consider the way that it betrays me and delivers to me the unwanted experience and behavior of mental illness, I thereby consider my body as an object, an "it" in contrast to "I" the subject. This pattern fits the idea that mental illness is caused by a "broken brain."[24]

Neglect of broader contexts. Corollary to this objectifying focus on the body as the site of mental illness, the inside-out model neglects the social, environmental, and relational contexts within which mental health problems emerge. To be sure, the inside-out model does not entirely ignore the "social determinants of mental health," but it renders them external to the essential site of mental illness, which is the inner mind and the body. Social and environmental factors are understood as risk factors or stressors that trigger vulnerabilities in brain circuits and mental processes, but the problem remains *within* the affected individual, who then is stigmatized for not bearing up under this stress.[25]

Individualistic focus of therapy. Fourth, the inside-out model overwhelmingly prioritizes treatments and therapies that focus on the individual. This is true of all medication treatment for mental illness, as well as somatic treatments such as electroconvulsive therapy (ECT) that by nature are dispensed to individual bodies. But psychotherapies likewise tend to focus on the individual. Clients present to therapists as individuals. They are diagnosed as individuals. Though psychotherapeutic approaches recognize how relationships contribute to mental health challenges, they tend to treat such challenges as reflecting, at root, problems in an individual's thinking or be-

24. See, for example, Nancy C. Andreasen, *The Broken Brain: The Biological Revolution in Psychiatry* (New York: Harper & Row, 1984).

25. Tanya Luhrmann describes how unhoused women in Chicago would often resist public services that required diagnoses of psychotic disorders because of the perception that this would mean that they lacked the strength to survive on the streets. See Tanya Marie Luhrmann, "'The Street Will Drive You Crazy': Why Homeless Psychotic Women in the Institutional Circuit in the United States Often Say No to Offers of Help," *American Journal of Psychiatry* 165 (2008): 15-20.

havior. As Ann's comments at the beginning of the chapter suggest, this focus on the individual often fails to address what is really going on in the case of mental health challenges.

The tyranny of self-vigilance. Even in the absence of mental health problems, the inside-out approach leads to a way of life characterized by vigilant, introspective attention to the self. Taylor rightly points out that one can care for the self without necessarily committing to introspection. One can simply care for one's body and one's personal projects.[26] The inside-out approach, however, encourages an inward, introspective posture. If mental illness is inside me, then mental health must be inside me too, in my inner self and its associated brain and body. As such, to care for the self requires focusing on my own experience and the state of my body. This is not entirely wrong. Christian faith encourages loving care of the body and cultivation of the inner life, as we will explore in future chapters. But this introspective focus can also fold us in on ourselves, hindering us from focusing on others, including God, whom we are called to love. "Those who want to save their life," Jesus said, "will lose it" (Matt. 16:25).

Toward a Psychology of Self in Relation

The inside-out approach, as named above, relies on the image of an interior self that is distinct from the external world and is closely related to the brain. But in addition to the philosophical and sociological voices noted above, prominent voices throughout the history of clinical psychiatry and psychology have argued that relationships and the lived world are so central to the experience of self that there is no self apart from the relationships that constitute it. Here, by way of illustration, I consider one such strain of thought and research centered on psychological object-relations and attachment theory.

Sigmund Freud is often credited with disrupting the modern account of a unified, transparent self that serves as the seat of our thought, emotion, and action. Listening to and creatively interpreting the experience of the upper-class citizens of Vienna who came to him for "psycho-analysis," Freud believed that humans were motivated primarily by the need to satisfy innate drives, particularly for sexual gratification, and that the function of the mind was to facilitate drive satisfaction while navigating relationships and social expectations and prohibitions. Though Freud's categories

26. Taylor, *Sources of the Self*, 131.

of mind shifted over time, he is most known for the distinction between the conscious mind and the unconscious mind, which operates outside of awareness, as well as for his description of a structure of ego (or "I") which negotiates between the competing demands of the drive-satisfaction-oriented id (or "it") and the restrictive, rule-oriented superego (or "over-I").[27] Freud understood relationships, particularly early relationships with parents, to be central to the development of mind, though primarily as vehicles for drive-satisfaction (i.e., the infant at the mother's breast) or as sources of prohibition and punishment (e.g., the threatened punishment from a boy's father that prevents consummation of sexual union with the mother in the "Oedipus complex," and that eventually leads the boy to identify with his father).

Psychiatrists, psychologists, and other thinkers working after Freud, however, began to wonder whether Freud had misunderstood humans' basic motivations. Clinician-researchers W. R. D. Fairbairn, Harry Guntrip, Donald Winnicott, and others wondered whether humans are motivated not so much to relieve pent-up desires for sexual satisfaction and perhaps for death as to connect with other humans. For these "object relations" theorists, human connection does not serve as a means to the end of drive satisfaction but rather constitutes the primary human need, the thing on which human development depends. These theorists revised Freud's theories to describe how relationships could be internalized as parts, or objects, of mental life. In object relations theory, the concept of the self as interior space remains, but the self's content is populated by objects (that is, people or mental representations of people) internalized from relationships and community.[28]

Object relations theorists like Winnicott and Fairbairn contributed to the rise of attachment theory, which has proved a more stable foundation for empirical studies of how relationships contribute to the development of the self. Psychiatrist John Bowlby, alarmed by the poor psychological and physical health of children and youth separated from their families in early childhood, posited that attachment to caregivers plays a central role in the development of the self.[29]

---

27. Sigmund Freud, *The Ego and the Id*, trans. James Strachey, in *The Standard Edition of the Complete Psychological Works of Sigmund Freud* (London: Hogarth, 1966), 19:1–66; Stephen A. Mitchell and Margaret J. Black, *Freud and Beyond: A History of Modern Psychoanalytic Thought* (New York: Basic Books, 1995).

28. Jay R. Greenberg and Stephen A. Mitchell, *Object Relations in Psychoanalytic Theory* (Cambridge: Harvard University Press, 1983), 151–230.

29. John Bowlby, *Attachment and Loss*, vol. 1, *Attachment* (New York, Basic Books, 1969);

Researchers Mary Ainsworth and Mary Main then developed a framework by which to apply Bowlby's observations to mental life. Ainsworth and Main observed thousands of children's interactions with significant attachment figures (mothers, fathers, or others who serve primary caregiving roles in a child's life) and identified four attachment patterns. When parents respond to children in consistent, attuned, empathic ways—validating and mirroring emotion, providing comfort when comfort is desired, and allowing exploration and separation when the child initiates these—children most often develop *secure* attachment, a pattern that correlates with having a stable self-identity, recognizing and acknowledging emotion, and forming close and healthy relationships. When parents respond to children erratically and unpredictably—providing comfort and acknowledging the child's experience at times but at other times ignoring or dismissing the child, or not allowing the child to separate from the parent—children are more likely to develop *resistant or ambivalent* attachment, a pattern characterized by emotional lability and preoccupation with the parent's location and feelings, and later in life by fears of abandonment in relationships, especially romantic relationships. When parents respond to children by punishing or shaming their expressions of emotion (e.g., "Don't cry, or I'll give you something to cry about!"), children may develop *avoidant* attachment, a pattern characterized by difficulty feeling, acknowledging, or displaying emotion. Later in life, those affected by this pattern may get stuck living at the level of the head rather than the heart and thereby struggle to form and sustain close relationships. Of most concern, when parents are abusive, threatening, or emotionally unavailable—often as a result of their own trauma or mental health crises—children are put at risk for *disorganized* attachment, a pattern characterized by extremes of emotion, stereotyped and bizarre behavior, and strong defensive responses when they perceive threats to safety.[30]

The attachment patterns developed in childhood correlate strongly with patterns of attachment in adulthood, which can be measured with a structured interview called the Adult Attachment Interview (AAI).[31] In studies of mothers and fathers across the world not selected from clinical samples, around 60 percent display secure attachment, around 25 percent display dismissing

Robert Karen, *Becoming Attached: First Relationships and How They Affect Our Capacity to Love* (New York: Oxford University Press, 1998).

30. David J. Wallin, *Attachment in Psychotherapy* (New York: Guilford, 2007), 84-98.

31. Erik Hesse, "The Adult Attachment Interview: Protocol, Method of Analysis, and Empirical Studies," in *Handbook of Attachment: Theory, Research, and Clinical Applications*, ed. Jude Cassidy and Philip R. Shaver (New York: Guilford, 2008), 552-98.

attachment (correlated with avoidant attachment in childhood), around 10 percent display preoccupied attachment (correlated with resistant/ambivalent attachment in childhood), and approximately 15 percent display unresolved experiences of trauma or cannot be classified. Although mental health problems can follow any pattern of attachment, they occur more frequently among people with insecure or disorganized attachment styles. In studies of adults in mental health treatment settings, 21 percent display secure attachment, 23 percent display dismissing attachment, 13 percent display preoccupied attachment, and 43 percent—nearly half—display unresolved experiences of trauma or cannot be classified.[32]

Following the groundbreaking work on attachment by Bowlby, Ainsworth, and Main, subsequent researchers have investigated how relationships affect the developing brain, the experience of self, and psychological health. In his work *Affect Regulation and the Origin of the Self* (1994), neuropsychologist Allan Schore reviews and summarizes a wide array of research related to brain development to show that "the early social environment, mediated by the primary caregiver, directly influences the evolution of structures in the brain that are responsible for the future socioemotional development of the child."[33] For instance, the nature and quality of a child's affective bonds, especially with a primary caregiver, influence the development of the region of the brain known as the orbitofrontal cortex, which is important for regulating and processing emotion. Early in infancy, Schore argues, positive, attuned face-to-face interactions between a child and a caregiver foster positive affect between the two and stimulate the growth of brain circuits that facilitate further positive affect as well as play and exploration. Later, attuned caregiver-child interactions stimulate the growth of a parallel brain circuit that enables a child to inhibit and regulate emotion, including shame. High-quality early child-caregiver interactions facilitate the integration of these two brain systems along with other neurodevelopmental processes, thereby fostering the development of a stable self capable of forming and sustaining positive relationships with others.[34]

Psychoanalyst Peter Fonagy developed the concept of "mentalization" as centrally important for development of the psychological self.[35] Mentaliza-

32. Marian J. Bakermans-Kranenburg and Marinus H. van IJzendoorn, "The First 10,000 Adult Attachment Interviews: Distributions of Adult Attachment Representations in Clinical and Non-clinical Groups," *Attachment and Human Development* 11 (2009): 223-63.

33. Allan Schore, *Affect Regulation and the Origin of the Self: The Neurobiology of Emotional Development* (New York: Routledge, 2016), 62.

34. Schore, *Affect Regulation*, 65-67.

35. Peter Fonagy et al., *Affect Regulation, Mentalization, and the Development of the Self* (New York: Other, 2002).

tion is the process of "keeping the mind in mind." Developing infants, Fonagy argues, come to experience themselves as minds insofar as early caregivers, in repeated face-to-face interactions, attend to the infant's mental experience. Such attention anticipates and stimulates in the infant capacities for self-presence and self-reflection, which help the infant to regulate emotion. Seeing her toddler fall and skin his knee, for example, an attuned mother might run to the crying child, hold and comfort him, and assume a facial expression that reflects the child's distress and conveys to the child, "You are hurt, and I feel that with you." In addition, by exaggerating the expression in a way that conveys a genuine but calm concern, the mother marks the experience, communicating that although she understands the child's feelings, she is not overwhelmed. She conveys to the child, "You are hurt, I feel that with you, *and* I know that you will be OK."[36] Fonagy holds that these attuned interactions, repeated tens of thousands of times in a healthy parent-child relationship, enable the child to grow as a physical agent (aware of the limits of her body, beginning in the first months of life), as a social agent (able from the first months of life to engage with others and to recognize some degree of separation between self and others), as a teleological agent (able to act for goals, starting around seven to nine months old), as an intentional agent (able to recognize and to attribute desires and goals that are distinct from the action they generate, around two years of age), and as autobiographical selves (able to comprehend and to represent the way that mind states link with each other—that is, showing a "theory of mind"—around four to five years of age).[37]

Fonagy's theory of mentalization resonates with the interpersonal neurobiology of psychiatrist Daniel Siegel. Siegel draws on the theory of nonlinear dynamics of complex systems (complexity theory) to describe the mind as "an embodied and relational process that regulates the flow of energy and information."[38] Siegel frames healthy psychological function as "the integration of energy and information within the nervous system and between people" (8). Shared experience in interpersonal relationships, particularly when the relationships are "mind-minded" and allow those who relate to "feel felt," facilitates integration that gives rise to healthy neuronal development, effective regulation of emotion, and ultimately fulfilling relationships. Though experienced "self-states" may be fragmented and disorganized (355-57), important

---

36. Fonagy et al., *Affect Regulation*, 175–81.
37. Fonagy et al., *Affect Regulation*, 203–51.
38. Daniel Siegel, *The Developing Mind: How Relationships and the Brain Interact to Shape Who We Are*, 2nd ed. (New York: Guilford, 2012), 2. Subsequent page references are given in parentheses in the text.

forms of integration—integration of conscious experience, integration of left and right hemispheres, integration of cortex with subcortical areas and brainstem, integration of implicit and explicit memory, integration of across time through narrative, integration of the self across social contexts, integration of the self in relationship, integration of the self in the context of finitude and death, and "transpirational" integration across all domains—contribute to a stable sense of self across time (379-87).

These theorists have contributed to what is by now a voluminous body of research from a variety of methodological approaches showing that mental health and mental illness are intimately related to social and interpersonal relationships, particularly early relationships and intimate relationships among romantic partners or family members. Among adults, secure attachment patterns are associated with ease in forming and maintaining meaningful relationships. Dismissing attachment patterns are associated with difficulty being emotionally available, and with diagnoses such as antisocial personality disorder, substance use disorders, and anorexia nervosa. Preoccupied attachment patterns are associated with internalizing disorders such as borderline personality disorder. In addition, unresolved trauma is associated, not surprisingly, with post-traumatic stress disorder.[39]

Psychological exploration of trauma vividly demonstrates how relationships are central to the development of self and to the experience of self. Two modern mental disorders that are identified in part by a fragile or unstable sense of self correlate strongly with early childhood trauma. Those who live with borderline personality disorder (BPD), which is characterized by a "pervasive pattern of instability of interpersonal relationships, self-image, and affects," and defined in part by a "markedly and persistently unstable self-image or sense of self," are more than thirteen times as likely to report a history of childhood sexual abuse as those without BPD.[40] Among those who live with dissociative identity disorder (DID), which is characterized by "two or more distinct personality states" involving "marked discontinuity in sense of self and sense of agency," 90 percent suffered childhood abuse and neglect.[41] In these disorders, abusive early relationships impair the person's ability to de-

39. Bakermans-Kranenburg and van IJzendoorn, "First 10,000 Interviews," 2009.

40. C. Porter et al., "Childhood Adversity and Borderline Personality Disorder: A Meta-analysis," *Acta Psychiatrica Scandinavica* 141 (2020): 6-20.

41. *DSM-5-TR*, 333; Daphne Simeon and Frank Putnam, "Pathological Dissociation in the National Comorbidity Survey Replication (NCS-R): Prevalence, Morbidity, Comorbidity, and Childhood Maltreatment," *Journal of Trauma and Dissociation* (2022): 1-14, https://doi.org/10.1080/15299732.2022.2064580.

velop as an agent in the world who can successfully navigate complex relationships and social situations. Because the world is fragmented and unreliable, the self also is fragmented and unreliable.

Beyond these two particularly trauma-associated disorders, trauma contributes to a wide variety of adverse psychological and somatic health outcomes. The Adverse Childhood Experiences (ACE) Study was a landmark epidemiological study among 9,508 California adults in the 1990s that identified seven adverse childhood experiences (physical abuse, sexual abuse, psychological abuse, substance abuse in household, mental illness in household, mother treated violently, criminal behavior in household) and examined whether individuals who reported these experiences were at risk of adverse health outcomes later in life. The study findings were striking and alarming. Adverse childhood experiences (ACEs) correlated strongly with the development of depression, suicide attempts, problematic substance use, risky sexual activity, and a number of medical conditions such as ischemic heart disease, cancer, and diabetes. Furthermore, one's overall risk of medical and mental health problems increased with the number of ACEs experienced.[42]

An Outside-In View of Mental Health Problems

These currents of research that emphasize the importance of relationships and social context for mental health and mental illness are well known within psychology and psychiatry, but their insights have not displaced the inside-out approach to mental illness. Adherents of the inside-out view acknowledge that factors in the external world such as abusive relationships, homelessness, and trauma affect the development and perpetuation of mental health problems. But these social determinants or social correlates of mental health have their effect, within this model, as risk factors for mental illness, which still develops *inside* the affected person. Childhood psychological abuse may well cause depression, the thought goes, but that is because living with psychological abuse floods the body with stress hormones, overwhelms the body's normal mood-regulating systems, exploits genetic susceptibilities, and eventually results in the neurochemical cascade associated with a major depressive episode. Psychological abuse may cause the mental disorder, but the disorder itself remains in-

42. Vincent J. Felitti et al., "Relationship of Childhood Abuse and Household Dysfunction to Many of the Leading Causes of Death in Adults: The Adverse Childhood Experiences (ACE) Study," *American Journal of Preventive Medicine* 14 (1998): 245–58.

side the individual. The experience of mental illness reflects and displays what is happening within an individual's neural circuits or core thought processes.

But what if we turn this model inside out? What if we recenter the site of what is wrong from inside the person to outside the person, to his or her (past and present) relationships, community, and culture? In this way of thinking—and staying with the association between psychological abuse and depression—the site of what is wrong is not the brain or the body, with psychological abuse contributing as a risk factor for an internal pathology. Rather, the site of what is wrong is the past or present abusive relationship. Depression, in all its experiential, behavioral, and neurobiological manifestations, is a response to that wrong thing outside the person. It is a way of operating in a particular context. This response will of course involve brain circuits, since we are embodied creatures, but the circuits are not the site of the problem. The problem is psychological abuse. The brain circuits, for the most part, are just doing their job, helping a person to meet life's opportunities and challenges as they come. Specific genes or other physiological processes might affect these circuits in ways that increase the likelihood that one will respond to chronic psychological abuse with the experience that corresponds to the diagnosis of major depression. But this would not prove that "mental disorders are biological disorders involving brain circuits that implicate specific domains of cognition, emotion, or behavior," as one version of the inside-out model would claim.[43] It would only mean that biology affects a person's response to social conditions. In the inside-out view, the experience and behavior of mental illness signifies internal (biological, neural) states that may be influenced by external (social, relational) risk factors. In the outside-in view, by contrast, the experience and behavior of mental illness signifies external (social, relational) states, with internal (biological, neural) factors affecting a person's response. In the inside-out view, mental disorders are individual (and possibly biological) disorders that show up in relationships, community, and culture. In the outside-in view, mental disorders are relational, communal, or cultural disorders that show up in the life (including the biology and neurology) of an individual.

The inside-out and outside-in views have very different implications for how clinicians, communities, and people with mental illness respond to the experience of mental disorders (see table 2).

43. Thomas Insel, "Transforming Diagnosis," National Institute of Mental Health, April 29, 2013, https://psychrights.org/2013/130429NIMHTransformingDiagnosis.htm.

Table 2. *Comparison of the Inside-Out and Outside-In Views of Mental Health Problems*

	Inside-Out View	Outside-In View
Root cause of mental health problems	Dysfunction in the body (e.g., brain circuits) or internal mental experience	Deprivations, threats, and challenges in the world
Role of the body	Its dysfunction gives rise to mental disorders	Its states affect a person's response to deprivations, threats, and challenges
Role of the external world	Deprivations, threats, and challenges render a person vulnerable to bodily dysfunction	A person experiences distress responding to deprivations, threats, and challenges
Markers of successful diagnosis	Diagnoses isolate and identify biological roots of particular mental disorders (e.g., Huntington's disease)	Diagnoses identify patterns of response to deprivation, threat, and challenge (e.g., demoralization, complex PTSD) and suggest ways to respond helpfully
Focus of research	Understanding the normal and abnormal operation of brain circuits that correlate with mental health problems (along with associated therapeutic responses)	Understanding how social and relational deprivations, threats, and challenges give rise to mental health problems (along with associated therapeutic responses)
Site of research	Basic science laboratory, functional neuroimaging, psychology laboratory	Community
Goal of treatment	Correct underlying causes of dysfunctional biological processes insofar as possible	Remedy deprivations, threats, and challenges when possible, help to adapt successfully when not

In the outside-in view, mental disorders stem from deprivations, threats, and challenges in the world, with body and brain states affecting a person's response to these deprivations, threats, and challenges. Successful diagnoses identify patterns of response to deprivation, threat, and challenge with sufficient precision to guide therapeutic responses that are helpful in the patient's context. Mental health research, focused on lived experience and often focused on communities and relational systems, seeks to understand how social and relational deprivations, threats, and challenges give rise to mental health problems. The most successful mental health treatments prevent mental disorders by eliminating unjust and harmful deprivations and threats and promote successful adaptation to the ordinary challenges of human life.

The outside-in view of mental disorder is not compatible with the Cartesian-Lockean vision of the punctual self that gives rise to the inside-out view because it does not view the mind (the "I" who thinks and acts) and the self (the "me" that is present when I attend to myself) as spaces constituted by interiority and privacy. Rather, it views the mind as the ability to perceive and make sense of both the external world and the body (the lived world) and to organize responses that help the self to adapt to them and to regulate threats and challenges as far as this is possible. The self is the experience of that organized response, but there is nothing intrinsically interior about either mind or self. Mind and self are not interior spaces to be tended. Rather, they are practical abilities to be cultivated. This resonates with Daniel Siegel's definition of mind as "an embodied and relational process that regulates the flow of energy and information." Siegel elaborates,

> If we ask, "where is the mind?" we can say that its regulatory functions are embodied in the nervous system and embedded in our interpersonal relationships. This emergent process of both the neural and the interpersonal locates the mind within the physiological and relational frame of reality. The mind develops in the interaction of at least these two facets of our human lives.[44]

Regarding the mind as a practical skill rather than an interior space effectively collapses the inside-outside distinction that funds the inside-out view of mental disorders. It removes the barrier that otherwise has to be crossed for things to get from external reality into the mind, because mind *encompasses*

44. Siegel, *Developing Mind*, 2, 7.

external reality in its sensing, perceiving, and regulating activity. It is not that the laptop on which I am typing somehow must be transported into my mind through my senses. Rather, my mind *just is* the regulative process by which I attend to everything in my present experience—the sound of rain outside, my grumbling and empty stomach, and my books and laptop at hand—and coordinate a response to what I judge to be the most pressing needs and goals before me.[45]

Mind and Body in Aquinas

Daniel Siegel derives his view of the mind as "an embodied and relational process that regulates the flow of energy and information" from complexity theory, but the view can point us back to the thought of Thomas Aquinas.[46] Though Aquinas considered Augustine a theological authority, unlike Augustine he focused less on how the mind knows itself than on how the mind apprehends the world. Aquinas turned outward, to the world of the senses. Like Aristotle, Aquinas held that ordinary knowing relies on sensory experience, and that "in the present state of life, in which the soul is united to a passible body, it is impossible for our intellect to understand anything actually, except by turning to [the composite of sense experience]."[47]

In his theory of the rational soul as the substantial form of the human person, Aquinas offers an account of human experience that undermines the self-body

---

45. Though I do not ascribe to the radical behaviorist roots of acceptance and commitment therapy (ACT), this account of the "outside-in" approach bears resemblances to the functional contextualism that is central to ACT. ACT theorists Steven Hayes, Kirk Strosahl, and Kelly Wilson argue that the focus on mechanism within modern psychology is unhelpful because it gives clinicians a false sense of objectivity, as if "the elements of the machine [of the mind] can seemingly be observed dispassionately, much as a spark plug sitting on a table can be examined." But it is more fruitful, they argue, to focus not on the form of private experience but rather the *functions* of behavior, including private experience, in particular contexts. ACT therapists always seek to understand the context within which particular forms of experience and behavior are intelligible, and how changing context may help to predict and to influence this experience and behavior. See Steven Hayes, Kirk Strosahl, and Kelly Wilson, *Acceptance and Commitment Therapy: An Experiential Approach to Behavior Change* (New York: Guilford, 1999), 18–26, quotation 23.

46. Siegel, *Developing Mind*, 2.

47. *STh* Ia q. 84 a. 7 *resp.* See Robert Pasnau, *Thomas Aquinas on Human Nature: A Philosophical Study of* Summa Theologiae *Ia 75–89* (New York: Cambridge University Press, 2002), 278–95.

dualism of Descartes and, by extension, the machine metaphor. For Descartes, body and mind (soul) are different kinds of things. The body is *res extensa*, material stuff extended in space. The mind is *res cogitans*, the immaterial stuff of knowledge and consciousness. Descartes thought the senses were important for knowledge, but he also thought the mind could rightly think of the body as something different from and outside of itself—leading to self-body dualism.

Aquinas, by contrast, understood the human being not as a mind-body duality but as a mind-body unity, in which the mind knows particular things by means of the bodily senses, which depend on the body's existence and function. The body is not for Aquinas a machine that feeds information to the mind or soul. Rather, body and soul, fitted for each other, know and act in union. For Aquinas most of human life, including dimensions of thinking, such as sensation, perception, basic emotional responses, and working memory, depend on the body and cannot occur apart from the body (*STh* Ia q. 84 a. 7; q. 85 a. 1). It is only as the soul apprehends universal forms and abstract truths of reason—as we move from a perception of *this* concrete stone to apprehending "stone" in the abstract—that the soul operates in a way that does not depend on the body for its function, since only an immaterial faculty can apprehend what is immaterial and universal (*STh* Ia q. 75, a. 2; q. 75 a 5; q. 76 a. 1).[48]

For Aquinas, the soul always operates at the nexus of two dimensions that, together, affect it. There is first the dimension of the body, which supports the soul's operations and is, as previously stated, the living material of which the soul is the life. Changes in the body—including dysfunctions of the body's usual processes—will affect the soul's operation. But there is, second, the dimension of the world—including the world of other human beings. The soul is always open, always seeking reality as it presents itself and conforming to the reality that it senses and perceives. Sitting in front of a laptop computer late in an afternoon, my soul, as Aquinas describes it, does not simply regard the laptop screen and the words on it. Rather, I have absorbed the form of the computer and the words; they have become part of me. Aquinas affirms Aristotle's dictum that "the soul is in a way all the things that exist," elaborating that the soul is configured to receive the forms of all things: sensible things through the senses, intelligible things through the intellect.[49]

48. See also James D. Madden, *Mind, Matter, and Nature: A Thomistic Proposal for the Philosophy of Mind* (Washington, DC: Catholic University of America Press, 2013), 265-74; and Adam Wood, *Thomas Aquinas on the Immateriality of the Human Intellect* (Washington, DC: Catholic University of America Press, 2020).
49. Aristotle, *De Anima* 3.8 (431b); from Aristotle, *De Anima (On the Soul)*, trans. Hugh

If the soul (or mind) is in a way all the things that exist, and if even rationality is linked to the inherently social practices of language and symbolization, then we no longer can regard mental health problems as interior problems of individuals.[50] Rather, mental health problems are rips in the fabric of the lived world. They are forms of social, cultural, interpersonal, relational brokenness displayed in the lived experience of an embodied creature. That they are felt by individuals does not mean that they are essentially internal to individuals.[51]

Toward a Biosocial and Ecological Understanding of Mental Health Problems

In chapter 2 and this chapter, drawing on Aquinas and others, I have argued that though we are creatures of earth, we cannot be reduced to creatures of earth. While it is true that our behavior and much of our experience happens in our

---

Lawson-Tancred (New York: Penguin Books, 1986); Aquinas, *Commentary on Aristotle's* De Anima 3.13.13-113; *STh* Ia q. 84 a. 2 *obj2, ad2*.

50. Herbert McCabe, drawing on Aquinas as well as on Ludwig Wittgenstein, argues that even rational thought is intrinsically social, because it is made possible and conditioned by language. "Society is not the product of individual people," McCabe argues. "Rather, individual people are the product of society." Social contract theories that posit that society was formed by individuals seeking mutual support and protection are incoherent, McCabe argues, because they suppose "these individuals to be already in possession of what only society could provide—institutions such as language, contract, agreement, and so on." It is socially constructed language that makes possible the exercise of rationality and, consequently, individuals. "Rationality," McCabe argues, "is a special way of being in a group. It is because there is some form of linguistic community that there are rational individuals or 'persons.' . . . The individual, you might say, is the way in which a linguistic community develops itself historically." Herbert McCabe, *The Good Life: Ethics and the Pursuit of Happiness*, ed. Brian Davies (London: Continuum, 2005), 26, 28. While Aquinas would not agree that individual people are *only* the product of society—such a claim is hard to square with Aquinas's teaching on the divine impartation of the rational soul—McCabe captures well how the content of what we apprehend can shape and construct the way that we experience and interpret ourselves.

51. Bringing Thomas's theory of the person into conversation with the thought of Karol Wojtyła (later Pope John Paul II) and Charles Sanders Peirce, Adrian Reimers argues that the soul is a twofold sign. It is a sign of the body and so linked to the material world. And it is a sign of the immaterial world of concepts and forms. It always exists within that dual signification. My present mental experience intimately reflects the operation of my body: when my body is rested and nourished, I am capable of writing clearly, and when it is not, I struggle. But it also reflects, signifies, the world as I engage it. See Adrian J. Reimers, *The Soul of the Person: A Contemporary Philosophical Psychology* (Washington, DC: Catholic University of America Press, 2006).

bodies, understanding human life requires much more than observation of our material dimension. It also involves appreciation of how our bodies are configured, the efficient causes that brought this configuration about, and the ends or goals toward which we are tending. Christian faith, agreeing with important insights from psychological science, affirms that humans are configured for relationship and for love. We are embodied creatures who find ourselves in and therefore *find our selves* through the relationships that form us.

I have argued that this affirmation—that we are relational creatures of earth, *biosocial* creatures—should lead us to appreciate the biosocial and ecological character of mental health and mental illness. While many in the mental health world also advocate for holistic views of mental health and illness, I offer an account grounded in a distinctively Christian approach to the human person. Mental health care is dominated by an inside-out view of mental health and mental illness, in which mental health problems start on the inside (in the brain or in the interior self) and show up in the outside world of relationship, community, and culture. This view has important Christian roots and should not be discarded entirely, but all too often it reinforces problematic and isolating conceptions of mental illness as a problem of individuals, and it pathologizes appropriate reactions to difficult and hostile social and relational experiences. These patterns lead clinicians to ignore or disregard their patients' social worlds. As an alternative, I have proposed an outside-in view of mental health problems, in which mental health problems *start* in problems of relationship, community, and culture, and then show up inside a person's experience and in the structure and function of the body.

To be clear, I do not seek to discard the inside-out approach entirely. Each of these approaches has a place in reckoning with the complex experience and behavior of mental illness. Sometimes, as in the case of Alzheimer's type neurocognitive disorder or alcohol-induced psychotic disorder, an inside-out approach that focuses on how changes to the body affect experience and behavior is indispensable (though the outside-in approach may still be fruitful). Sometimes, as in the case of complex post-traumatic stress disorder and generalized anxiety disorder, an outside-in approach that focuses on how someone is responding to relational, communal, and cultural challenges is essential (though the inside-out approach may still be fruitful). The point is not to choose categorically one approach over the other but rather to consider which approach fits best in a given situation. Often, both will be fruitful in different ways.

That said, it is difficult to hold the inside-out and outside-in perspectives in view at the same time. I find it useful to consider the analogy with a figure-

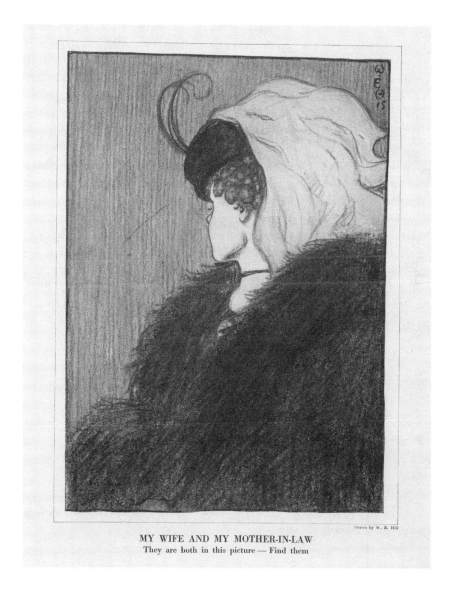

MY WIFE AND MY MOTHER-IN-LAW
They are both in this picture — Find them

Figure 4. The challenge of balancing an inside-out and outside-in perspective (W. E. Hill, "My wife and my mother-in-law. They are both in this picture—find them," 1915, Library of Congress)

ground gestalt image as displayed in figure 4. In this image, one can see a younger woman looking to the left and away, or alternatively an older woman looking to the left and down, but most people find it very difficult to see both the younger and older woman *at the same time*. Our minds, observing the same sensory input, naturally fix on one interpretation or the other: one approach will dominate as the figure and the other will recede to the imperceptible ground. Analogously, in my experience, we naturally fix on either an inside-out view of mental illness *or* an outside-in view, in a way that occludes the other perspective.[52]

When I see patients or supervise students and psychiatry residents, therefore, I ask them to consider which of these views provides a best fit in a given situation. How might an inside-out view of a person's challenges illuminate the situation and facilitate possibilities for growth and freedom? Conversely, how might an outside-in view similarly help? Which of these views fits best? By asking these questions, we challenge the privilege and dominance of inside-out ways of seeing within psychiatry and psychology. We also summon a more holistic, biosocial, and ecological approach to mental health care that befits the nature of humans as embodied creatures of earth who love, who grow, and who *find our selves* in relationship.

52. R. D. Laing drew on the same image to argue that the psychiatrist can view patients (and patients can view themselves) as "organisms" comprised of "*it*-processes" or as "person[s] seen . . . as responsible, as capable of choice, . . . as self-acting agent[s]." See R. D. Laing, *The Divided Self* (New York: Pantheon Books, 1960), 18–21.

From Shame to Security

Our Worth, Desirability, and Loveliness Are in God

> If I say, "Surely the darkness shall cover me,
>   and the light around me become night,"
> even the darkness is not dark to you;
>   the night is as bright as the day,
>   for darkness is as light to you.
>
> —*Psalm 139:11–12*

Contrary to the machine metaphor, human beings are intrinsically and irreducibly relational beings. We are creatures of earth who love, who grow, and who find ourselves in relationship. In the last chapter, I discussed the importance of a relational understanding of mental health and mental illness that attends to our relationships with others and with the world around us. As humans, we are not meant to be alone. We need the love, care, and support of others. We need to live in neighborhoods, communities, and institutions that are cultivated to promote, not to prevent, our flourishing.

This relational understanding of mental health and mental illness challenges the individualism, internalism, dualism, and technicism of the machine metaphor. But as discussed in the last chapter, the relational character of human life is widely appreciated by many mental health clinicians and by theoretical perspectives such as attachment and object relations theory. Any psychiatrist or other mental health clinician who endeavors to treat mental illness without inquiring about patients' social and relational world, and who does not encourage healthy relationship building and social support, is arguably not fulfilling their professional obligations according to the standards of modern mental health care.

What happens, though, when problems are too deep and great for even the highest-quality mental health care to handle? What about those who live or work in pervasively hostile environments that are destructive and inconsistent with health and flourishing? What happens if someone is estranged from family members and everyone else and has no easy prospects for social support outside of a possible relationship with a therapist? What happens when the black dog of depression has made it impossible to feel the love and support of others even when it is being offered? What happens when someone feels utterly, achingly alone?

In this case, Christian faith offers radical hope that modern psychiatry and psychology, on their own terms, cannot. Christian faith does not affirm only that we were created in and for relationship with others. It affirms that we were created in and for relationship with God. Christian faith furthermore affirms that God is faithful to maintain God's end of that relationship. God knows and loves every human being even and *especially* when someone is unable to feel or to reciprocate that love. This is not a psychological but an *ontological* truth. Our deepest identity as human beings is that we are known and loved by God. We are not bundles of cells, adrift in the world, alone until someone or something directs love to us. We are already sites of God's presence and love.[1] God holds us in existence, knows us, and loves us, and that—not anything we have done or not done, not anything else that we are or are not—is the deepest truth of who we are.

In this chapter and the next, I will flesh out this claim as it relates to Scripture and Christian thought, drawing on Thomas Aquinas as a guide. In chapter 5, I will argue that humans are known and loved by God in three overlapping modes, each more personal and intimate: humans are God's good creatures; humans are created in God's image; and humans are enfolded by the Holy Spirit into the person of Jesus, and therefore into the triune God's innermost life of love. In this chapter, in order to better account for why these affirmations are such good news, and why they are relevant to mental health problems and mental health care, I will first explore shame, an ever-present reality of human experience that affects clinicians as well as those who seek mental health care. Shame is important to this story not only because it often co-occurs with mental health problems, either as cause or unfortunate consequence, but also because it is a sign of present or feared disconnection and isolation rather than of connection and belonging. Christian communities and Christian practices can contribute to the overcoming of shame, but they can also cause and perpetuate shame. Any faithful engagement with mental

---

1. Norman Wirzba, *From Nature to Creation: A Christian Vision for Understanding and Loving Our World* (Grand Rapids: Baker Academic, 2015), 19.

health care, then, must come to terms with shame's reality and seek healthy ways to overcome it.

Engaging Shame

Shame is the elephant in the room in nearly any setting in which humans seek each other's approval or fear each other's judgment—which is to say, nearly any context of human life. Shame operates—sometimes visibly, sometimes invisibly—not only in clinic rooms but also in classrooms, church sanctuaries, offices, kitchen tables, living rooms, and bedrooms. In the world of mental health care, it affects not only those who seek mental health care but clinicians also, with distorting and sometimes devastating consequences.

Shame is difficult to speak about. In part, this is due to disagreement about what shame is. Among the academic disciplines, cultural anthropologists, sociologists, theologians, philosophers, and psychologists all have distinct ways of understanding and describing shame.[2] Even within modern psychology, there is considerable debate about the nature and function of shame. Psychoanalytic clinicians and thinkers, drawing on and modifying the ideas of Sigmund Freud and his followers, were among the first within the modern clinical disciplines to write about shame.[3] Helen Block Lewis made an important contribution to the field when she distinguished shame, which involves negative feelings and judgments about one's *self*, from guilt, which involves negative feelings and judgments about one's particular *actions*: "Shame is *about* the self; guilt involves activity *of* the self."[4] If guilt says, "what I did was wrong or bad," then shame says, "*I* am wrong or bad." Guilt, while unpleasant, is an adaptive and socially constructive emotion: if I feel guilty about something that I have done, I can acknowledge the wrong, seek repair and restitution, and restore damaged relationships. But shame, because it is more free-floating and more deeply ingrained in the self, is more damaging and destructive. Shame prompts us to hide from others and to guard ourselves from relationships in which we are vulnerable. It prompts us to disparage ourselves and possibly others also, with no clear paths to restoration and healing.

2. Stephen Pattison, *Shame: Theory, Therapy, Theology* (Cambridge: Cambridge University Press, 2000), 39-64.

3. Leon Wurmser, *The Mask of Shame* (Baltimore: Johns Hopkins University Press, 1981).

4. Helen Block Lewis, "Shame and Guilt in Neurosis," *Psychoanalytic Review* 58 (1971): 419-38, quotation 425; June Price Tangney and Ronda L. Dearing, *Shame and Guilt* (New York: Guilford, 2002).

Other psychological theorists, drawing remotely on René Descartes's and Baruch Spinoza's account of primary passions and affects and more proximately on the emotion classification of Charles Darwin, have sought to further identify how shame relates to other emotions by engaging it behaviorally and phenomenologically. Psychologist Silvan Tomkins proposed a system of nine primary affects, understood as biological mechanisms underlying the feeling or experience of emotion, and argued that shame-humiliation is a painful, biologically programmed affect, characterized behaviorally by averted and downcast eyes and slumped neck and shoulders, that serves to attenuate or to block the affects of interest-excitement or enjoyment-joy, even when the interest- or enjoyment-producing stimuli are still present. Someone, for example, might experience interest or enjoyment in gazing at the body of a stranger but would be inhibited from doing this by the affect of shame-humiliation.[5] Drawing on Tomkins's theory, Donald Nathanson argues that shame triggers four characteristic responses that he describes as the "compass of shame": withdrawal, attacking oneself (including masochistic deference and conformity), narcissistic avoidance, and attacking others (humiliated rage).[6]

Other researchers have found Tomkins's and Nathanson's account of shame to be insufficiently attentive to the way that shame is related to negative judgments about the self, though their theories diverge into two camps. Some theorists have argued that shame follows from a global evaluation that one's self (and not just one's actions) has fallen short of one's standards, rules, and goals.[7] Shame is therefore a secondary, self-conscious emotion that emerges later in development and requires some capacity for self-reflection and self-awareness—more akin to embarrassment and pride than to the primary, unreflective emotions such as joy, fear, anger, disgust, and surprise.[8] Other theorists, however, have argued that shame emerges

5. Silvan Tomkins, "The Varieties of Shame and Its Magnification," in *Exploring Affect: The Selected Writings of Silvan S. Tomkins*, ed. E. Virginia Demos (Cambridge: Cambridge University Press, 1995), 397–410; Donald L. Nathanson, *Shame and Pride: Affect, Sex, and the Birth of the Self* (New York: Norton, 1992), 134–49. Nathanson, a student of Tomkins, distinguishes affect (a biological system), feeling (the awareness of an affect), emotion (the combination of affects with memories and the affects that these memories trigger, i.e., biography) and mood (a persistent state of emotion). "Whereas affect is biology, emotion is biography" (50).

6. Nathanson, *Shame and Pride*, 305–77.

7. Michael Lewis, *Shame: The Exposed Self* (New York: Free Press, 1992), 74–76.

8. Lewis, *Shame*, 84–97. Of note, Aquinas would not have characterized joy (*gaudium*) as a primary emotion in this sense, as joy marks the attainment of a higher good and not just a sensual good (*STh* IaIIae q. 31 a. 3).

much earlier in development. Researchers in interpersonal neurobiology and relational psychotherapy have proposed that shame begins not as cognitive belief ("I am bad" or "I am incompetent") but rather as the experience of an infant or toddler who, seeking the warmth of connection and attunement with a close caregiver, finds that connection rebuffed, without a means of repair.[9] Shame, in the formulation of therapist Patricia DeYoung, is "an experience of one's felt sense of self disintegrating in relation to a dysregulating other."[10] In the view of Allan Schore, Patricia DeYoung, and others, children (and adults) who seek connection but do not find it feel an aching neediness that they learn to hate and perhaps to disown. Children and adults form beliefs about themselves in response to this primitive ache for unrequited connection, to make sense of it and even to compensate for it. If the problem is essentially with *me*—with my unlovability, or my incompetence, or my badness—then I no longer have to wonder why I feel so ashamed, though I also have no path forward.

In each of these theories, however, shame is understood to be an emotion that involves negative bodily sensations and associated beliefs about the unworthiness, incompetence, or undesirability of the self.[11] In this way, it is distinct not only from guilt, as described above, but also from shyness and embarrassment (which are often not accompanied by beliefs about the self's undesirability and incompetence). Though shame often follows from humiliation, it is not the same: humiliation entails that one has been brought low and denigrated by someone else, but it is possible to endure humiliation without the subjective experience of shame.[12]

---

9. Allan Schore, "Early Shame Experiences and Infant Brain Development," in *Shame: Interpersonal Behavior, Psychopathology, and Culture*, ed. Paul Gilbert and Bernice Andrews (New York: Oxford University Press, 1998), 57–77.

10. Patricia A. DeYoung, *Understanding and Treating Chronic Shame: A Relational/Neurobiological Approach* (New York: Routledge, 2015), xiii.

11. Paul Gilbert, "What Is Shame? Some Core Issues and Controversies," in Gilbert and Andrews, *Shame*, 3–38.

12. Lewis, *Shame*, 79–83, 110–14. Of note, Aquinas engages shame (*verecundia*) in the *Summa theologiae* but does not engage it with the depth of other writers surveyed in this section. Aquinas defines shame as a kind of emotion (passion), specifically "fear of a base action." It is not a virtue but is a "praiseworthy passion" since it helps to protect against following through with the base action. It is fear both of vice and of the disgrace that accompanies vice, and it is felt most acutely when one is worried about being judged by others whom one respects. In some ways, shame is achievement because it signifies an intact capacity to recoil from wrong, but it is most desirable to live a form of life where shame is not necessary because no action is base (*STh* IIaIIae q. 144).

Shame, Stigma, and Mental Health Care

Shame magnifies and compounds the felt experience of mental health problems. As mentioned in the introduction, Ann vividly describes the way that shame about psychological struggle was a pervasive part of life in her North Carolina hometown:

> [Shame] didn't show up at church, except in the sense that no one was going to talk about it. But that was a whole town. It was a whole neighborhood. We were post-World War II. These men come home from the war and they're starting their families. Every house in our little part of town, at least one parent was an alcoholic or had mental health issues, was hiding in the bedroom.
>
> You knew which houses you could go into and which you couldn't, because you didn't know what was going on or who wasn't feeling well. My mother talked about these other people. They talked about her. In that sense, the secrets were the root of that shame. That if you can't talk about it, then there must be something wrong. It's just bad. Weak. Something wrong with these people.[13]

Research confirms that shame is associated with a wide variety of common mental health problems. Shame, more than guilt, is associated with the development of depressive symptoms and anxiety symptoms.[14] It is an underappreciated but important contributor to some forms of post-traumatic stress disorder (PTSD), particularly PTSD that is associated with moral injury, and may be particularly important in the association between PTSD and suicide.[15]

---

13. Personal interview, June 3, 2022.

14. For depressive symptoms, see Sangmoon Kim, Ryan Thibodeau, and Randall S. Jorgensen, "Shame, Guilt, and Depressive Symptoms: A Meta-analytic Review," *Psychological Bulletin* 137 (2011): 68–96. In this meta-analysis of 108 studies engaging 22,411 participants, shame was associated with a moderate to large effect size ($r = 0.43$), and guilt was associated with a smaller, moderate effect size ($r = 0.28$). For anxiety symptoms, see Diana-Mirela Cândea and Aurora Szentagotai-Tăta, "Shame-Proneness, Guilt-Proneness, and Anxiety Symptoms: A Meta-analysis," *Journal of Anxiety Disorders* 58 (2018): 78–106.

15. Judith Lewis Herman, "Posttraumatic Stress Disorder as a Shame Disorder," in *Shame in the Therapy Hour*, ed. Ronda L. Dearing and June Price Tangney (Washington, DC: American Psychological Association, 2011), 261–75; Mel Singer, "Shame, Guilt, Self-Hatred and Remorse in the Psychotherapy of Vietnam Combat Veterans Who Committed Atrocities," *American Journal of Psychotherapy* 58 (2004): 377–85; Katherine C. Cunningham et al.,

It is associated with substance use issues and is closely tied with the origin and manifestation of borderline personality disorder.[16] To be sure, not all mental illness is related to shame, and many people do not experience shame connected to their mental health challenges. But shame is the elephant in many therapy rooms, an exceedingly common but often unacknowledged power that pervades the lives of clinicians and patients alike. It is powerful because it often goes unnamed and sometimes even unrecognized. Unrecognized "by-passed shame," as Helen Block Lewis called it, can too often show up as chronic anger (often, but by no means exclusively, in men) or as chronic depression (often, but by no means exclusively, in women), or both.[17]

The problem with chronic shame is that unlike guilt for specific actions, which points the way to restitution and repair, shame often causes us to withdraw from and to avoid the very relationships that would lead to its healing. The bodily postures associated with shame, as affect theorists have pointed out, include downcast eyes, tight facial muscles, and slumped posture. People who live with chronic shame tend to withdraw from relationships or to hide their vulnerability within relationships. We do things to blunt the feeling of shame, which may include unhelpful pain-reducing behaviors involving alcohol and drugs, sex, or risk-taking. We go to great lengths to achieve the approval of others, even though no achievement-based approval is ever quite enough. We make others the enemy, attacking others in order to transform shame into the more palatable and action-directed emotion of anger. Or we attack ourselves, sabotaging long-sought plans and projects and perhaps even considering suicide.

Shame crops up within mental health care in complex ways. People often seek mental health care in part because chronic shame has led to depression, anxiety, addiction, trauma, pain in relationships, or thwarted goals and projects. Others have experienced shame as a result of the challenges associated with mental illness—as when someone with bipolar disorder, forced to withdraw from college courses after hospitalization for acute mania, feels shame for not living up to her own and her family's expectations for academic perfor-

---

"Shame as a Mediator between Posttraumatic Stress Disorder Symptoms and Suicidal Ideation among Veterans," *Journal of Affective Disorders* 243 (2019): 216-19.

16. Ronda L. Dearing, Jeffrey Stuewig, and June Price Tangney, "On the Importance of Distinguishing Shame from Guilt: Relations to Problematic Alcohol and Drug Use," *Addictive Behaviors* 30 (2005): 1392-1404; Tzipi Buchman-Wildbaum et al., "Shame in Borderline Personality Disorder: Meta-analysis," *Journal of Personality Disorders* 35, supp. A. (2021): 149-61.

17. Lewis, *Shame*, 119-62.

mance. Either way—whether shame is the cause of mental health challenges, or the consequence, or both—shame is a potent force that perpetuates suffering and inhibits recovery.

At its best, good mental health care provides a context in which shame can be named and felt where it exists, in a way that points toward healing. But it does not always work this way. Many people experience mental health care to be the occasion for shame, and even the *cause* of shame, rather than a way for shame to be healed. Many people who seek mental health care, no doubt as well as many clinicians, carry deep-seated convictions not just that mental illness *is* associated with shame, as a matter of fact, but beyond that, that mental illness *ought to be* associated with shame. They believe that mental illness does indeed reflect core unworthiness, incompetence, or un-desirability of the self, and that the shame associated with mental illness is therefore justified. If clinicians perpetuate or promote these convictions in the context of mental health care—as, for instance, when a clinician be-rates a patient for relapsing on substances, not taking medications, or not following recommendations—then mental health care is itself experienced as shaming. Patients who feel shamed in therapy may well leave treatment and never return.

Even for those who do continue to seek treatment, the possibility that mental health care might be shaming forms (and deforms) modern mental health care in several ways. Rather than serving as a healing path for naming and overcoming shame, modern mental health care is often a complex set of strat-egies for avoiding shame. Even mentioning the word "shame," particularly if it is not done in the context of a trusting therapeutic relationship, can awaken feelings of shame and can be interpreted as shaming. Perhaps for this reason, it is more common for clinicians and mental health advocacy organizations to speak of stigma rather than shame. The National Alliance on Mental Illness (NAMI) and other advocacy groups, for example, often speak of the need to confront stigma associated with mental illness:

> NAMI condemns all acts of stigma and discrimination directed against people living with mental illness, whether by intent, ignorance, or insen-sitivity. Epithets, nicknames, jokes, advertisements, and slurs that refer to individuals with mental illness in a stigmatizing way are cruel. NAMI considers acts of stigma to be discrimination. Stigma reflects prejudice, de-humanizes people with mental illness, trivializes their legitimate concerns, and is a significant barrier to effective delivery of mental health services. Because of stigma, individuals and families are often afraid to seek help;

health care providers are often poorly trained to refer people to mental health professionals and/or mental health practitioners, and services are too often inadequately funded.[18]

In the advocacy world, stigma is widely embraced as an enemy to be confronted, but it carries different meanings. Primarily it refers to bias, discrimination, and negative judgments made about people who live with mental illness because of their illness. But it also refers to the feelings that are associated with these negative judgments: the US Surgeon General's 1999 report that first described stigma as a public health problem speaks of "feelings of stigma and shame,"[19] and the most recent NAMI Public Policy Platform, while never mentioning shame, refers to the need for "relief from guilt and stigma."[20]

Confronting stigma is important, but stigma is not shame, and it is important not to conflate the two. Stigma, as sociologist Erving Goffman classically described it, is a negative social judgment that something about a person is "deeply discrediting," denoting a shortcoming or failure to live as a "whole and usual" person. When this judgment is internalized—when stigmatized people agree that something about their identity is defiling—then "shame becomes a central possibility." But stigma is not shame and need not lead to shame. One may, for example, seek the company of others who bear the same stigma in order to find solidarity and support.[21] One may even interpret marks of stigma as gifts, as when the apostle Paul boasted that "I carry the marks [literally, *stigmata*] of Jesus branded on my body" (Gal. 6:17). Furthermore, as good as it would be to eliminate discrimination and overt negative social practices related to mental illness, this would not eliminate shame associated with mental illness, particularly shame that stems from early dehumanizing or invalidating relationships. At worst, focusing on stigma can be a way of avoiding talking about shame.

18. "Public Policy Platform of the National Alliance on Mental Illness," National Alliance on Mental Illness, 12th ed., December 2016, https://www.nami.org/Advocacy/Policy-Platform.

19. US Department of Health and Human Services, *Mental Health: A Report of the Surgeon General* (Rockville, MD: US Department of Health and Human Services, Substance Abuse and Mental Health Services Administration, Center for Mental Health Services, National Institutes of Health, National Institute of Mental Health, 1999), 84.

20. "Public Policy Platform of the National Alliance on Mental Illness," 6.

21. Erving Goffman, *Stigma: Notes on the Management of Spoiled Identity* (Englewood Cliffs, NJ: Prentice-Hall, 1963), 3, 7, 19–31.

Focusing on stigma, however, is far from the only way that modern mental health care displaces and avoids shame. All of the deforming aspects of mental health care discussed in chapter 1—individualism, self-symptom dualism, self-body dualism, technicism, and commodification—can be understood as strategies by which clinicians and patients collude to avoid shame. Individualism, the assumption that mental disorders occur in individuals rather than in shared social space, may indeed intensify shame by persuading people with mental illness that the problem is within them, but it also may paradoxically shield people from the need to explore how past and present relationships have contributed to shame, pointing instead to the need for cognitive-behavioral or medication interventions. Self-symptom dualism and self-body dualism, by enabling the unwanted experience and behavior of mental illness to be externalized as symptoms that are located within the body, allow shame to be displaced and externalized. Technicism enables the focus of mental health care to be on finding the right technique to reduce unwanted symptoms, in a way that prevents shame from being named and felt. And commodification places the shame-bearing consumer in the role of market agent, shifting the responsibility for recovery onto the provider or the service.

The Shame of Clinicians

All of this is made more complex by the fact that shame does not operate only in those who seek mental health care. It also operates in the lives and work of mental health clinicians, affecting the way that clinicians approach patients and themselves. This is first of all because clinicians are human beings who carry burdens of shame just like anyone else. Some clinicians have found effective ways to name, to understand, and to partially heal our own shame, and some have not. But whatever vulnerabilities clinicians carry with us are put to the test in the context of mental health practice. Most clinicians want to believe that what we are doing is important. We want to be valued and to be considered competent by patients, by colleagues, and by the systems in which we work. Usually, we like to be liked. When we are valued, liked, and considered competent, we thrive. Most clinicians link how *we* are doing with how our patients respond to the treatments we offer. If our patients are getting well, doing better, and valuing the services that we offer, then all is well. We value ourselves, and unless our models of treatment are somehow threatening to other clinicians, we find more often than not that colleagues and systems value us also.

Unfortunately, patients do not always get better—at least not in the ways that we predict. Treatments do not always work. Patients and family members do not always like us. When that happens, clinicians commonly experience shame at the prospect of being dismissed, devalued, and judged incompetent by patients, by colleagues, and by the systems in which we work. Even the prospect that such failure *might* happen can invoke potent feelings of prospective shame.

Clinicians, like patients, respond in various ways. Sometimes we recognize shame for what it is, acknowledge it, and engage in meaningful relationships in which shame can be overcome. But often we seek other solutions. Rather than blaming ourselves, we may displace shame and instead hold someone or something else responsible for our patients' not getting better. We may blame the systems in which we work: *if only I were free to practice like I want and not to be under the thumb of managers and insurance companies, things would be much better.* We may blame the technologies and techniques that we are using: *this medication doesn't work that well anyway.* We may blame patients for not doing what we advise, or for sabotaging their own recovery.

Or we may internalize and rationalize shame by blaming ourselves: *I do not know enough; I am not skilled enough; I am not experienced enough for this work.* Such self-blaming rationalizations may seem to offer little comfort, but at least they provide a way to make sense of painful feeling. Self-blaming also leads to practical responses, some adaptive and some not. We resolve to try harder: to read more, to get better supervision, to attend more conferences. We focus our energy on areas where we feel more competent, such as research or teaching or administration (and this can work in reverse also, where researchers who are feeling shame related to their research can divert energy to clinical care). We associate with colleagues who are most likely to value and to praise us. Or we find ways to disengage. We focus our energy on applying a technique accurately, basing our self-worth on the proper application of the technique, rather than on how our patients are doing as a result of the technique. Any failure is simply a known feature of the technique (such as neurostimulation, or a particular school of manualized psychotherapy) rather than a failure of ourselves as clinicians. Or we simply try to fly under the radar, hoping not to be discovered, doing the minimal work necessary to avoid discovery of our own incompetence, and not risking anything more. Or we self-medicate with alcohol or opioids—and so on. Compounded over months and years, these strategies to avoid shame—from overengagement, to blaming others, to emphasis on technique, to disengagement—can lead to clinician burnout.

CHAPTER 4

Naked and Ashamed: Shame in Biblical Perspective

The Bible is not a psychology textbook, and Scripture does not provide a comprehensive account of shame. But shame is inextricably tied up with sin and broken relationships. In chapter 2, we encountered the affirmation of Genesis 2 that humans are creatures of dust, *adam* from *adamah*, and formed for relationship. The culmination of the creation story of Genesis 2 is a beautiful picture of vulnerable creatures of dust, held in a web of divine and human relationship: "and the man and his wife were both naked, and were not ashamed" (Gen. 2:25).

But this healthy, vulnerable relational connection did not last long. The text immediately introduces an additional character, the serpent, who addresses the woman and begins to sow doubt about the security of her relationship with God, and God's intentions toward her:

> Now the serpent was more crafty than any other wild animal that the LORD God had made. He said to the woman, "Did God say, 'You shall not eat from any tree in the garden'?"
>
> The woman said to the serpent, "We may eat of the fruit of the trees in the garden; but God said, 'You shall not eat of the fruit of the tree that is in the middle of the garden, nor shall you touch it, or you shall die.'"
>
> But the serpent said to the woman, "You will not die; for God knows that when you eat of it your eyes will be opened, and you will be like God, knowing good and evil."
>
> So when the woman saw that the tree was good for food, and that it was a delight to the eyes, and that the tree was to be desired to make one wise, she took of its fruit and ate; and she also gave some to her husband, who was with her, and he ate. Then the eyes of both were opened, and they knew that they were naked; and they sewed fig leaves together and made loincloths for themselves.
>
> They heard the sound of the LORD God walking in the garden at the time of the evening breeze, and the man and his wife hid themselves from the presence of the LORD God among the trees of the garden. But the LORD God called to the man, and said to him, "Where are you?"
>
> He said, "I heard the sound of you in the garden, and I was afraid, because I was naked; and I hid myself." (Gen. 3:1-10)

In this account of the first human sin, all of the salient features of shame are present. The serpent's words prompt the couple to question God's statement that they will die and then to eat from the tree of knowledge of good and evil, which God has explicitly commanded them not to do. Their nakedness and vulnerability become not a blessing but a curse. Punishing and hiding themselves from each other, they sew together abrasive fig leaves to cover the most intimate parts of their bodies, and then hide from God. Found by God and unable to hide any longer, they admit eating of the tree but resort to blaming each other and the serpent for what had happened (Gen. 3:11-13).

Christians often assume that these broken relationships are due entirely to the humans' disobedience in eating the forbidden fruit. But it is possible to see the disobedience as, in part, the result of relational fracturing. As Curt Thompson observes, the crafty serpent's initial question was on first glance easy to answer: God had *not* forbidden the humans to eat from any tree in the garden. But the question sowed the seed of doubt in the woman, encouraging her to question *by herself* whether God indeed intended her best interest, and ultimately leading her to trust her own judgment about the nutritional, aesthetic, and wisdom-imparting qualities of the fruit over God's counterintuitive prohibition. The relational disconnection at the core of shame started *before*, not after, the consumption of the fruit.[22]

Elaine Heath, relating this story to the dynamics of childhood sexual abuse, takes this observation even further. Drawing from Saint Irenaeus of Lyons's view that Adam and Eve were psychologically and spiritually like children, she argues that having no prior experience of death or evil, they had no reason not to trust the serpent and would not have had any personal experience of death. The crafty serpent, then, played the role of a groomer, exploiting their childlike vulnerability and tricking them into doing something that seemed at the time to be right but that immediately revealed itself to be a terrible wrong. The first humans were sinned *against* before they sinned, hurling them into a cycle of shame and sin that only intensified in the coming generations.[23]

Despite being deceived, the first humans—and by extension all of humankind, now under the condition of sin—bore terrible consequences, including patriarchal domination (3:16), difficult toil (3:17-18), physical death (3:19), and exile from the garden (3:22-24). The relationship of the man and woman was perhaps never fully repaired: having previously referred to his wife by the intimate term *ishah*, connoting her profound connection to him as "bone of

---

22. Curt Thompson, *The Soul of Shame: Retelling the Stories We Believe about Ourselves* (Downers Grove, IL: InterVarsity Press, 2015), 100-107.

23. Elaine Heath, *Healing the Wounds of Sexual Abuse: Reading the Bible with Survivors* (Grand Rapids: Brazos, 2019), 13-24; Irenaeus, *Against Heresies* 3.22.4.

my bones and flesh of my flesh," the first man now names her by reference not to himself but to her motherhood and offspring: *havvah*, Eve, the mother of all living (3:20). But even in this text, God does not allow shame and separation to have the last word. God replaces their self-made, abrasive fig leaf coverings with more comfortable and durable protection: "and the LORD God made garments of skins for the man and for his wife, and clothed them" (3:21). Even in their shame, God was providing for their needs.

Healing Shame

Shame is foundational to the biblical narrative and is an ever-present part of human life, sitting at the root of many mental health problems and interacting in complex ways with mental health care. What, then, is needed for the healing of shame? If shame is at root a relational problem that (at least in part) stems from the experience of dysregulating or invalidating relationships, manifests in beliefs that the self is worthless, incompetent, or undesirable, and leads to withdrawal from and distortion of relationships, then shame can be healed only in relationship.

But what kind of relationship? Mental health clinicians often place a great deal of importance on the clinician-patient relationship, because that is what we have to offer. Indeed, the strength and quality of the therapeutic relationship is an important contributor to the outcomes of mental health treatment. The strength of the alliance between psychotherapists and patients may matter more for the clinical outcome than the particular form of psychotherapy that is being employed.[24] The therapeutic alliance plays an underappreciated but vital role in outcomes related to psychiatric medication use.[25] Healthy therapeutic relationships can be highly effective in ameliorating the effects of chronic shame. A healthy therapeutic relationship, rather than denying or avoiding shame, may actually welcome feelings of shame into the room, as chronic

---

24. Bruce E. Wampold and Zac E. Imel, *The Great Psychotherapy Debate: The Evidence for What Makes Psychotherapy Work*, 2nd ed. (New York: Routledge, 2015).

25. C. Jason Mallo and David L. Mintz, "Teaching All the Evidence Bases: Reintegrating Psychodynamic Aspects of Prescribing into Psychopharmacology Training," *Psychodynamic Psychiatry* 13 (2008): 13–38; David L. Mintz and David F. Flynn, "How (Not What) to Prescribe: Nonpharmacologic Aspects of Psychopharmacology," *Psychiatric Clinics of North America* 35 (2012): 143–65; Warren A. Kinghorn and Abraham M. Nussbaum, *Prescribing Together: A Relational Guide to Psychopharmacology* (Arlington, VA: American Psychiatric Association, 2021).

shame comes to the surface in the context of the therapeutic relationship—but it will not perpetuate shame. Within a therapeutic relationship, there is an opportunity to "give shame light and air," allowing shame to be disclosed, felt, named, and ultimately reduced in the context of a healing, attuned connection.[26] A healthy therapeutic relationship can provide space for vulnerability, in which someone who bears shame opens to another and discovers, in the place of judgment and ostracism, a stance of acceptance and love. Gradually, in the context of this attuned connection, there is the opportunity to challenge the core beliefs that are associated with shame.

But, of course, not everyone has access to a relationship with a therapist, and most people seeking outpatient mental health care will spend no more than an hour per week, and often considerably less, in direct contact with their therapist or psychiatrist.[27] Ultimately these clinician-patient relationships have value insofar as they allow other relationships to be inhabited differently—relationships with family members, with coworkers, with supervisors, with acquaintances, and with ourselves. It is within these other relationships that we are held, loved, and healed—or that we are belittled, shamed, and even dehumanized. A healthy therapist-patient relationship can go a long way toward relieving shame and experiences that are associated with it, including depression and anxiety. But it is within other relationships that most of life is lived. Many clinicians and researchers therefore quite rightly believe that shame is healed within networks of secure, loving relationships in which vulnerability is reciprocated by love and not by ostracism or judgment.

To this point, a Christian response to shame could be completely answered by the core insights of the previous two chapters: as creatures of earth who love, grow, and who find ourselves in relationship, we need healthy, loving relationships to heal from shame. To be sure, this is a place to start. If healthy relationships were seen as the core of mental health, rather than as helpful additional resources for what is fundamentally an individual matter, this would challenge the individualistic assumptions of modern mental health care and would force clinical systems to be more communally oriented. But while Christian faith will always affirm the importance of healthy and loving human relationships, Christian faith does not stop there, because human

26. DeYoung, *Understanding and Treating Chronic Shame*, 116-35.

27. Traditional psychoanalysis, involving up to five sessions per week, is clearly an exception, as are inpatient treatment and partial hospitalization treatment models. In these contexts, the relationship between clinician and patient may become deeper and richer, commensurate with the amount of direct time spent together.

relationships can and do fail. Because we are vulnerable creatures of earth, human relationships are always contingent and vulnerable. Even secure human connections can be severed through death, disease, or displacement. Many people, through no fault of their own, do not have access to healthy and secure networks of relationship. Furthermore, because shame is fueled by the fear of ostracism and isolation—*if they only knew the truth about me, I would be cut off*—then it is possible to reject the very forms of relationship that can lead to healing.

Beyond the vulnerability and fragility of relationships, a driver of shame is the assumption of existential aloneness, the core belief that if stripped of the roles, responsibilities, and relationships that we value, that we would be completely and totally alone. Healthy human relationships can remove this experience of aloneness, but they cannot eliminate its future possibility.

In the face of the vulnerability and fragility of human relationships and the specter of existential aloneness, Christian faith offers a deeper antidote for shame that we will explore in detail in the next chapter. Christian faith teaches that our worth and desirability, our *loveliness*, is ours by virtue of being creatures of a God who loves us first, prior to any of our love for God or for each other. The deepest truth of who we are as human beings is that we are known and loved by God.

CHAPTER 5

From Bare Existence to Beloved Existence

We Are Known and Loved by God, Made in the Image of God,
Held in the Life of the Son

> Even before a word is on my tongue,
> O LORD, you know it completely.
> You hem me in, behind and before,
> and lay your hand upon me.
>
> —*Psalm 139:4-5*

> It's good that you exist; it's good that you are in this world!
>
> —*Josef Pieper,* Faith, Hope, Love[1]

Stigma and shame hang like a cloud over many experiences of mental health challenge. Clinicians, advocates, and those who live with mental illness seek to overcome stigma by normalizing psychological distress, by encouraging mental health care-seeking, and by working to dismantle stigmatizing systems. Likewise, we seek to engage and overcome shame by cultivating trusting therapeutic relationships in which healthy and safe vulnerability is possible and that lead to trusting, affirming relationships in other areas of life. But what happens when human relationships, therapeutic and otherwise, fail? In this case, Christians strongly affirm that our deepest and fullest identity is found in our status as good creatures of God, who knows us and loves us more deeply than we love and know ourselves.

---

1. Josef Pieper, "On Love," in *Faith, Hope, Love* (San Francisco: Ignatius, 1997), 163-64.

God's love for us is displayed in three overlapping ways, each more specific than the last, and in this chapter, we will consider each of them. First, we are known and loved by God as creatures. Second, we are known and loved by God as those who are formed in God's image. Third, though God does not force this upon us, all humans are invited by the Holy Spirit into the life of the Son of God, Jesus Christ, and known and loved within the core of the life of the triune God, held and known within the intimate love of the Father for the Son.

"And Indeed, It Was Very Good": The Grace of Being a Creature

Mental health challenges such as major depression are often characterized by a deep sense that a previously familiar world has become hostile and unintelligible, that in place of meaning and purpose there is confusion, emptiness, and disappointment. Novelist William Styron describes it so poignantly:

> What I had begun to discover is that, mysteriously and in ways that are totally remote from normal experience, the gray drizzle of horror induced by depression takes on the quality of physical pain. But it is not an immediately identifiable pain, like that of a broken limb. It may be more accurate to say that despair, owing to some evil trick played upon the sick brain by the inhabiting psyche, comes to resemble the discomfort of being imprisoned in a fiercely overheated room. And because no breeze stirs this caldron, because there is no escape from this smothering confinement, it is entirely natural that the victim begins to think ceaselessly of oblivion.[2]

This sense is not new to human nature or to biblical faith. The writers of Scripture, particularly within the Psalms, speak in ways that would very possibly, in our time, be interpreted as symptoms of major depression. Take, for example, Psalm 13:

> How long, O LORD? Will you forget me forever?
>   How long will you hide your face from me?
> How long must I bear pain in my soul
>   and have sorrow in my heart all day long? (Ps. 13:1–2)

---

2. William Styron, *Darkness Visible: A Memoir of Madness* (New York: Vintage, 1992), 50.

Or Psalm 88:

> O LORD, why do you cast me off?
>> Why do you hide your face from me?
> Wretched and close to death from my youth up,
>> I suffer your terrors; I am desperate.
> Your wrath has swept over me;
>> your dread assaults destroy me.
> They surround me like a flood all day long;
>> from all sides they close in on me (Ps. 88:14–17).

Or the book of Lamentations:

> I am one who has seen affliction
>> under the rod of God's wrath;
> he has driven and brought me
>> into darkness without any light;
> against me alone he turns his hand,
>> again and again, all day long.
> He has made my flesh and my skin waste away,
>> and broken my bones;
> he has besieged and enveloped me
>> with bitterness and tribulation;
> he has made me sit in darkness
>> like the dead of long ago.
> He has walled me about so that I cannot escape;
>> he has put heavy chains on me;
> though I call and cry for help,
>> he shuts out my prayer;
> he has blocked my ways with hewn stones,
>> he has made my paths crooked.
> He is a bear lying in wait for me,
>> a lion in hiding;
> he led me off my way and tore me to pieces;
>> he has made me desolate;
> he bent his bow and set me
>> as a mark for his arrow.
> He shot into my vitals
>> the arrows of his quiver;

> I have become the laughingstock of all my people,
>> the object of their taunt-songs all day long.
> He has filled me with bitterness,
>> he has sated me with wormwood.
> He has made my teeth grind on gravel,
>> and made me cower in ashes;
> my soul is bereft of peace;
>> I have forgotten what happiness is. (Lam. 3:1–17)

Each of these biblical writers gives voice to the anguish that resonates with contemporary experiences of depression and severe anxiety. Many of my patients, over the years, have found these bleak texts of Scripture to be powerful and even comforting, as they see their own experience articulated in the Bible itself, and as the shame associated with not being able to "just get over it" begins to abate. Ann, whose story we encountered in the introduction, speaks of the way that biblical stories were profoundly helpful for her own journey with depression:

> I think of a lot of Old Testament stories. The whole wilderness wandering section of Scripture. The delivery of the Israelites from their prison of labor, hard labor and being forced to make bricks. . . . I really felt like I had been in prison. Mentally, emotionally, spiritually, even in a really small place. A lot of the Old Testament stories came just alive and made so much sense to me from my experience. It gave me imagery. Then, as far as New Testament stories, it was little things like disciples in the prison, and the singing and praising, and the doors were flying open.[3]

There is a difference, though, between these biblical texts and modern experiences of depression, anxiety, and serious mental illness. To understand why, we have to take a step back. Most humans in Western societies live as what Charles Taylor, drawing on Max Weber, refers to as "bounded" or "buffered" selves within a "disenchanted" world. To be buffered is to live with the assumption that "thoughts, etc., occur in minds; minds are (grosso modo) only human; and they are bounded: they are inward spaces."[4] Furthermore,

---

3. Personal interview, June 3, 2022. In *Dust in the Blood: A Theology of Life with Depression* (Collegeville, MN: Liturgical Press, 2022), Jessica Coblentz also resonates with the image of depression as a wilderness experience, drawing especially on the experience of Hagar.
4. Charles Taylor, *A Secular Age* (Cambridge: Belknap, 2007), 31.

buffered selves are constituted by the assumption that meanings are assigned within this inward space of the mind: everything in the world has meaning only insofar as it has been assigned meaning by my mind or another's mind. Taylor argues that this assumption that meaning is in the mind makes self-body dualism intelligible with respect to the experience of depression or melancholy:

> A modern [person] is feeling depressed, melancholy. He is told: it's just your body chemistry, you're hungry, or there is a hormone malfunction, or whatever. Straightaway, he feels relieved. He can take a distance from this feeling, which is *ipso facto* declared not justified. Things [in the world] don't really have this meaning; it just feels this way, which is the result of a causal action utterly unrelated to the meanings of things. This step of disengagement depends on our modern mind/body distinction, and the relegation of the physical to being "just" a contingent cause of the psychic.[5]

But this was not the experiential world of the biblical writers or of the earliest readers of Scripture. They lived, rather, as "porous" selves in an enchanted world. They experienced themselves as immersed in a world permeated by gods, good and evil spiritual forces, and charged physical objects, such as relics of saints, that conveyed spiritual and moral power. In the enchanted world, meanings are not created and found only in the mind. They are already present in the spiritual and moral forces at work all around. The self, moreover, is not buffered (insulated, defended) but porous to these forces. Possession by demons or malevolent forces was a terrifying possibility, not a psychological metaphor. And in contrast to the idea of depression as an internal mental state, melancholy *just is* an excess of black bile:

> Black bile is not the cause of melancholy, it embodies, it *is* melancholy. The emotional life is porous here again; it doesn't simply exist in an inner, mental space. Our vulnerability to the evil, the inwardly destructive, extends to more than just spirits which are malevolent. It goes beyond them to things which have no wills, but are nevertheless redolent with evil meanings.[6]

What difference does this shift from the porous self to the buffered self make for the experience of mental health problems, and for reading these

---

5. Taylor, *A Secular Age*, 37; bracketed text added for clarity.
6. Taylor, *A Secular Age*, 32, 37.

anguished biblical texts? For the porous selves of the psalmists, for whom the pervasiveness of spiritual forces was unquestioned, God's felt absence (Ps. 13) or God's perceived infliction of pain (Ps. 88; Lam. 3) was devastatingly painful. But the flip side was that even in God's felt absence, God was still a subject of address. The psalmists and the writer of Lamentations, steeped and formed in the liturgical, political, and cultural life of Israel, cried out to a God who was presumed to be an ever-present, even if at times experientially absent, part of their world.

In our disenchanted secular age, this assumed presence of God—or the assumption that anything outside of our minds means anything—cannot be taken for granted. As buffered, bounded selves, inoculated to the world of spiritual forces, we perceive ourselves as meaning-inventing machines who are subject to ultimately meaningless patterns and laws of nature. This opens new, bleak possibilities for the felt experience of depression and other mental health problems. No longer is despair experienced (necessarily) within the context of a self that cannot but think of itself as connected to forces that transcend the self. Rather, there is the possibility of ultimate meaninglessness. If when depressed we feel totally and completely alone, that may be because we *are* totally and completely alone in a meaningless universe. To find meaning in depression, like the man in Taylor's example we might turn to the closest authority structures that we have, that of modern science, and fix on a biological chemical imbalance as an explanation for our experience. But because this naturalistic explanation cannot admit of some higher purpose or meaning to human life—neurotransmitters just *are*—they cannot ultimately impart meaning. It falls to someone who is depressed, often within the context of a therapeutic relationship, to find a story, any story, that will make sense of one's experience.

A Christian approach, however, begins in a radically different place, not with nature but with creation. The first affirmation of Scripture is that "in the beginning, God created" (Gen. 1:1). The point of the poetical account of creation in Genesis 1 is that all of creation is formed and breathed by God, including humans who (as we will explore below) are uniquely made "in the image of God."

But that is not all. God is not indifferent to God's creation. We are told that upon each day of creation, God saw the work of that day as "good" (*tob*, "beautiful," "pleasant," "fair" [Gen. 1:4, 10, 12, 18, 25]). At the conclusion of the sixth day, "God saw everything that he had made, and indeed, it was very good" (Gen. 1:31). And then God finished the work by resting on the seventh day and inaugurating the Sabbath, God's delighted rest in God's creation.

The first and second accounts of the creation in Genesis offer a foundational contrast to the modern idea of nature as purposeless mechanism—including the part of nature that is human beings. God is not a distant designer who sets the world spinning and then leaves the scene, or who governs only by impersonal laws. Rather, God knows the creation in intimate detail. God speaks all that is—including "every living creature that moves, of every kind" (Gen. 1:21)—into existence. With respect to human beings, as we will explore further below, God created humankind "in his image," blessed the first humans, and called them to service and stewardship (Gen. 1:27-30). The creation narrative of Genesis 2, though different in language and detail, follows the same threefold pattern. God forms the first man (*adam*) from the dust of the ground (*adamah*). God breathes into him the breath or spirit (*ruah*) of life, upon which the man becomes a living being (*nephesh*). God blesses the man by planting a garden in Eden containing "every tree that is pleasant to the sight and good for food" and placing the man in it (Gen. 2:9). And having placed the man in the garden, God calls him "to till it and to keep it" (Gen. 2:15).

But God does not simply know God's creation. God also *loves* God's creation. Relative to many other texts of Scripture, it may seem that Genesis 1 and 2 do not speak strongly of God's love, since the characteristic words translated as "love" in the Old Testament (such as *hesed*) never appear in Genesis 1-11. But the text of Genesis 1 tells us that after God created, "God saw everything that he had made, and indeed, it was very good" (1:31).

Norman Wirzba argues that because the Genesis account not only describes the fact that God created but also provides insight into God's perspective on the creation, we also are invited to inhabit "God's mode of perception," according to which every creature is a material manifestation of God's creative love:

> Looking out onto that first Sabbath sunrise, God sees the hospitable love that "makes room" for what is not God to be and to flourish. Divine love is the action that brings creation into being, which means that *God sees each creature and his own love at the same time*. Seeing the night and the day, the water and the dry land, the fish of the sea and the birds of the air, and the creeping things and wild animals of the earth, God also sees the divine love that desires each and every thing to be the unique thing that it is. In other words, a tree, when seen by God, is never simply a vertical log with varying kinds of foliage or some amount of lumber. A tree is also, and more fundamentally, an incarnation of God's love—made visible, tactile, and fragrant

as a giant redwood or cedar of Lebanon. Perceiving the diverse forms of creation *and* the love that holds and sustains them in their being, God "rests."[7]

God's rest on the seventh day, Wirzba emphasizes, is not an escape: indeed, "it couldn't be, because God's world is saturated and sustained by love, and love results in *relationship* rather than alienation, *hospitality* rather than separation."[8]

Drawing on Thomas Aquinas, Josef Pieper argues that this affirmation—"indeed, it was very good"—captures the heart of all human and divine love:

> Is there any meaning at all to the universal question: What is the "nature of love?" . . . My tentative answer to this question runs as follows: In every conceivable case love signifies much the same as approval. This is first of all to be taken in the literal sense of the word's root: loving someone or something means finding him or it *probus*, the Latin word for "good." It is a way of turning to him or it and saying, "It's good that you exist; it's good that you are in this world!"[9]

Quoting a contemporary, Pieper terms love "an act of partisanship for the existence of the beloved,"[10] and he makes clear that love in this sense is not based on any capacity or attribute but rather purely on the fact that the beloved exists: "For what the lover gazing upon his beloved says and means is *not*: How good that you are *so* (so clever, useful, capable, skillful), but: It's good that you are; how wonderful that you exist!"[11] Aquinas joyfully affirms that "God loves everything that exists"—infusing and creating the goodness in things as God loves them (*STh* Ia q. 20 a. 2 *resp.*).[12]

It's good that you exist. It's good that you are in this world. This affirmation of ineradicable belovedness, the movement from bare existence to beloved ex-

---

7. Norman Wirzba, *From Nature to Creation: A Christian Vision for Understanding and Loving Our World* (Grand Rapids: Baker Academic, 2015), 75.

8. Wirzba, *From Nature to Creation*, 75.

9. Pieper, "On Love," 163-64.

10. Pieper, "On Love," 168, quoting Alexander Pfander.

11. Pieper, "On Love," 170.

12. Étienne Gilson makes clear how an account of creation as manifestation of God's love is different from the machine metaphor: "The universe, as represented by St. Thomas, is not a mass of inert bodies passively moved by a force which passes through them, but a collection of active beings each enjoying the efficacy delegated to it by God along with actual being. At the first beginnings of a world like this, we have to place not so much a force being exercised as an infinite goodness being communicated. Love is the unfathomable source of all causality." See Étienne Gilson, *The Christian Philosophy of St. Thomas Aquinas*, trans. L. K. Shook (Notre Dame: University of Notre Dame Press, 1994), 183.

istence, makes all the difference for the way that humans grow, develop, and flourish. Writing in the middle of the twentieth century, Pieper mentions the sobering observations of René Spitz, an Austrian-American psychiatrist who documented that children raised in institutions for orphans and separated children that provided for their basic needs for food, shelter, clothing, and hygiene, but in which there was little interpersonal warmth and relationship, developed startling rates of illness, depression, and even death.[13] Borrowing from sociologist and psychoanalyst Erich Fromm's use of the scriptural image of "milk and honey," Pieper comments that these children were provided the milk—the basic requirements of bodily life—but not the honey of "the sweetness of life and the happiness of existing." But a proper understanding of creation requires both:

> Augustine says in the last chapter of his *Confessions*, "We see things because they exist; but they exist because Thou seest them." There is an analogous principle at work in our context: Because God wills and affirms things, man and the universe as a whole, therefore and solely for this reason they are good, which is to say, lovable and affirmable, to us also.[14]

The movement from bare existence to beloved existence sets the stage for everything that follows in the biblical story. In the creation narrative of Proverbs 8:22-31, Woman Wisdom, interpreted by some as the first of God's creatures and by others (including Thomas Aquinas) as a personification of the second person of the Trinity,[15] exults at being "beside [the Lord] like a master worker" (or, alternatively, "like a little child") in the work of creation,

> And I was daily his delight
>   Rejoicing before him always,
> Rejoicing in his inhabited world
>   And delighting in the human race (Prov. 8:30-31).

Even Job, in his anguish, was able to cry to God,

> You clothed me with skin and flesh,
>   And knit me together with bones and sinews

13. René Spitz, "Hospitalism," *Psychoanalytic Study of the Child* 2 (1946): 113-17.
14. Pieper, "On Love," 174-75, 178.
15. For the former interpretation, see David Kelsey, *Eccentric Existence: A Theological Anthropology* (Louisville: Westminster John Knox, 2009), 163, and for the latter, see Aquinas, *Summa contra Gentiles* 4.11.18-19; 4.12.

> You have granted me life and steadfast love,
>> And your care has preserved my spirit (Job 10:11–12).

The Psalms, particularly the text from Psalm 139 that appeared at the beginning of this chapter, also speak repeatedly of God's providential care for creation and special regard for human beings:

> O LORD, you have searched me and known me.
> You know when I sit down and when I rise up;
>> you discern my thoughts from far away.
> You search out my path and my lying down,
>> and are acquainted with all my ways.
> Even before a word is on my tongue,
>> O LORD, you know it completely.
> You hem me in, behind and before,
>> and lay your hand upon me. (Ps. 139:1–5)

Because the entire creation is known and loved by God, bearing beloved existence beyond bare existence, it is not meaningless, never to be engaged as purposeless mechanism. In the world of Scripture, God inhabits and pervades all of it:

> You have made the moon to mark the seasons;
>> the sun knows its time for setting;
> You make darkness, and it is night,
>> when all of the animals of the forest come creeping out.
> The young lions roar for their prey,
>> seeking their food from God.
> When the sun rises, they withdraw
>> and lie down in their dens.
> People go out to their work
>> and to their labor until the evening.
> O LORD, how manifold are your works!
>> In wisdom you have made them all;
>> The earth is full of your creatures. (Ps. 104:19–24)

Intimately guided by God, the creation is then oriented back to God: "The heavens are telling the glory of God; / and the firmament proclaims his handiwork" (Ps. 19:1). Aquinas draws on this language in affirming that "the entire universe, with all its parts, is ordained toward God as its end, inasmuch as it imitates, as it were, and shows forth the Divine goodness, to the glory of God" (*STh* Ia q. 65 a. 2 *resp.*). Étienne Gilson, summarizing Aquinas's stance toward the creation, emphasizes that for Aquinas the world is a "sacred universe":

> The Thomistic universe is a world of beings, each one of which gives testimony to God by the very fact that it is. All things therein are not of the same rank. There are glorious beings like the angels, noble ones like men, and more modest beings like beasts, plants and minerals. Of all these beings there is not one which does not bear witness that God is the supreme act-of-being. Like the highest of the angels, the humble blade of grass bears this resemblance to God. The world of St. Thomas is one where it is a marvelous thing to be born. It is a sacred world.

Gilson goes on to say that every fiber of this world is sustained and upheld by "the intimate presence of a God whose supreme actuality preserves it in its own actual existence."[16]

"In His Own Image God Made Humankind": The Grace of Being Human

Humans are a part of God's good creation, but humans are also unique among creatures in that humans are noted in Scripture to be created in the image of God. This is first affirmed of humanity in Genesis 1, as noted above: "Then God said, 'Let us make humanity in our image, according to our likeness'" (Gen. 1:26). It is then reaffirmed in Genesis 5:1 ("When God created humankind, he made them in the likeness of God") and Genesis 9:6 ("Whoever sheds the blood of a human, by a human shall that person's blood be shed; for in his own image God made humankind"). Two New Testament texts directly refer to humans as created in God's image and likeness: James 3:9 ("With [the tongue] we bless the Lord and Father, and with it we curse those who are made in the likeness [*kath' homoiōsin*] of God") and, more ambiguously, 1 Corinthians 11:7 ("For a man ought not to have his head veiled, since he is the image [*eikōn*] and reflection [glory, *doxa*] of God").

The concept of the image of God, or *imago Dei*, has long been associated with human uniqueness and human dignity and in the modern era has often been cited as the ground for treating vulnerable humans with dignity and respect. The Pseudo-Clementine literature of the early church, for example,

---

16. Gilson, *Christian Philosophy of St. Thomas Aquinas*, 101.

states that "you should do good to and pay honor and reverence to man, who is made in the image of God: . . . minister food to the hungry, drink to the thirsty, clothing to the naked, hospitality to the stranger, and necessary things to the prisoner."[17] The affirmation that all humans are made in the image of God was central to the attempts of Dominican friar and priest Bartolomé de Las Casas to protect indigenous peoples in the New World from colonial abuses. Martin Luther King Jr., continuing a tradition of drawing on the *imago Dei* to defend the rights and freedom of Black Americans and of those on the socioeconomic margins, drew on the *imago Dei* frequently to ground human dignity:

> Deeply woven into the fiber of our religious tradition is the conviction that men are made in the image of God and that they are souls of infinite metaphysical value. If we accept this as a profound moral fact, we cannot be content to see men hungry, to see them victimized with ill health, when we have the means to help them. In the final analysis, the rich must not ignore the poor because both rich and poor are tied together.[18]

In that respect, the teaching that humans are made in the image of God remains a powerful endorsement of all humans' identity before God and of the need for all human beings, including those who live with mental illness, to be treated with respect and dignity.

But not always. As John Kilner makes clear, when certain humans are denied the status of bearing the image of God, then the concept of the image of God can paradoxically contribute to mistreatment, oppression, and dehumanization. Christian interpreters of Scripture have often associated the image of God with human attributes or capacities that humans are thought to share with God. Kilner succinctly identifies these attributes and capacities—all of which he takes to be misunderstandings—as *reason, righteousness, rulership*, and *relationship*.[19] Many Christian theologians, including Augustine and Aquinas, have located the *imago Dei* in that which distinguishes humans from other animals and have often centered the *imago* on intellect and reason: humans image God in our endowment with "a certain form of the illuminated

17. Pseudo-Clementine, *Recognitions* 5.23; quoted in John Kilner, *Dignity and Destiny: Humanity in the Image of God* (Grand Rapids: Eerdmans, 2015), 8.

18. Martin Luther King Jr., *Where Do We Go from Here: Chaos or Community?* (Boston: Beacon, 1968), 180; quoted in Richard W. Wills, *Martin Luther King Jr. and the Image of God* (New York: Oxford University Press, 2009), 26–27.

19. Kilner, *Dignity and Destiny*, 177–230.

mind," as Augustine put it.[20] An equally notable tradition, particularly within Reformed Protestantism, adds to the *imago Dei* the expectation of righteousness and holiness: in the words of the Westminster Confession of Faith (1642), "After God had made all other creatures, he created man, male and female, with reasonable and immortal souls, endued with knowledge, righteousness, and true holiness after his own image."[21] More recently, the insight of modern scholars that the Hebrew word for image, *tselem*, often referred to a statue of a king placed in a public space to reflect that king's dominion,[22] has led to an interpretation that the image of God is centrally linked to the exercise of dominion over the creation, and especially over other animals.[23] Still other interpreters have argued that humans are most like the triune God in our relationships with God and with each other.[24]

Kilner argues persuasively that interpreting the image of God as reason, righteousness, rulership, or relationship—at least if these concepts are understood as capacities that must be displayed for the image to be actualized—is not supported by a close reading of the few biblical texts that explicitly reference the image of God. These common capacity-based interpretations can also be damaging for people who live with mental illness. To be clear, reason, moral agency, leadership and authority, and relationship are important for human life and human community. But when these goods are identified as what it means to be made in the image of God, it is tempting to assume that those who do not display these goods or capacities, either permanently or temporarily, may somehow bear God's image either not at all or to a lesser degree. If the image of God is associated with human dignity, it follows that people may be subjugated and mistreated who do not display these attributes or who in the light of histories of marginalization and exploitation are not *thought* to display these attributes. Indeed, mistreatment and oppression of women, colonized populations, people with disabilities (including in the thought of Adolf Hit-

20. Augustine, *Unfinished Literal Commentary on Genesis* 57-62; *Literal Commentary on Genesis* 3.29-31; 6.20-22; Aquinas, *STh* Ia q. 93 a. 2. Quotation is from Augustine, *Literal Commentary on Genesis* 3.30, from Augustine, *On Genesis*, trans. Edmund Hill, OP (Hyde Park, NY: New City Press, 2002), 234.

21. Westminster Confession of Faith 4.2.

22. Allen Verhey, *Reading the Bible in the Strange World of Medicine* (Grand Rapids: Eerdmans, 2003), 86.

23. See David Gushee, *The Sacredness of Human Life: Why an Ancient Biblical Vision Is Key to the World's Future* (Grand Rapids: Eerdmans, 2013), 46-47, who criticizes this view.

24. Stanley J. Grenz, *Theology for the Community of God* (Grand Rapids: Eerdmans, 2000), 178-80.

ler), and of Black Americans during and after the time of enslavement have often been correlated with claims that in some way these people fail to display capacities that are associated with God's image.[25]

Capacity-based accounts of human dignity always fail individual human persons who do not display the capacities that are most valued. People who live with mental illness or disability often bear the brunt of this failure. Humans have various degrees of capacity to exercise the use of reason, but if rationality is understood as a marker of those individuals who bear God's image, then persons with intellectual disability, dementia, or chronic psychosis will be at risk of being devalued and perhaps dehumanized. Humans have various degrees of capacity for emotional warmth and attunement, but if this is understood as a marker of those individuals who bear God's image, persons with autism or severe depression may be judged deficient.[26] Attributing human dignity to capacities always places humans who do not display these capacities at risk of exclusion and dehumanization.

The good news, as Kilner argues, is that these capacity-based accounts of the *imago Dei* are not supported by a close reading of the biblical texts. Of the three texts that explicitly reference the image or likeness of God, or both, in Genesis, none explicitly link the image to any capacity, including language or rationality, and Genesis 9:6 clearly ascribes the image to humans after the fall into sin described in Genesis 3. Furthermore, James 3:9 identifies those whom we *curse*—surely those whom we perceive to have fallen deeply short of perfection—as bearing the likeness of God.[27] So there is no biblical requirement to ground the status of being made in the image of God—or to ground human worth, human value, or human personhood—in any capacities that an individual human might bear. We are not said to be made in God's image because we can think, because we can use language, because we can relate warmly to others, because we can adhere

25. Kilner, *Dignity and Destiny*, 17–37. Kilner observes that in his manifesto *Mein Kampf*, Hitler referred to stronger members of society as "images of the Lord" and weaker members as "deformities" of the image to be "cleansed" from society (20).

26. D. Dixon Kinser, "Reimagining Relationship: What Autism Reveals about What It Means to Relate to God," DMin thesis, Duke University, 2021.

27. Kilner, *Dignity and Destiny*, 128. Note that in this section I do not distinguish between "image" and "likeness," despite the precedent of Irenaeus and many who have followed after him, including Aquinas. I follow Kilner's argument that "image" [*tselem*] and "likeness" [*demuth*] are mostly used interchangeably in the Hebrew Bible and that their appearance together, for example, in Genesis 1:26, is an example of Hebrew parallel construction rather than of theological or philosophical distinction. As described below, Kilner argues that the participation in divine life that Irenaeus and his successors denoted by likeness is better represented in Scripture through the concept of glory (*doxa*); Kilner, *Dignity and Destiny*, 62.

to social norms and expectations, because we are righteous, or because we can exercise authority. We are made in God's image, rather, because God has created us so, in love. We are God's creatures, known and loved by God. No matter how much we struggle with psychological pain and behaviors that are damaging to ourselves and to others, we continue to be made in God's image. That we are made in the *imago Dei* is given in creation and not dependent on capacities.

But there is more to the truth that we are made in God's image. When the texts of the Old Testament and the New Testament refer to the image of God, they almost never—with the possible exception of 1 Corinthians 11:7—refer to humans as a whole as the image of God. They speak of humans being created and formed *in* or *according to* God's—and often, more specifically, Christ's—image or likeness (Rom. 8:29; 1 Cor. 15:49; 2 Cor. 3:18; Eph. 4:24; Col. 3:10; James 3:9). But the New Testament writers consistently refer to Jesus *as* the image of God. Jesus is "the image [*eikōn*] of the invisible God" (Col. 1:15); the "image [*eikōn*] of God" (2 Cor. 4:4); the "reflection of God's glory and the exact imprint [*charaktēr*] of God's very being" (Heb. 1:3). "Whoever has seen me," Jesus told Philip, "has seen the Father" (John 14:9). All humans are created *in* the image of God, but Jesus *is* the image of God.[28]

Linking the *imago Dei* firmly to the person of Jesus helps us to avoid capacity-based interpretations of God's image and also opens exciting new horizons for understanding who humans are and who we are called to be. Before Jesus descended to us "in the likeness of sinful flesh" (Rom. 8:3), we were created in the likeness of the sinless life of the Son, the second person of the Trinity who is for us the perfect image of the triune God.[29]

This leads to two affirmations about the image. First, if each human is made in the image of God, and if the perfect image of God is Christ, then every human continues to hold what Kilner calls a "special connection" with Christ and therefore with the triune God, in a way that is unrelated to capacity and not diminished or effaced by sin.[30] There is no human state of affairs—including no form of mental illness and no substance use problem—that can take

---

28. See *STh* Ia q. 35 a. 2.

29. Because Jesus is the perfect image of the triune God, it would be inaccurate to say that humans are made in the image of Christ only and not of the triune God as a whole. Aquinas specifically considers this possibility and rejects it for two reasons: first, if the Son perfectly images the Father, then "it would follow of necessity if man were made in the likeness of the Son that he is made to the likeness of the Father"; and second, that in Genesis, God (Aquinas assumes the Father) states, "Let us make man to our own image and likeness," which implies that humans are made in the image of the whole Trinity (*STh* Ia q. 93 a. 5 *ad4*).

30. Kilner, *Dignity and Destiny*, xi.

CHAPTER 5

that away. Just as psychiatrist Harry Stack Sullivan memorably commented that "we are all much more simply human than otherwise, be we happy and successful, contented and detached, miserable and mentally disordered, or whatever," the Christian can joyfully affirm that "we are all made in the image of God, be we happy and successful, contented and detached, miserable and mentally disordered, or whatever."[31]

The affirmation that humans made in the image of God maintain a special connection with Christ regardless of capacity or circumstance helps us to see how the doctrine of the *imago Dei* helps us to read other texts of the New Testament. When Jesus tells his disciples that "just as you [came to the assistance of] one of the least of these who are members of my family, you did it to me" (Matt. 25:40), he is affirming not only that the hungry and thirsty, the stranger, the naked, the sick, and the incarcerated continue to bear a special connection with him but that to come to their aid is to come to the aid of Jesus himself.[32]

Slightly earlier in Matthew's Gospel, the affirmation of this special connection helps to make sense of Jesus's response to some Pharisees who "went and plotted to entrap him in what he said":

So they sent their disciples to him, along with the Herodians, saying, "Teacher, we know that you are sincere, and teach the way of God in accordance with truth, and show deference to no one; for you do not regard people with partiality. Tell us, then, what you think. Is it lawful to pay taxes to the emperor, or not?"

But Jesus, aware of their malice, said, "Why are you putting me to the test, you hypocrites? Show me the coin used for the tax." And they brought him a denarius. Then he said to them, "Whose head is this, and whose title?"

They answered, "The emperor's."

Then he said to them, "Give therefore to the emperor the things that are the emperor's, and to God the things that are God's." When they heard this, they were amazed; and they left him and went away. (Matt. 22:15–22)

31. Harry Stack Sullivan, *Conceptions of Modern Psychiatry* (Washington, DC: The William Alanson White Psychiatric Foundation, 1948), 7.
32. While there is some debate among New Testament scholars about whether the members of Jesus's family (literally, "brothers") mentioned in this text are specifically Jesus's disciples or all humans, it is important to note that this text has been important for Christian care of the sick, including the non-Christian sick, across Christian history. See Gary Ferngren, *Medicine and Health Care in Early Christianity* (Baltimore: Johns Hopkins University Press, 2009), 97–104.

Jesus and his questioners both knew that to encourage tax avoidance was to invite the wrath of the Romans, while to support Roman taxation was a tangible sign of submitting to the emperor's claim to be Lord. Jesus responds by asking whose image (*eikōn*) is on the coins that will be paid in taxes. Since the coins bear the emperor's image, the emperor can claim them for his own, and so it is appropriate to pay taxes. But Jesus's hearers would have understood the larger question that did not have to be spoken: whose image is inscribed on you? If humans are made in the image of God, then God and not Caesar is properly Lord, and so it is important to "give . . . to God the things that are God's" (Matt. 22:21).

Humans, then, bear a special connection to God by virtue of having been created in God's image and cannot lose that status. There is no human being who does not continue to bear God's image. But the affirmation that humans are made in God's image also entails a call to grow into that image more and more, to "clothe [ourselves] with the new self, created according to the likeness of God in true righteousness and holiness" (Eph. 4:24). Kilner argues that this call to be conformed to the image of God in which we are made—that is, to participate in the life of Christ—does not mean that the image of God itself increases or decreases in us in relation to our devotion or holiness. The perfect image of God is Christ and cannot be corrupted or destroyed. But Scripture does allow that by conforming to the image of God in Christ, we grow in "glory" (*doxa*): "And all of us, with unveiled faces, seeing the glory [*doxa*] of the Lord as though reflected in a mirror, are being transformed into the same image [*eikōn*] from one degree of glory [*doxa*] to another; for this comes from the Lord, the Spirit" (2 Cor. 3:18). As we draw closer to Christ and therefore participate more fully in the life of the triune God, the image does not increase in us, but the glory of Christ's life does.[33]

The biblical concept of the image of God, then, can be interpreted both as declaration and as call. The biblical texts declare that humanity is made in the image of God, and they utilize this concept in ways that do not link the image to capacities but that do link the image to the expectation that humans will be treated with dignity (e.g., Gen. 9:6; James 3:9). God has created all humans according to God's image and in doing so has conferred upon all humans—without regard to capacities or abilities—a dignity and value that cannot be taken away. But having been created in the image of God, humans are called to live into that image—to become more like the image according to which we were created. If that were identical to a call to become more rational, more

---

33. Kilner, *Dignity and Destiny*, 62-69.

relational, more righteous, or more regal, it would disempower those who live with mental illness and also project as godlike those human qualities that are most desired and admired in modern culture. But that is not the biblical teaching. Rather, because Christ is the image of God, if we wish to grow more deeply into God's image, we will look to the person and life of Jesus.[34]

"Your Life Is Hidden with Christ in God": The Grace of Being Held in Jesus's Life

In a chapter on our identity as humans, it may seem strange and even inappropriate to speak of Jesus as a core foundation of human identity. First, most contemporary humans—those who do not claim Christian faith—do not recognize any special status for Jesus among humans, except perhaps as a great religious teacher or prophet. Even among Christians, Jesus is often celebrated more for what he has done for humans (paying the debt of sin, bridging the way to God) or for the moral example of his life and his teaching than for the way that Jesus forms and defines who humans are. But the good news of Christian faith is that Jesus is not just an exemplary leader whom we are called to imitate. For those who will accept the invitation, Jesus is the life in which we are called to participate. The writer of Colossians puts it this way:

> For in [Christ] the whole fullness of deity dwells bodily, and you have come to fullness in him, who is the head of every ruler and authority. In him also you were circumcised with a spiritual circumcision, by putting off the body

34. Thomas Aquinas offers a detailed interpretation of the *imago Dei* in *STh* Ia q. 93, describing the *imago* as the "end" (*finis*) or "term" (*terminus*) of the production of humans. Following Augustine, Aquinas holds that the *imago* is found most properly in the knowing and loving acts of the mind. Because of this, some disability-conscious critics, including Kilner, cite Aquinas as an example of locating the *imago Dei* in rationality in a way that contributes to the marginalization of persons with intellectual disability or certain forms of mental illness; e.g., Kilner, *Dignity and Destiny*, 19. This is an oversimplification and misreading of Aquinas's nuanced account. Aquinas not only affirms that all humans are made in the image of God, but also makes clear that persons with what would now be called intellectual disability or serious mental illness are endowed with the rational faculty of the soul and are to be treated with respect and dignity. I provide more detail about Aquinas's account of the *imago Dei*, and how his account can be defended against disability critiques, in the appendix to this book. Nonetheless, because Aquinas's account can so easily be (mis)interpreted to reinforce intellectualist hierarchies of value, I have chosen to place it in the background, rather than the foreground, of this section.

of flesh in the circumcision of Christ; when you were buried with him in baptism, you were also raised with him through faith in the power of God, who raised him from the dead. And when you were dead in trespasses and the uncircumcision of your flesh, God made you alive together with him. (Col. 2:9-13)

You have come to fullness in him; in him you were circumcised; you were buried with him; you were also raised with him. The letter to the Colossians makes clear that Jesus, the "image of God, the firstborn of all creation" (Col. 1:15), is also the one in whom we find our identity. We are to "live [our] lives in him" (Col. 2:6). Shortly later, the writer sums this up with exacting succinctness: "for you have died, and your life is hidden with Christ in God" (Col. 3:3).

As God's good creatures, all humans are visible manifestations of God's love, known and loved as those who are created in God's image and likeness. God further invites us, by grace, to live into that love by living into Jesus himself, and to be held in the life of the Son.[35]

Jesus, the Image to Which We Are Called to Conform

Throughout the New Testament, Jesus is held up as the one life that his disciples and followers are summoned to emulate (e.g., 1 Cor. 11:1; Eph. 5:1; Phil. 2:5-11; 1 Thess. 1:6; Heb. 12:1-2; 1 Pet. 3:20-21). Thomas Aquinas described Jesus as the bearer of all the virtues, the model that humans are to follow (*In I Sent.* d. 14 q. 2 a. 2),[36] and the paradigm life in which the habits of intellectual excellence, moral excellence, and excellence in relation to the life of God are most fully displayed (*STh* IIIa q. 7 a. 2 *resp.*). Insofar as mental health, in our time, names the goods of a well-lived life that embodies intellectual and moral virtue, it is fair to say that Jesus serves for Christians as a model for mental health. But just what sort of life is it to which we are called to conform? We must necessarily be selective here but will focus on four dimensions of Jesus's

---

35. Christian life of course requires and entails much more than what can be said here: baptism, the other sacraments, repentance from sin, participation in the church, and so on. Yet all authentic Christian discipleship, including these things, draws us into deeper participation in Christ's life.

36. Cf. Jean-Pierre Torrell, *Saint Thomas Aquinas*, vol. 2, *Spiritual Master*, trans. Robert Royal (Washington, DC: Catholic University of America Press, 2003), 60; Frederick Christian Bauerschmidt, *Thomas Aquinas: Faith, Reason, and Following Christ* (New York: Oxford University Press, 2013), 179-227.

life that are particularly relevant for those who live with mental illness: the beloved Jesus, the sent Jesus, the wounded and crucified Jesus, and the resurrected and ascended Jesus.

The beloved Jesus. Before all else, the Father loves the Son. Reporting on Jesus's baptism in the Jordan by John, all three of the synoptic gospel narratives report that the Holy Spirit descended on Jesus like a dove and that "a voice came from heaven, 'You are my Son, the Beloved; with you I am well pleased'" (Mark 1:11). Later, not in a river valley but on the top of a high mountain, a voice "from the cloud" proclaimed to Jesus's disciples, "This is my Son, the Beloved; listen to him" (Mark 9:7). The life into which we are called is a beloved life.

The sent Jesus. Just before giving the Holy Spirit to his disciples, the Gospel of John reports that the risen Jesus told his disciples, "Peace be with you. As the Father has sent me, so I send you" (John 20:21). One of John's most central themes is that the known and beloved Son is sent for the healing and restoring of God's beloved world (3:16-17). The Son is sent "that the world might be saved through him" (3:17). He "speaks the words of God" and "gives the Spirit without measure" (3:34). He testifies in word and sign to the Father's will (5:36-47; 7:28-29; 10:36-37). He makes the Father's name known to his disciples, "that the love with which you have loved me may be in them, and I in them" (17:26). In the Gospel of John and elsewhere in Scripture, the beloved Son is the sent Son, who then sends his beloved disciples into the world that they may participate in his life.

But into what was the Son sent? For people who live with mental illness, who have been shamed because they do not conform to current social standards of "reason, righteousness, rulership, and relationship," the good news of the gospel is that "we do not have a high priest who is unable to sympathize with our weaknesses, but we have one who in every respect has been tested as we are, yet without sin" (Heb. 4:15). Christian faith holds that Jesus's earthly life was always righteous, lived without sin. But in that sinless life, he nonetheless bore stigma, including the stigma of being labeled as someone who is mentally ill. Early in his ministry, the Gospel of Mark reports that Jesus was preaching and healing near his hometown in Galilee when a great crowd gathered around him. But "when his family heard it, they went out to restrain him, for people were saying, 'He has gone out of his mind'" (Mark 3:21).[37] Though we cannot conclude from the text that Jesus ever met criteria

---

37. The Greek word here, *existēmi*, means literally "to be beside oneself" or "to be removed from a standing or fixed position." In certain New Testament passages, including

for what would today be called a mental disorder, the text does tell us that Jesus knew what it meant to bear the stigma of ascribed madness. Those who had known him the longest, and who loved him the best, attempted to restrain him. Similarly, in the Gospel of John, some of Jesus's hearers speculated that "he has a demon and is out of his mind" (John 10:20).[38]

As the text above from Hebrews alludes, and as the gospel narratives of Jesus's temptation make clear, the sent Jesus was also one who bore temptation. He knew hunger, and he knew what it was like to be tempted to satisfy that hunger with food that would have distracted from his mission. Shown "all the kingdoms of the world and their splendor" (Matt. 4:8), he knew what it was like to be tempted to pursue power for its own sake. Dared to jump from the pinnacle of the temple, the highest point in Jerusalem, he knew what it was like to be tempted to prove that he was loved by the Father rather than simply to rest assured in that unbreakable fact. The writer of Hebrews emphasizes that this was for us, including for those of us who live with mental illness:

> Since, therefore, the children share flesh and blood, he himself likewise shared the same things, so that through death he might destroy the one who has the power of death, that is, the devil, and free those who all their lives were held in slavery by the fear of death. For it is clear that he did not

in the Gospel of Mark, it signifies astonishment but not necessarily a failure of reason or presence of madness (Mark 2:12; 5:42; 6:51; cf. Matt. 12:23; Luke 2:57; 8:56; 24:22; Acts 2:7, 12). But in this context, it signifies concern that Jesus was possessed by Beelzebul (Mark 3:22). Jesus's family may have sought to restrain him because they were concerned that somehow Jesus's own actions were threatening (perhaps by misjudging the danger of the crowd, from whom his disciples had recently removed him so that he wouldn't be crushed), or they may have wanted to protect him from violence by the authorities. Either way, the situation bears marked resemblance to the way that mental health crises are managed today.

38. Reflecting on recent debates in biblical scholarship, Joanna Collicutt points out that in Mark 3, John 20, and other texts, Jesus is regarded as "mad," with debate among his hearers about whether this represents "divine madness," and therefore the root of subversive and apocalyptic wisdom, or "simple madness." She takes this point further by suggesting that even much later in his ministry, at the time of his passion, Jesus may have been regarded by the Jewish and Roman authorities as mad (with either simple or divine madness that threatened the ruling order), which may account for why Jesus was executed but his followers were not. She argues that Jesus's madness is central to understanding the gospel: "To understand the rationality of Jesus's *madness*—what Paul calls God's wise foolishness (1 Cor. 1:25)—one must, as far as is possible, inhabit it. In this we may find that *mad* people, *mad* ways of thinking, and *mad* times in life can be unexpectedly helpful" (49–50). See Joanna Collicutt, "Jesus and Madness," in *The Bible and Mental Health*, ed. Christopher C. H. Cook and Isabelle Hamley (London: SCM, 2020), 34–53.

come to help angels, but the descendants of Abraham. Therefore he had to become like his brothers and sisters in every respect, so that he might be a merciful and faithful high priest in the service of God, to make a sacrifice of atonement for the sins of the people. Because he himself was tested by what he suffered, he is able to help those who are being tested. (Heb. 2:14–18)

Jesus did not bear stigma and temptation for its own sake. He did so because it was only by "becoming like his brothers and sisters in every respect" that he is able to reach us in our deepest places of wound, isolation, shame, and suffering. The sent Jesus is not only the bearer of stigma and temptation but also the bearer of healing and reconciliation.

Ann describes how healing it has been for her to understand Jesus's keen and compassionate way of engaging those who suffer. Reflecting on Jesus's healing of the woman who had been unable to stand straight for eighteen years (Luke 13:10–17), Ann says,

Jesus called her forward and said to her, "Woman, you are set free from your infirmity." He put his hands on her and immediately she straightened up. I keyed in on the eighteen years. I keyed in that she was crippled by a spirit, bent over and couldn't straighten up, so she couldn't see ahead.

[As someone who lives with depression] I go, "Oh, I know what that feels like." Someone who's never experienced any kind of crippling spirit, trauma, be it some sort of disaster or some sort of debilitating illness or something that puts you in that position, then you can't appreciate how Jesus can *see*. That's what he saw. He could see people trapped in prison, in their own selves and the need to be freed. To me, I just feel like over the years, Jesus, the spirit, the counselor, my brother, he comes to me and he says, "Come here." It's that acceptance of you, "Yeah. You've been crippled for eighteen years. Let's do something about that. Let's work together on this. Come here."

That's the way it always feels like to me when encountering Christ, Jesus, the man, the healer, the one who can see straight through you and read all your bullshit.[39]

The wounded and crucified Jesus. The stigma that Jesus bore during his ministry, including from his family in Galilee, was never greater than in the ritual humiliation that he endured at the hands of the Romans, sanctioned by

39. Personal interview, June 3, 2022.

the religious leaders and authorities in Jerusalem at the time. Every feature of Jesus's treatment from the time of the trial before Pilate was calculated to inflict not only physical pain and discomfort but also psychological torment and humiliation. He was clothed in grotesque imitations of royal garb and summarily mocked for having claimed that he was a king. He was stripped naked and hung to die on a piece of wood, in full public display. He was taunted by his executioners, by others in the crowd, and even by those who were being crucified with him.

Jesus's resurrection on the third day marked God's triumph over death and over all the powers that oppose the reign of God and that led to his crucifixion. But the resurrected Jesus remained the wounded and crucified Jesus. As Shelly Rambo makes clear in a haunting reading of John 20, the resurrected Jesus appeared to the disciples in the upper room in a simultaneously spectral and fleshly manner—and then promptly shows them his wounds. In this text, it is Jesus's wounds, not his appearance per se, that most clearly demonstrate that he has returned in fleshly form, and they can only be apprehended by fleshly contact. When Thomas, learning later of Jesus's appearance, comments to others that he will believe only by touching Jesus's wounds, the ghostly Jesus again walks through a locked door and commands Thomas not just to touch his wounds but to plunge his hand into his ribs. "The nearer you get to the wounds, things will begin to stir within," Rambo says, and to know Jesus after the resurrection requires the hard path of "wound-work": not just knowing about Jesus's wounds, not just theorizing them, but *touching* them in a way that demands that we are aware of our own places of wound.[40] The life into which we are called is a wounded and crucified life.[41]

The resurrected and ascended Jesus. The life into which we are called is a life that knows stigma and temptation, that knows humiliation and wounds, that knows death itself. That is good news for those of us in our time who bear scars of shame, wound, stigma, and temptation. Jesus knows those things also. But that is of course not the end of the Christian story. God raised Jesus from the dead, and in doing so "disarmed the rulers and authorities and made a public ex-

40. Shelly Rambo, *Resurrecting Wounds: Living in the Afterlife of Trauma* (Waco, TX: Baylor University Press, 2017), 87, 92.

41. Aquinas states in his lectures on the Gospel of John that it was the site of his encounter with Jesus's wounds, when he became only the second disciple after Peter to speak of Jesus as God, that "Thomas quickly became a good theologian by professing a true faith"; *Lectura super Ioannem*, chap. 20, lect. 6; translation from Thomas Aquinas, *Commentary on the Gospel of John, Chapters 9–21*, trans. Fr. Fabian R. Larcher, OP (Lander, WY: The Aquinas Institute for the Study of Sacred Doctrine, 2013).

ample of them" (Col. 2:15). And then this resurrected Jesus ascended to the right hand of the Father (Rom. 8:34; Eph. 1:20; Acts 7:55–56; Col. 3:1; Heb. 12:2).

As Shelly Rambo's work makes clear, Jesus's resurrection and ascension do not erase the marks of his wounding and crucifixion. The resurrected and ascended Jesus is still the wounded and crucified Jesus. Resurrection is not a denial of wounds. But it is an affirmation that wounds, and the death that they signify, do not have the last word.

Jesus, the Life in Which We Are Held

What, then, is our relationship to the life of the beloved, sent, wounded, crucified, resurrected, ascended Jesus? It is that we are held within it. We are known and loved by God, not simply as God's good creatures, created in God's image; we are known and loved by God *in* the life of God's Son.

Paul speaks of this relationship in his letters to the Galatians and to the Romans:

> But when the fullness of time had come, God sent his Son, born of a woman, born under the law, in order to redeem those who were under the law, so that we might receive adoption as children. And because you are children, God has sent the Spirit of his Son into our hearts, crying, "Abba! Father!" So you are no longer a slave but a child, and if a child, then also an heir, through God. (Gal. 4:4–7)

> For all who are led by the Spirit of God are children of God. For you did not receive a spirit of slavery to fall back into fear, but you have received a spirit of adoption. When we cry, "Abba! Father!" it is that very Spirit bearing witness with our spirit that we are children of God, and if children, then heirs, heirs of God and joint heirs with Christ—if, in fact, we suffer with him so that we may also be glorified with him. (Rom. 8:14–17)

In each of these texts, Paul is speaking of what sets Christians free from bondage: in Galatians, from bondage to the "elemental spirits of the world," including the law (Gal. 3:23–4:3); in Romans, from bondage to "the law of sin and of death" (Rom. 8:1). There is a similar Trinitarian architecture in each of these texts. God the Father sends the Spirit into our hearts, the centers of our animating desire. This Holy Spirit, referred to in Romans as the *pneuma tou theou* (Spirit of God [Rom. 8:14]) and in Galatians as the *pneuma tou huiou*

(Spirit of the Son [Gal. 4:6]), is God's breath, now breathed from within us. And from *within* our hearts, God's breath says, "Abba! Father!" a familial and perhaps even intimate term that can only be properly uttered by the beloved Son. The logic here is that the Spirit, sent by the Father, enables us to speak to the Father as the beloved Son speaks to his Father. We do so not just *alongside* the Son but *in* the Son, as the Spirit of the Son is in us. We are not simply absorbed into Christ, losing our individuality—Romans makes clear that our spirit remains distinct from God's Spirit, and that we are "joint heirs" with Christ—but it is nonetheless *in* Christ that we now find our adoptive identity. We are held tightly in the dance of love that is the Trinity, addressing the Father through the Spirit in the Son and loved *as* the Son in the Spirit by the Father. The Spirit holds us gently but decisively in Christ's life, bringing us into the very life of God. And in this is the promise of resurrection: Aquinas affirms that "our Savior the Lord Jesus Christ, in order to save his people from their sins, . . . showed unto us in his own person the way of truth, whereby we may attain to the [beatitude] of eternal life by rising again" (*STh* IIIa *proem.*).[42]

It is from this place—held by the Spirit in the life of the Son—that we can best appreciate faith, hope, and love, the dispositions that Aquinas called the theological virtues. As we will explore in chapter 8, Thomas taught that all of these begin in God. None are attainable through human effort alone. Faith for Aquinas (though Paul interpreted the concept more broadly) is the God-given capacity of the intellect to apprehend truths of God—truths like the nature of God as Trinity—that cannot be attained through reason alone (*STh* IIaIIae q. 4 a. 1 *resp.*). Hope is the God-given capacity of the will to cast ourselves onto the promise of a future that only God can make possible, even when this future seems far distant (*STh* IIaIIae q. 17 a. 1 *resp.*, a. 5 *resp.*). Love or charity is God's love, given to us, by which we might love God and the things of God in return: we love because he first loved us (1 John 4:19) (*STh* IIaIIae q. 24 a. 2). Held in Jesus's life, faith, hope, and love become possibilities that are attainable, though not by our own effort. We are able to display them only because God has adopted us as God's children.

---

42. Torrell translates a portion of Aquinas's commentary on Ephesians that captures the heart of this truth: "when we are loved by God, it is not because of ourselves; we are loved because of Him who is beloved of the Father. . . . Now the Son is by nature similar to the Father, and that is why he is loved by him in the first place. He is by nature and in the most excellent manner the Beloved of the Father. As to us, we are sons by adoption in the degree to which we are in conformity with the Son [by nature]; that is why we have a certain participation in God's love"; *In ad Eph.* I, 6, lect. 2, n. 16, in Torrell, *Saint Thomas Aquinas*, 2:79.

Engaging Mental Health Care as Those Who Are Known and Loved by God

Our deepest identity as humans is that we are known and loved by God. We are known and loved by God as God's good creatures. We are known and loved by God as those created in God's image, which is to say, in the Son. For those who accept the invitation to be adopted into Jesus's beloved, sent, wounded, crucified, resurrected, ascended life, we are held in the life of the Son, known and loved by God as the Father loves the Son, "hidden with Christ in God."

What are the implications of this for living with mental illness and for engaging mental health care? The fact that we are known and loved by God—even if we believe it to be true—is not a panacea, not a quick cure, not a get-out-of-depression-free or get-out-of-addiction-free card. Mental health problems are always much more complicated than that, involving bodily states of affairs, larger networks of relationships, ongoing trials and challenges, and deeply ingrained habits of feeling, thinking, and behaving, of only some of which are we consciously aware. It would be naive to assume that the statement "God loves you" would instantly cure someone of any complex pattern of mental illness.

But it is a place to start. Like warm ocean waves that slowly but inexorably reshape an entire coastline, the awareness that the deepest truth about our lives is that we are known and loved by God can slowly erode and reshape the bulwark foundations of shame that contribute to or perpetuate many forms of anxiety, depression, addiction, and other common manifestations of mental illness. When shame says, "you are not enough," the good news of Jesus says, "you are loved and known by God." When shame says, "if others knew the full truth about you, you would be ostracized," the good news of Jesus says, "you are loved and known by God." When shame says, "you need to hide," or "you need to fight back," or "you need to disappear," the good news of Jesus says, "you are loved and known by God." "There is no fear in love," writes John, "but perfect love casts out fear; for fear has to do with punishment; whoever fears has not reached perfection in love. We love because he first loved us" (1 John 4:18-19). To those of us who in shame take on what we believe to be the work of God, punishing ourselves because we believe wholeheartedly that God would punish us, the good news of Jesus says, "you are loved and known by God." And no matter who we are, the good news of Jesus says, "you are not alone. No matter who you are or what you have done, God knows you and loves you and wants to hold you in the wounded, resurrected, ascended life of Jesus."

From Mental Health to Participation in Blessing

We Are Summoned on a Journey to God

> Where can I go from your spirit?
>> Or where can I flee from your presence?
> If I ascend to heaven, you are there;
>> if I make my bed in Sheol, you are there.
> If I take the wings of the morning
>> and settle at the farthest limits of the sea,
> even there your hand shall lead me,
>> and your right hand shall hold me fast.
>
> *—Psalm 139:7–11*

In the previous chapters, we have considered some important dimensions regarding who humans are, as this relates to engaging mental health care. Before all else, humans are loved and known by God, good creatures of God who are created in God's image and invited by grace to participate in the life of Jesus. We are also creatures of earth who love, grow, and become who we are in relationship. We are biosocial and ecological creatures, and all of our experience and behavior—including experience and behavior that comes to be labeled mental illness—takes place at the interface of our bodies, other bodies, our environment, and the cultures in which we participate.

We are also always on a journey. We do not stay still. Our lives are always *about* something. We find ourselves drawn to certain people and places. We pursue certain tasks and goals. We find ourselves to be on the move.

Thomas Aquinas captured this inevitable aboutness of life when he characterized humans in this life as wayfarers who are on a journey. Living in a culture where pilgrimage to holy sites was an important manifestation of piety, Aquinas cast all of human life in this world as a kind of pilgrimage from

God, as source and Creator, to God, as fulfillment and goal. In the end, when humans stand in the presence of God in eternity, humans are *comprehensores*, those who have attained the journey's end, where there is nothing left to desire. But for now, until then, we are *viatores*, wayfarers.

This image of the human as wayfarer is centrally useful for practical discernment about engaging mental health care. It is a frame within which to consider human life as a whole and to ask specific questions about mental health and mental illness. Specifically, if we are on a journey, where are we going? What gets in the way? What natural and grace-given endowments do we have as aids and helps for the journey? What does it look like to journey well? And, centrally, what is needed for the journey?

The end or goal of mental health care is often understood as mental health. But what is mental health? In this chapter, I outline several prominent ways that mental health is understood in the clinical mental health disciplines, drawing on perspectives in modern research psychology, psychoanalysis, and mindfulness-oriented approaches. I then explore Thomas Aquinas's approach to this question, which frames all of human life as an ongoing quest for *beatitudo*—happiness, fulfillment, flourishing, or what I prefer to render as "participation in blessing." Because we are wayfarers and not machines, because the meaning of our lives is not something that we freely self-create or that is arbitrarily assigned to us but rather that is an inherent aspect of our creatureliness, we *just are* the kind of creatures who seek *beatitudo*. We cannot help but do so, in all of our action. And because *beatitudo* is found and secured ultimately in God, then God—love of God, union with God, grace-enabled participation in God's life—is the goal of our journey. We are pilgrims seeking *beatitudo*, wayfarers on a journey to God.

What Is Mental Health?

One of the curious things about modern mental health care is that clinicians and researchers spend much more time talking and thinking about specific mental disorders, and how to treat them, than talking and thinking about the nature of mental health. I was halfway through my third year of residency training in psychiatry, and in my seventh year of clinical training overall, before anyone asked me in a formal teaching context to consider the questions, What is health? and What is mental health? Mental health care enacts a curious conspiracy of silence regarding mental health, the concept that supposedly stands at the center of our work. It is not that individual clinicians do not have operating concepts of mental health that inform and guide our work. It is rather that if we articulate these working concepts too broadly, we open ourselves to disagreement when the moral commitments that are implicit within them become explicit. It is easier to remain silent about health, and vocal about disorders and their treatment.

That said, different psychological researchers and theorists have attempted to describe and to define "mental health" over the last half century, with illuminating results. First, building on mid-twentieth-century thinkers such as Erik Erikson, Carl Rogers, and Abraham Maslow, and on the survey work of Marie Jahoda, researchers have attempted to define mental health using empirical paradigms.[1] Ed Diener and colleagues have framed mental health as subjective well-being, which includes the presence of positive emotion and affect, the relative absence of negative emotion and affect, self-reported overall life satisfaction, and satisfaction with particular domains of life.[2] Carol Ryff and Corey Keyes argue that flourishing includes positive relationships, living with purpose and meaning, and connecting positively to society.[3] Martin Seligman has proposed a fivefold characterization of human flourishing as positive emotion, engagement, positive relationships, meaning, and accomplishment. Tyler VanderWeele has proposed mental and physical health as domains of flourishing along with happiness and life satisfaction, meaning and purpose, character and virtue, close social relationships, and financial and material stability.[4]

---

1. Marie Jahoda, *Current Concepts of Positive Mental Health: A Report to the Staff Director, Jack R. Ewalt*, Joint Commission on Mental Illness and Health Monograph Series 1 (New York: Basic Books, 1958), 1.

2. Ed Diener, "Subjective Well-Being." *Psychological Bulletin* 95 (1984): 542–75; Warner Wilson, "Correlates of Avowed Happiness," *Psychological Bulletin* 67 (1967): 294–306; Norman M. Bradburn, *The Structure of Psychological Well-Being* (Chicago: Aldine, 1969); Ed Diener, "Subjective Well-Being: The Science of Happiness and a Proposal for a National Index," *American Psychologist* 55 (2000): 34–43.

3. Carol D. Ryff, "Happiness Is Everything, or Is It? Explorations on the Meaning of Psychological Well-Being," *Journal of Personality and Social Psychology* 57 (1989): 1069–81; Carol D. Ryff and Burton H. Singer, "Know Thyself and Become What You Are: A Eudaimonic Approach to Psychological Well-Being," *Journal of Happiness Studies* 9 (2008): 13–39; Carol D. Ryff and Corey Lee M. Keyes, "The Structure of Psychological Well-Being Revisited," *Journal of Personality and Social Psychology* 69 (1995): 719–27; see also Richard M. Ryan and Edward L. Deci, "On Happiness and Human Potentials: A Review of Research on Hedonic and Eudaimonic Well-Being," *Annual Review of Psychology* 52 (2001): 141–66.

4. Martin E. P. Seligman, *Flourish: A Visionary New Understanding of Happiness and Well-Being* (New York: Free Press, 2011), 16–29; Tyler J. VanderWeele, "On the Promotion of Human Flourishing," *Proceedings of the National Academy of Sciences* 114 (2017): 8148–56.

Second, mental health is framed in overlapping but distinct ways by modern psychodynamic clinicians like Nancy McWilliams and the other authors of the *Psychodynamic Diagnostic Manual* (PDM), a guide to clinical formulation and diagnosis that reflects a psychodynamic (broadly Freudian and post-Freudian) approach to psychotherapy.[5] Focused primarily on the context of individuals in psychotherapy, the *PDM* draws together a number of psychodynamic resources to describe the shape of a "healthy personality." Such a personality, in the *PDM*'s language, is able

- to view self and others in complex, stable, and accurate ways (identity);
- to maintain intimate, stable, and satisfying relationships (object relations);
- to experience in self and perceive in others the full range of age-expected affects (affect tolerance);
- to regulate impulses and affects in ways that foster adaptation and satisfaction, with flexibility in using defenses or coping strategies (affect regulation);
- to function according to a consistent and mature moral sensibility (superego integration, ideal self-concept, ego ideal);
- to appreciate, if not necessarily to conform to, conventional notions of what is realistic (reality testing);
- to respond to stress resourcefully and to recover from painful events without undue difficulty (ego strength and resilience).[6]

Mental health is described in a third way by clinicians and researchers who draw on eastern meditative and contemplative traditions for conceptual and practical resources. Drawing on the work of clinicians such as Jon Kabat-Zinn,[7] on attachment theory, and on neurobiology, psychiatrist Daniel Siegel writes of human well-being as characterized by flexible, context-dependent integration that avoids the lethal poles of excessive psychological rigidity and psychological chaos. Healthy integration for Siegel is *flexible, adaptive, coherent, energized, and stable* (FACES) and is characterized by eight principal domains: the integration of *consciousness* (in a mindful way that aids regulation of emotion and clear decision-making), *horizontal* integration (between the

5. PDM Task Force, *Psychodynamic Diagnostic Manual* (Silver Spring, MD: Alliance of Psychoanalytic Organizations, 2006).

6. PDM Task Force, *Psychodynamic Diagnostic Manual*, 20–23.

7. Jon Kabat-Zinn, *Full Catastrophe Living: Using the Wisdom of Your Body and Mind to Face Stress, Pain, and Illness*, 15th anniv. ed. (New York: Delta, 2005).

holistic, context-focused right brain and the logical, linear, task-focused left brain), *vertical* integration (of the brain with the body), *memory* integration (of past, present, and future), *narrative* integration (of one's life as a coherent story), *state* integration (in a way that does not push away or deny basic human needs for closeness, relationship, mastery, and so on), *interpersonal* integration (that allows for flexible, realistic relationships with others), and *temporal* integration (that accepts human finitude and mortality, and prepares us for eventual death).[8]

Seven themes emerge from these diverse methodological and theoretical approaches to mental health.

· Personal and bodily **security**
· **Positive regard** for oneself and one's life
· The capacity for a **full range of emotion**
· The capacity for **finding meaning**
· Purposeful and engaging **activity**
· The capacity for intimate and fulfilling **interpersonal relationships**
· The ability to **respond flexibly and creatively** to challenges

First, for modern researchers and clinicians, mental health requires *personal and bodily security*. Though deprivation, neglect, and trauma can provide important contexts for personal growth, these are not generally conducive to well-being itself. Second, mental health involves *positive regard for oneself and one's life*. This doesn't mean that we are happy with ourselves all of the time, or don't seek to change, but it means that the mentally healthy person will have a basic sense of self-worth that makes this self-discontent constructive and bearable. Third, mental health involves *the capacity for a full range of emotion*—not just the capacity for happiness but also the capacity for negative emotions like anger and sadness when these are appropriate. Fourth, mental health involves the *capacity for finding meaning*—that is, the ability to make sense of particular situations and experiences in light of a larger context and story that gives one a way to go on. Fifth, mental health involves *meaningful and engaging activity*. Sixth, mental health involves the *capacity for intimate and fulfilling interpersonal relationships*. Seventh, mental health involves the

8. Daniel Siegel, *Mindsight: The New Science of Personal Transformation* (New York: Bantam, 2011), 64-76. For a slightly different ordering, see Daniel J. Siegel, *The Developing Mind: How Relationships and the Brain Interact to Shape Who We Are*, 2nd ed. (New York: Guilford, 2012), 379-87.

ability to respond flexibly and creatively to challenges. A psychologically healthy person is not insulated from challenge and hardship but rather is able to confront challenges and hardships with emotional, cognitive, and interpersonal flexibility, responding creatively and adaptively in the present moment in a way that promotes learning, healthy reliance on others, and ultimately confidence in one's ability to confront such challenges in the future. This is all consistent with the World Health Organization's description of mental health as "a state of mental well-being that enables people to cope with the stresses of life, realize their abilities, learn well and work well, and contribute to their community."[9]

What does Aquinas's thought, and Christian theology more broadly, have to add to this list? The first word is that it is a good list. Each of the seven attributes of mental health listed here is a Christian good, encouraged and supported by Aquinas's vision of the human as a wayfarer. It is also worth noting that this list shows the inadequacy of the machine metaphor as a model for mental health care. It is possible to keep a machine secure. It is possible to program a machine to exhibit a defined array of responses. It is increasingly possible for artificial intelligence platforms to display what others perceive as meaning-making, purposeful activity, the capacity for interpersonal relationships, and so on. But the frame of reference for judging whether these goods have been realized—for example, deciding when a relationship is intimate, or whether a set of emotional responses is contextually adequate—is distinctively human and cannot be reduced to mechanistic language. An appreciation of what it means for *human beings* to be mentally healthy—even apart from any specifically theological consideration—shows that the machine metaphor cannot adequately ground mental health care.

---

9. "Mental Health," World Health Organization, June 17, 2022, https://www.who.int/news-room/fact-sheets/detail/mental-health-strengthening-our-response. Accessed August 26, 2023. Of note, this formulation has been challenged by those who suggest that for people in environments of extreme deprivation or challenge, mental health may be present without well-being. A recent working group proposed an alternative WHO definition more focused on flexibility than well-being: "Mental health is a dynamic state of internal equilibrium which enables individuals to use their abilities in harmony with universal values of society. Basic cognitive and social skills; ability to recognize, express and modulate one's own emotions, as well as empathize with others; flexibility and ability to cope with adverse life events and function in social roles; and harmonious relationship between body and mind represent important components of mental health which contribute, to varying degrees, to the state of internal equilibrium." See Silvana Galderisi et al., "Toward a New Definition of Mental Health," *World Psychiatry* 14 (2015): 231–33. These shifting definitions point to the elusiveness and instability of the concept that is supposedly the central goal of mental health care.

Aquinas, though, does more than beckon us to appreciate this list. He encourages us to ask deeper questions of it, especially about how these goods are related to each other and how any of them can be pursued and realized in a sustainable way over the course of a lifetime (and beyond). Before engaging these questions, however, it is necessary to introduce the basic contours of his thought on *beatitudo*.

"Who Satisfies Your Desire with Good Things":
Aquinas on *Beatitudo*

When I wake in the morning, I engage in several ordinary tasks that I do not think much about. I prepare a pot of coffee and then breakfast. I shower and dress for the day. I check my email. All of these actions, however automatic and mindless, both deliver a certain degree of intrinsic pleasure and also meet certain immediate desires and needs. I am sleepy and so drink coffee; hungry and so eat breakfast; unkempt and so shower and dress; curious and so (regrettably) check email. But beyond this immediate satisfaction of desire, they are also for other things. I eat, drink, bathe, dress, and even check email in order that I can then engage in the events of the day: spending time with my family, seeing patients, spending time with students and colleagues, attending meetings, attending church services, responding to more and more email, washing dishes, exercising, taking my son to his soccer practice. Many of these daily activities bring intrinsic pleasure, and some (did I mention email?) do not; but they, too, are done not only for themselves, but for a complex web of broader goods and goals, which may stand alongside or even in tension with each other.[10] I care for patients in order, hopefully, to help them to live more freely and wholly, and also because the Department of Veterans Affairs pays me to do so, and this money supports me and my family. I spend time with students because I want to participate in their formation as faithful pastors, clinicians, and scholars, and also because in doing so, I gain some status and respect within my academic institution as a capable teacher and educator. I take my son to soccer practice not only to connect more fully with him but also to support my wife and to share the everyday responsibilities of parenting.

---

10. Of course, there are additional practices, including spiritual practices like prayer, meditation, and Bible reading, that I would *like* to say that I do every morning, but alas, I cannot.

But even these larger goals and aspirations, however honorable or dishonorable, do not stand alone. They take shape within an even broader matrix of commitments and values that collectively orient the kind of person that I aspire to be. I spend time with my children in order that they might become capable and strong young adults who can form meaningful relationships and pursue life-affirming vocations and in order that I might be a father of whom both my wife and children can be proud. I teach at a university and write books like this in order that I might somehow participate in the church's faithfulness to the gospel as it relates to health and health care. At least I would *like* to think that these are the commitments that drive my everyday actions. But I may, of course, be mistaken or may be reluctant to reckon with other commitments that might stand alongside these stated aspirations. Perhaps I spend time with my children not only to contribute to their formation as persons but also in order not to feel lonely, and to gain the respect of my peers as a good dad. Perhaps I am writing this book not only to participate in the church's faithfulness to the gospel but also to try to gain status and respect as an author and expert in faith and mental health, with the material and reputational rewards that follow, or simply to overcome my own feelings of inadequacy. My reasons for acting as I do may not always be clear, even and especially to me.

Thomas Aquinas structured his entire account of why humans act as we do, and how to live wholly and fully, with the assumption that our action is always *for* something. No human action or even state of being stands alone. It is always directed toward something else. Following Aristotle, Aquinas held that the end of an activity, the goal toward which it is directed, is what makes it the kind of activity that it is. We are familiar with this kind of goal-identified, or teleological, way of describing our behavior and that of others. Take, for instance, the example of a man who places his right hand over his left chest. This behavioral description alone does not help us to make sense of his behavior; we also need to know the context and also the aims that he is seeking to pursue. If he is standing at attention and looking at the American flag while a band is playing the national anthem, we might say that he is saluting the flag. If he is standing at a triage desk in an emergency department just after the triage nurse has asked him about his reason for presentation, we might say that he is identifying the location of his pain. If he has just finished an invigorating workout and is seeking to gauge his heart rate, we might say that he is monitoring his heart rate. The physical behavior may look identical, but the context of the behavior and, even more, the intention with which the man engages in the behavior is what makes it the kind of action that it is.

Aquinas believed that we go through life in this way, intending certain goals and defining our lives by the goals that we pursue. Although not all of our behaviors are *consciously* intentional in the sense that we have identified a particular end to pursue and chosen to move toward that end, nonetheless we become who we are in virtue of the kinds of goals that we pursue. And we cannot *not* pursue goals. Living creatures just are the kind of beings who act for ends that are particular to their nature.[11] All living creatures, including plants, move in ways that fit their needs for nutrition, growth, and reproduction, as when a tree extends its branches to catch a patch of full sunlight. All animal creatures, including humans, are endowed with basic capacities for sensation, perception, working memory, and appraisal of threat and danger, and so are capable of more complex forms of goal-pursuit that often involve sophisticated social displays.[12] As I write this, two hummingbirds are jockeying for position at a feeder just outside my screen porch. The less dominant hummingbird is both drawn to the food in the feeder as a source of nutrition and keenly able to judge the presence of its competitor. Its approach to the feeder is guided by these twin appraisals of reward and threat. Many animals, including hummingbirds, are capable of complex forms of mentality and sociality, as they pursue goals that are particular to their created natures. But Aquinas believed that humans stand alone in not only pursuing goals but being able to reflect in language on the goals that we pursue. Further, humans are unique in being able to pursue not just particular goals, like finding food at a feeder without being attacked, but also abstract goals like justice and human rights.[13] This deliberate pursuit of ends, which is specific to humans, is properly called human action, rather than simply action or behaviors performed by humans.[14]

Aquinas held not only that we are the kind of creatures who act for ends or goals but also that we find ourselves drawn by desire toward even broader ends, and that therefore the ends for which we act have a kind of directedness to them. Brushing my teeth this morning delivered a certain degree of satisfaction, but I brushed my teeth primarily *in order to* be socially presentable and *in order to* promote my overall health. Being socially presentable and physically

---

11. Herbert McCabe, *On Aquinas*, ed. Brian Davies (London: Continuum, 2009), 29-40; Paul Wadell, *The Primacy of Love: An Introduction to the Ethics of Thomas Aquinas* (Eugene, OR: Wipf & Stock, 1992), 29-36; Rebecca Konyndyk DeYoung, Colleen McCluskey, and Christina Van Dyke, *Aquinas's Ethics: Metaphysical Foundations, Moral Theory, and Theological Context* (Notre Dame: University of Notre Dame Press, 2009), 70-73.

12. See *STh* Ia q. 78 a. 1.

13. McCabe, *On Aquinas*, 29-40.

14. See *STh* IaIIae q. 1 a. 1 *resp.*

healthy also delivers some satisfaction, but they also are not the ultimate goals of my life. I pursue them *in order that* I might fulfill my vocations as father, husband, psychiatrist, professor, church member, and so on.

There is much to be said for the simple joy of finding a place for oneself in the world and being content with that. As David Kelsey has emphasized, the biblical wisdom literature celebrates the goodness of the quotidian, the joy of everyday, routine life before God, without assuming that this quotidian life should be denigrated in favor of some higher degree of actualization.[15] "I know that there is nothing better for [those who work] than to be happy and enjoy themselves as long as they live," says Qoheleth. "Moreover, it is God's gift that all should eat and drink and take pleasure in all their toil" (Eccles. 3:12-13). In a culture that is always calling us to produce more, consume more, achieve more, work more, there is a deep grace in settling into our lives as gifts of God, without a constant restless striving for more. There is deep grace in taking joy in being a caregiver, a friend, a spouse, a coach, a teacher, an encourager, a gardener, or any other good form of life. But Aquinas warns us that if any of these things are pursued for their own sake, as if the happiness of our lives depends on them, then sooner or later we will end up disappointed. Not only can friends move away, jobs disappear, and health challenges impair our ability to pursue these activities, but there is always a "something more" that beckons us not just to take joy in everyday life but to look to God "who satisfies you with good as long as you live" (Ps. 103:5).[16] "As the soul is the life of the body," Aquinas quotes Augustine, "so God is man's life of happiness: of whom it is written, 'Happy is that people whose God is the Lord'" (*STh* IaIIae q. 2 a. 8 *sed contra*, quoting Ps. 144:15). Focused on this something more, we do not leave behind the goodness and joy of everyday life, but we do place it in the broader context of life before God.

Aquinas believed that we move through our lives pursuing ends that point to a series of other ends, that collectively point to whatever would leave us with our desires fully and completely satisfied. He called this state of satisfaction *beatitudo*, which as above is often translated "happiness" or "flourishing." *Beatitudo* is Aquinas's Latin word for Aristotle's Greek *eudaimonia*, which is also generally translated as "happiness" or "human flourishing." Aquinas believed that we are naturally drawn to desire *beatitudo*, the state in which all our desires will be satisfied and that there is nothing left to be desired. All

---

15. David Kelsey, *Eccentric Existence: A Theological Anthropology* (Louisville: Westminster John Knox, 2009), 201-14.

16. Quoted in *STh* IaIIae q. 2 a. 8 *resp.*

of our actions, Aquinas held, are ultimately directed toward *beatitudo*—even mundane activities like brushing our teeth (*STh* IaIIae q. 1 aa. 4–7).

But in what, Aquinas asks, does true *beatitudo* consist? Here Aquinas begins not only to name but to relativize the seven modern goods of mental health. He answers this question by first naming eight things that are genuine goods but that do not bring perfect wholeness and contentment. He begins by considering four extrinsic goods that arise from outside of one's own embodied experience. First, he states, happiness does not consist in *wealth*, since wealth is never an end in itself but is always *for* something else. "Natural wealth," like food, clothing, wheeled vehicles, and dwellings are for the natural needs and wants that they are meant to satisfy; "artificial wealth," like money, is for the purchase of natural wealth, and so on (*STh* IaIIae q. 2 a. 1 *resp*.). Second, *beatitudo* does not consist in *honors* that one accrues, since these honors are not ends in themselves but are meant to attest to some excellence in the honored person; honors are *for* the excellence to which they refer (*STh* IaIIae q. 2 a. 2). Third, *beatitudo* does not consist in *fame or glory*, since glory can be deceptive, and at any rate, it makes no sense to base one's own happiness on the appraisal of others (*STh* IaIIae q. 2 a. 3). Fourth, *beatitudo* does not consist in *power*, since power exists in evil people, since power can corrupt the powerful, and since power is often acquired through fortune or external cause rather than as a result of a person's own desert or excellence (*STh* IaIIae q. 2 a. 4).

Having argued that happiness does not consist in these extrinsic goods, Aquinas considers whether *beatitudo* rather consists in goods that are *intrinsic* to the human person; and unlike many modern psychologists of happiness, he finds these goods insufficient also. First, *beatitudo* does not consist in physical or mental health. It does not consist in *bodily health* (literally, "the goods of the body," *bona corporis*) because the body exists not for itself but *for* the life (*anima*) constituted in and by that body: "all goods of the body are ordained to the goods of the soul [*bona animae*], as to their end" (*STh* IaIIae q. 2 a. 5). But neither does it consist in "mental health," if by that term is meant properly functioning reason and will, since reason and will are not *for* themselves but rather for whatever human life is for (*STh* IaIIae q. 2 a. 5). Second, *beatitudo* does not consist in *pleasure* or positive emotion. Pleasure is in fact a good to be pursued—Aquinas strongly affirms that "it comes to the same whether we desire good, or desire delight, which is nothing else than the appetite's rest in good" (*STh* IaIIae q. 2 a. 6 *ad1*)—but it is not the final end of human life, because pleasure is meant to *reflect* one's experience of encountering what is genuinely good. If one pursues pleasure for its own sake, one can forget that pleasure is not self-sustaining or self-generating but rather results from an encounter with what is genuinely good (*STh* IaIIae q. 2 a. 6 *resp.*). Third, *beatitudo* does not consist in any "good of the soul" (*bonum animae*), which Aquinas intends as a catch-all term for any psychological or spiritual capacity, virtue, skill, or activity of the human that is not externally derived and not clearly related to the body. While *beatitudo* will indeed be *displayed* in these capacities, virtues, and activities, these goods cannot constitute *beatitudo*, since like everything else on the list—external goods, bodily goods, positive emotions, and so on—these psychological and spiritual capacities are *for* something external to themselves. They find their fulfillment when they participate in this good, though they are not themselves the *source* of the good.

This would seem to be a pretty comprehensive list and that Aquinas leaves nothing capable of serving as the final end of human life, capable of constituting *beatitudo*. In a technical sense, he does not. No created good [*bonum creatum*], which is to say no thing, is capable of constituting *beatitudo*. One must look beyond things to the sustaining cause of all things. Ending the suspense, Aquinas writes that

> *beatitudo* is the perfect good, which lulls the appetite altogether; else it would not be the last end, if something yet remained to be desired. Now the object of the will, *i.e.*, of man's appetite, is the universal good; just as the object of the intellect is the universal true. Hence it is evident that naught can lull man's will, save the universal good. This is to be found, not in any creature, but in God alone; because every creature has goodness by participation. Wherefore God alone can satisfy the will of man, according to the words of Psalm 102:5, "who satisfies your desire with good things." Therefore God alone constitutes man's *beatitudo*. (*STh* IaIIae q. 2 a. 8 *resp.*)

God alone, that is, is the ultimate good capable of so satisfying human longing that there is nothing left to be desired. All other goods—including wealth, honor, fame, glory, physical health, mental health, positive emotion, pleasure, and anything else—are good insofar as they participate in God's goodness. All of these things are good when properly oriented to God, but none of them is the *highest* good that is capable of grounding and constituting *beatitudo*. In Aquinas's account, only God can do that.

Here it becomes clear that Aquinas's concept of *beatitudo* is difficult to render in English in a way that is not misleading. "Happiness" is partially true but misleading because of its strong connotation in our contemporary context with pleasure and positive emotion, which is not the most significant feature of *beatitudo*. "Flourishing" is partially true but misleading because it can easily be interpreted naturalistically, along the lines of Aristotle's concept of *eudaimonia*, without any reference to God as its source and sustainer. But for Aquinas *beatitudo* is found most perfectly in God, and in humans only by participation. Speaking of God's *beatitudo*, Aquinas defines *beatitudo* as "the perfect good of an intellectual nature, where an intellectual nature is one which (a) is capable of grasping its own satisfaction with the good that it possesses, (b) is capable of doing well or doing badly, and (c) is a master of its own actions."[17] God possesses and displays perfect *beatitudo*, and human *beatitudo* is properly a participation in God's *beatitudo*. For this reason, Reinhard Hütter renders *beatitudo* as "participation in divine happiness."[18]

Hütter's translation is admirably precise, but I will not use it in this book, focused on the relevance of Aquinas's thought for modern mental health care, because, again, of the way that "happiness" is so often reduced to positive emotion. Instead, I turn to the word traditionally used to translate the Greek term *makarios* in the "beatitudes" of Matthew 5:1-12 and used of God (as Aquinas notes) in 1 Timothy 6:15: *blessed*. God's *beatitudo* is God's blessedness, in which humans are invited to participate. When participated in by humans, God's blessedness takes the form of blessing for us—God's blessing of God's life. "Happiness," Josef Pieper affirms, "is essentially a gift."[19] For this reason, I will refer to this end that all humans pursue either simply as *beatitudo* or as "participation in blessing." To be *beatus* is to live well, with humble and expectant awareness that the heart of living well is seeking God as one's end, participating in the blessing of God's life and God's own blessedness.

Having established that *beatitudo*, participation in blessing, consists in union with God, Aquinas then turns to the things required for *beatitudo* and what *beatitudo* looks and feels like in a person's embodied life. He agrees with Aristotle

17. *STh* Ia q. 26 a. 1 *resp*. The quotation here is from *New English Translation of St. Thomas Aquinas's "Summa Theologiae,"* trans. Alfred Freddoso, available at: https://www3.nd.edu/~afreddos/summa-translation/TOC-part1.htm. Josef Pieper considers the objections of modern readers who might be disturbed that God's *beatitudo* is perfect and complete even when the world is full of evil. Far from rendering God distant from the suffering of creation, Pieper argues that God's *beatitudo* is a precondition for healing: "If God were not happy, or if His happiness depended upon what happened in the human realm and not on Himself alone, if his happiness were not beyond any conceivable possibility of disturbance; if there were not, in the Source of reality, this infinitely, inviolably sound Being—we would not be able even to conceive the idea of a possible healing of the empirical wounds of Creation." Pieper, *Happiness and Contemplation*, trans. Richard and Clara Winston (South Bend: St. Augustine's Press, 1998), 30.

18. Reinhard Hütter, *Bound for Beatitude: A Thomistic Study in Eschatology and Ethics* (Washington, DC: Catholic University of America Press, 2019), 6-15.

19. Pieper, *Happiness and Contemplation*, 25.

that *beatitudo* is not a static state but rather an activity or operation, a way of living well (*STh* IaIIac q. 3 a. 2). He furthermore argues that *beatitudo* requires the activity not only of the psychological capacities that humans share with other animals but also of the distinctively human capacities of intellect and will: the intellect apprehends God and the good things of God, and the will pursues them and, finding them, delights in them (*STh* IaIIae q. 3 aa. 3, 4; q. 4 aa. 1, 2).

Aquinas strongly asserts that "final and perfect participation in blessing" (*beatitudo ultima et perfecta*) results only from the contemplation of God in God's essence in the life to come (*STh* IaIIae q. 3 a. 8 *resp.*), but he affirms that in this life, humans are nonetheless capable of a good but "incomplete participation in blessing" (*beatitudo imperfecta*) that involves not only contemplation but also the right ordering of one's actions and emotions (*STh* IaIIae q. 3 a. 5 *resp.*; q. 5, a. 3). Both perfect and imperfect participation in blessing require not only an intellect that is oriented to God and to the things of God but also a will that pursues God and God's good things. Participation in blessing, after all, is an activity, and it would be pointless to speak of participation in blessing without the activity of the will in which it is displayed (*STh* IaIIae q. 4 a. 4; q. 5 a. 7). Both perfect and imperfect participation in blessing are *embodied* and are facilitated when the body does not get in the way of a person's pursuit of God (*STh* IaIIae q. 4 a. 6). But there are significant differences also. While Aquinas affirms that in the life to come, God will be so present to the wayfarer that neither external goods like food and shelter nor the company of friends are necessary for participation in blessing, he affirms also that both the goods necessary to meet basic human needs and interpersonal relationships are necessary for participation in blessing in this life (*STh* IaIIae q. 4 aa. 7, 8). While the imperfect *beatitudo* of this life can be lost through forgetfulness, sickness, or vice, the perfect *beatitudo* of the next life cannot be lost (*STh* IaIIae q. 5 a. 4 *resp.*). While the imperfect *beatitudo* of this life can be attained at least partially by a person's natural capacity to order his or her life in a way consistent with virtue, the perfect *beatitudo* of the next life is unattainable by human effort alone and requires the special and direct intervention of God (*STh* IaIIae q. 5 aa. 5, 6).

Aquinas's account of *beatitudo* is at heart a vision of profound freedom before God and among our fellow creatures. He believed that all humans were created with a basic capacity to choose between competing goods ("freedom of choice," or *liberum arbitrium*) that can never be taken away as long as the body is supporting basic psychological function. Even people who are physically constrained (e.g., incarcerated) or psychologically constrained (e.g., by substance use disorders) can choose one thing over another: to eat or not to eat, to speak or not to speak, and so on. But the journey of participation in blessing, because it aligns and draws on what is truly good and life-giving (ultimately God), is a journey of progressive freedom: not just freedom to choose among a wider range of options but freedom *for* that which is truly good.[20] Aquinas envisioned the path of participation in blessing as a journey of enlargement and psychological and spiritual opening to God and to God's creation. This vision of freedom and delight in God and God's creation is powerfully captured in Aquinas's prayer "For the Attainment of Heaven," in which he speaks of his hope for the end of his journey in the presence of God:

> O most bountiful Rewarder, endow my body
>> with beauty of splendor,
>> with swift responsiveness to all commands,
>> with complete subservience to the spirit,
>> and with freedom from all vulnerability.
> Add to these
>> an abundance of your riches,
>> a river of delights,
>> and a flood of other goods
> So that I may enjoy
>> Your solace above me,
>> a delightful garden beneath my feet,
>> the glorification of body and soul within me,
>> and the sweet companionship
>>> of people and angels around me.
> With you, most merciful Father,
>> may my mind attain
>>> the enlightenment of wisdom,
>> my desire
>>> what is truly desirable,
>> and my courage
>>> the praise of triumph. . . .
> Give me, O Lord my God,

---

20. Servais Pinckaers refers to this as the distinction between "freedom of indifference" and "freedom for excellence." See Servais Pinckaers, *The Sources of Christian Ethics*, trans. Mary Thomas Noble (Washington, DC: Catholic University of America Press, 1995), 327–99. See also Pinckaers, *Morality: The Catholic View*, trans. Michael Sherwin, OP (South Bend: Saint Augustine's, 2003), 65–81; Benedict M. Ashley, *Healing for Freedom: A Christian Perspective on Personhood and Psychotherapy* (Arlington, VA: Institute for the Psychological Sciences Press, 2013), 211–16.

that life without death
and that joy without sorrow
where there is
    the greatest freedom,
    unconfined security,
    secure tranquility,
    delightful happiness,
    happy eternity,
    eternal blessedness,
    the vision of truth,
    and praise, O God.
    Amen.[21]

Journeys have a feel to them. When my family travels to visit my parents in the South Carolina Lowcountry with its massive expanses of tidal estuaries and salt marshes, we know that we are nearing our destination when we begin to smell the earthy, sulfuric smell of the marshlands and feel the dense humidity of the coastal breeze. While newcomers to the area might find the smell of the marshes distasteful, it is for me an occasion for joy, as it signifies the successful conclusion of hours of travel, and homecoming to a place where many generations of my family have lived. The successful journey *feels* a certain way. In an analogous way, for Aquinas a successful journey is signified by a feeling of openness to God, by the capacity to delight in oneself and God's creatures, and by freedom to know and to do what is truly life-giving.

But freedom for Aquinas is more than the absence of constraint and more than feeling. Several years ago, I traveled to New York City for a speaking engagement and found myself alone on a sunny spring day near Bryant Park in midtown Manhattan with a couple of hours to spare. Though I do not visit often, I love New York, and in a sense, I was completely free. But I was not at home there. I did not know anyone, and, though I knew generally where I was in the city, it took a moderate effort to orient myself. I needed to consult a map to find the right subway lines and even to find my hotel. Other than my hotel room, I did not have access to any private spaces. I did not know the best spots for a cheap meal or for a quiet place to work. Everything required a great deal of conscious activity. In

21. Thomas Aquinas, "Qua ad Caelum Adspirat," in *The Aquinas Prayer Book: The Prayers and Hymns of St. Thomas Aquinas*, trans. and ed. Robert Anderson and Johann Moser (Manchester, NH: Sophia Institute Press, 2000), 52–57. I substituted "people" for "men" to translate Aquinas's *juxta de angelorum et hominum delectabili associatione*.

contrast, when I returned to North Carolina the following day, I effortlessly navigated from the airport to meet with a colleague at a local coffee shop, and then to the university library, and then home. I could get on with the business of the day without wondering at every step where I was. I not only had freedom to move, but I was at home, and so I knew *how* and *where* to move to attain particular goals.

For Aquinas, this capacity not only to act without external constraint but to act with skill and confidence is central to the freedom that comes with journeying well. To be free in this sense is to progressively become an *agens*, "agent," one who acts rather than one who is acted upon (*STh* IaIIae q. 1 a. 1 *resp.*). It is to be the originator, or *principium*, of what one does (*STh* IaIIae *proem.*). Agency, the capacity to be the originator of our own actions, is therefore for Aquinas a central good.

Aquinas and the Goods of Mental Health

For Aquinas, *beatitudo* or participation in blessing consists in pursuing God as the goal of the journey and, in the process, finding oneself progressively free to know and to act in a way that is consistent with what is true and good. How might Aquinas's concept of *beatitudo* help in making sense of the way that modern clinicians and researchers understand the seven orienting goods of modern mental health care?

First, Aquinas helps us to recognize that all of the dimensions of mental health outlined above are what we might call *experiential* goods. Experiential goods display either the capacity for or the actuality of happiness or flourishing. They are evident in the experience of the person who displays them. As such, they are all genuine goods that are consistent with Aquinas's vision of *beatitudo*. But Aquinas would argue that each of them is unsustainable if pursued for its own sake. Live a life consumed by the quest for personal and bodily security, Aquinas would say, and one will find oneself pursuing a life dedicated to control (see chapter 9). Live a life dedicated to purposeful activity, and one may find oneself chasing novelty and meaning without a clear sense of what purposes and ends will lead to fulfillment. Live a life focused on intimate and fulfilling relationships, and these relationships may take on such power that one cannot separate from them if they become unhealthy.

Beyond these experiential goods, Aquinas would encourage us to identify a different category of good, namely, that of *teleological* goods. Teleological goods are goods that, when pursued, enable the sustainable growth and display of experiential goods. They are the goods that we are to pursue in order to realize the experiential goods of positive self-regard, a full emotional repertoire, fulfilling relationships, and so on. As the discussion above makes clear, for Aquinas the only teleological good that can sustain *beatitudo* is God. God is the end of the wayfarer's journey, the pearl of great value (Matt. 13:45–46) who when pursued enables other good things.[22] "Strive first for the kingdom of God and his righteousness," Jesus said, "and all these things will be given to you as well" (Matt. 6:33).

Furthermore, Aquinas's concept of *beatitudo* helps us to see that there are at least three different types of experiential goods of mental health. Some goods are *preparatory* goods, important for mental health because they establish conditions that are conducive to flourishing. Most clinicians and researchers, for example, would agree that basic bodily security is important for mental health but would not equate security with mental health. Rather, security is important because it makes space for the other goods such as healthy and fulfilling relationships to emerge. Other goods are *operational* goods, in that they name the activity of living well. Operational goods on the list above include personal and engaging activity, (realized, not just potential) fulfilling interpersonal relationships, and (realized, not just potential) flexible adaptation to changing circumstances. Finally, some goods are *consummate* goods, in that they arise from a person's reflection on the well-lived life as a whole. Positive regard for one's life and meaning-making are examples of consummate goods. Table 4 shows how the seven goods of mental health listed above might be organized in overlapping ways into categories of preparatory, operational, and consummate goods.

Table 4. *Distinguishing the Seven Experiential Goods of Mental Health*

Preparatory Goods	Personal and bodily **security**
	The **capacity** for full range of emotion
	The capacity to seek **meaning** in one's life
	Access to intimate and fulfilling **interpersonal relationships**
	The **ability** to respond flexibly and creatively to challenges
Operational Goods	Purposeful and engaging **activity**
	Intimate and fulfilling **interpersonal relationships**
	Responding flexibly and creatively to challenges
	Seeking meaning in one's life
Consummate Goods	**Positive regard** for oneself and one's life
	Successfully finding meaning in one's life
	Enjoying intimate, fulfilling **interpersonal relationships**

22. Aquinas, *Commentary on the Gospel of Matthew* 1194–1195.

While Aquinas makes clear that true participation in blessing can be achieved only when God is pursued as one's highest good, this division of experiential goods helps to order the way that one might pursue them. Specifically, Aquinas's teaching would counsel that if we want to be mentally healthy, we will seek to secure the preparatory goods (e.g., bodily security) as much as it is in our power to do so and then primarily focus on the *activity* of the operational goods—always with the knowledge that these goods can't be pursued for their own sake as the highest end of life.

To be mentally healthy, Aquinas might say the following: Remember that only God can satisfy every desire and enable true participation in blessing. Keep participation in God's life as the goal. Care for and protect your body as a site where God dwells. As much as it depends on you, cultivate the capacity for thinking, feeling, and acting in a way that you are more and more open to the love and care of others and the love and care of God—which includes having unpleasant and negative emotions and reactions in the face of threats or obstacles to love. Keeping God as the goal, focus on the *activity* of responding creatively to challenges, building relationship with God and others, and taking things one step at a time. Trust the rest to God, knowing that perfect participation in blessing is not possible in this life. When things remain hard, when life doesn't make sense and negative thoughts and emotions outweigh the positive, don't give up. This is how the journey goes sometimes, and you are not alone. But when things seem to be going well, when you experience your life as satisfying and rich in meaning, accept this as a gift.

CHAPTER 7

From Bodily Feeling to Embodied Love

Our Thinking, Willing, and Feeling Are Guided by Our Loves

> O that you would kill the wicked, O God,
>> and that the bloodthirsty would depart from me—
> those who speak of you maliciously
>> and lift themselves up against you for evil!
> Do I not hate those who hate you, O LORD?
>> And do I not loathe those who rise up against you?
> I hate them with perfect hatred;
>> I count them my enemies.
>
> *—Psalm 139:19-22*

In the last chapter, we considered the goal of the journey, which for Aquinas is *beatitudo* or participation in blessing. But how are human beings shaped for the process of the journey? What capacities and endowments have been granted to human beings in creation that enable us to be wayfarers? In the *Summa theologiae*, Aquinas offers a detailed and fruitful account of human psychology that sometimes coheres with but often challenges the assumptions of modern mental health care. In this chapter, following Aquinas's account in the *Summa*, I will describe how the powers of intellect and will and our experience of emotion function to guide us through the journey. At their best, our intellect, will, and emotion help us to enjoy the freedom to pursue ends that are good and life-giving, and to love God and God's creatures more fully and deeply. Central to this freedom is the development of agency, the capacity to be the originator (*principium*) of our own activity.

172

Intellect, Will, and Action

To understand how this journey unfolds, Aquinas turns to the psychological theory of his time derived from the Greek philosophical tradition that he inherited, especially from Aristotle. He first distinguishes between the human capacities of intellect and will. Intellect is a set of capacities that broadly pertains to our ability to know and therefore pertains to what is true. Intellect is central to our being more than isolated, individual bodies that act only according to our natural form, as a rock is inclined to fall or as fire is inclined to rise. Intellect enables us to take the forms of other things into ourselves and therefore to exist in a network of relationships with things, with people, and with God. It allows us to be knowing creatures. Drawing on the work of Aristotle and the Eastern Christian thinker Pseudo-Dionysius the Areopagite, Aquinas goes so far as to say that "the soul of man is, in a way, all things by sense and intellect: and thereby, those things that have knowledge, in a way, approach to a likeness to God, in Whom all things pre-exist" (*STh* Ia q. 80 a. 1 *resp.*).[1]

Aquinas distinguishes between the speculative intellect, which deals with knowing things as they are, and the practical intellect, which deals with

---

1. See also Robert Edward Brennan, *Thomistic Psychology: A Philosophic Analysis of the Nature of Man* (New York: Macmillan, 1941), 25. In his focus on intellect, Aquinas is often accused by modern disability theorists of prioritizing a rationalist account of human excellence over and above a more authentically Christian relational account in a way that marginalizes people with intellectual disability (e.g., Hans S. Reinders, *Receiving the Gift of Friendship: Profound Disability, Theological Anthropology, and Ethics* [Grand Rapids: Eerdmans, 2008]; Reinders, "Life's Goodness: On Disability, Genetics, and 'Choice,'" in *Theology, Disability, and the New Genetics: Why Science Needs the Church*, ed. John Swinton and Brian Brock [London: T&T Clark, 2007], 163-81). While it is easy to read Aquinas this way, see the appendix to this book for how Aquinas's view can be defended. Additionally, it is important to note that in Aquinas's judgment, intellect and human relationship are related to each other. Though it is possible to be in relationship without any recognition of or present knowledge of the relationship—as may be so in cases of people in minimally conscious states or advanced dementia, for example, or alternatively may describe the way that many humans relate to God—nonetheless it is usually the case that relationship forms through some kind of awareness of another's presence and regard, which is possible through the work of knowing. No living relationship is possible unless at least one party to the relationship sustains this knowing work. In the usual course of human affairs, relationality presupposes some degree of intellectual capacity. To be sure, *how* this capacity is displayed will differ considerably from person to person. And with regard to the way that humans relate to God, Aquinas was quick to quote Saint Gregory that "since we know God imperfectly, thus we also name him imperfectly, as if stuttering" (*In I Sent.* d. 22 q. 1 a. 1; quoted in Jean-Pierre Torrell, *Saint Thomas Aquinas*, vol. 2, *Spiritual Master*, trans. Robert Royal [Washington, DC: Catholic University of America Press, 2003], 27).

knowing as it informs action—though he is careful to say that these are two dimensions of one power of knowing rather than distinct powers (*STh* Ia q. 79 a. 11 *resp.*). Speculative intellect broadly names the capacities to grasp first principles of logic (*intellectus*), to engage in deductive reasoning to draw conclusions from these first principles (reason or *ratio*) (*STh* Ia q. 79 aa. 8-9), and to encode abstract truths in memory (*memoria*) (*STh* Ia q. 79 aa. 6-7). Practical intellect broadly names the capacities to grasp first principles of ethics, such as that good is to be pursued and evil avoided, which supports the activity that Aquinas termed *synderesis* (*STh* Ia q. 79 a. 12), and to make judgments about particular acts (conscience, *conscientia*) (*STh* Ia q. 79 a. 13).

Will (*voluntas*) is a power distinct from intellect in that it is concerned not with knowing but with doing, and not with what is true in itself but with what is *good* for the life of the creature. Will, for Aquinas, is the appetite of the intellect. It is the motive power that directs us to pursue what the intellect identifies as good (for us), or to flee what the intellect identifies as evil (for us). If intellect supplies knowledge, then will supplies motivation to act on that knowledge. If my intellect identifies that it is Election Day and that my vote matters, then my will directs me to drive to the polling place and cast my ballot. If my intellect identifies that there is a strong chance of thunderstorms this afternoon and that a raincoat might help to protect me from getting drenched, my will directs me to pick up my raincoat before leaving home.

Aquinas posited a complex relationship between intellect (how we believe) and will (how we order activity in response). First, the intellect can move the will by identifying appropriate goals for the will to pursue (*STh* IaIIae q. 9 a. 1). However, because it is naturally directed toward the good in itself, the will can also move the intellect by directing the intellect to do its job well. "From this," Aquinas states, "we can easily understand why these powers include one another in their acts, because the intellect understands that the will wills, and the will wills the intellect to understand" (*STh* Ia q. 82 a. 4 *ad1*). Furthermore, just as it can move the intellect, the will can move itself when it wills not only to pursue a particular end that is perceived as good but also wills the means to achieve this end (*STh* IaIIae q. 9 a. 3 *resp.*).

In practice, Aquinas holds, the powers of intellect and will work together in a complex but orderly two-step that comprises the apparatus of practical reason. This two-step occurs constantly as we go about our ordinary life. Let us say, for example, that it is noon and that I recognize that it is lunchtime. I think of an eating spot on campus that serves delicious South Indian vegetarian food, and my intellect *determines* (rightly or wrongly) that this food would be good for me—that is, enjoyable and nourishing to my body. As my intellect has determined not only that Indian food would be good for me but also that this food is attainable, my will then orients me in the direction of this Indian food, *intending* that I will attempt to attain it (*STh* IaIIae q. 12). I then think about precisely *how* to attain this food. Would it be better to go now or after I have checked my morning email? Which route should I take to get there? How will I pay? Should I invite a colleague to accompany me? Through a process of *counsel*, the intellect determines the appropriate means, and through *consent*, the will ratifies these means (*STh* IaIIae qq. 14-15). Having set Indian food as a worthy goal for my action and determined the appropriate means, intellect and will then collaborate in *choosing* or *electing* this course of action: I say, with decision, "I'm going" (*STh* IaIIae q. 13). And then, in a final act of *command*, I leave my office and go to enjoy a delicious South Indian meal.[2]

The body and the senses are intimately involved in all of this. While Aquinas teaches that the immaterial angels also display intellect and will, they do so in very different ways (*STh* Ia qq. 54-59). Humans, though, engage the world around us through our senses, and sensory knowledge—knowledge, for example, of the Indian samosas that I enjoyed at lunch—requires the body. We travel through this life as bodies. We sense as bodies, we move as bodies, and we feel in our bodies. Even most of what we identify as "thinking" happens in our bodies.[3]

---

2. Eleonore Stump provides a helpfully clear account of this process in *Aquinas* (London: Routledge, 2003), 287-94.

3. Aquinas notably claims that the rational faculty of the soul, which enables humans to know universal forms rather than only particular sensible objects, is immaterial and does not depend on the body for its proper function. This faculty includes both the agent intellect, the abstracting agent that identifies the forms, and the passive intellect, which receives the forms identified by the agent intellect. It is clear from this that Aquinas is not a thoroughgoing materialist when it comes to the mind. But neither does he believe that the mind, if that refers to the process and experience of human psychological life, is disembodied. As I write this footnote, for example, I am thinking, but my thought is a complex and embodied activity. I see the screen on which I'm typing and occasionally press the backspace button to correct errors. I lose my train of thought and look back at the previous sentence to regain momentum. I think of a book that has illumined Aquinas's account of mind for me and picture its cover and typeface in my mind. I say a phrase aloud, discard it, and write a different one. All of these sensory and cognitive capacities—sensation, perception, memory of particular objects, emotional appraisal of particular objects, and so on—are common to humans and to other animals and so involve the body. It is only my capacity to discern in many books the common form of book, and to hold this in mind as an abstraction, that according to Aquinas does not involve the body—though as soon as I link the universal form of book to images of individual books, the body is necessary. For Aquinas, this had to do with a basic metaphysical commitment that material things could not know immaterial realities, and that nonhuman animals could therefore know only

The journey of the wayfarer is an embodied journey, and the human powers of intellect and will are deeply entwined with the body.

The body is critically important for the wayfarer's path in two ways. First, as detailed in chapter 2, the body is the configured matter that makes life, including psychological life, possible. Bodies often function similarly, and it is therefore possible to categorize certain features and aptitudes of human experience and behavior as normal in a statistical sense. But because all bodies are different, the particulars of psychological life will also be different. One person might have a particular aptitude for remembering the lyrics of songs heard in childhood, because of brain configurations related to acoustic and verbal memory. Another might have a particular aptitude for visualizing three-dimensional structures. Another might have a particular aptitude for empathy. A deaf person will have an experience of the world different from that of a hearing person, due to a different configuration of the body. We are creatures of earth, and we live in and as bodies.

But the body is not only a condition of our lived experience. It is also a finely tuned system by which we live in the world. A few years ago, my father-in-law gave my son his old Boy Scout compass, and my son was pleased to find that it still works. A compass is a simple but amazing instrument. Like the body, it must be crafted in a particular way for it to do its job: too much friction, too much imbalance, and the pin will not move. But even an old Boy Scout compass, set on a flat surface, will wobble and turn until the pin points to due north. Those few old bits of metal, simply designed and small enough to fit in a pocket, align themselves with the magnetic field of the earth.

In Aquinas's view, the living body is also attuned. Fearfully and wonderfully made, the body is not a machine and is vastly more complex than a Boy Scout compass. But informed by the soul (see chapter 2), it is capable of aligning not with the earth's magnetic field but with God, the object of its fulfillment, and with God's *ratio*, God's providential ordering of the world.[4] Aquinas is careful to specify that knowledge of God in God's essence is known in the present life only through the immaterial power of the intellect, and

---

particulars, not abstractions. My dog can intimately know my wife, my children, and me, but Aquinas believes that he knows us as individuals and does not use the abstract form of human being to understand us. And because God and God's law are immaterial, this means that only humans, among the animals, are given the capacities to know God and God's providential ordering of creation. See *STh* Ia q. 75, a. 2; q. 79.

4. God, that is, is the objective ultimate end of the rational creature; *beatitudo* is the subjective ultimate end. Reinhard Hütter, *Bound for Beatitude: A Thomistic Study in Eschatology and Ethics* (Washington, DC: Catholic University of America Press, 2019), 18–19.

then only imperfectly and with the special light of grace (*STh* Ia q. 12). But as the person is drawn toward *beatitudo* through knowing what is true and loving and moving toward what is good, the body participates in this knowing and loving. The journey begins to *feel* a certain way, as our bodies respond positively to people, places, and situations that we interpret as good for us and negatively to people, places, and situations that we interpret as harmful for us. Aquinas refers to these feelings that correspond to judgments of benefit or harm as passions. In modern mental health care, they are most often known as emotions.

Making Sense of Emotion

There is more to mental health than emotion, but emotion is never far from the surface of mental health care. People seek mental health care because of distressing or unwanted emotion, or sometimes by the *lack* of particular emotions when this is desired. Emotions that are experienced as negative, such as anger, fear, sadness, and shame, show up in the experience of nearly every clinic session of every mental health clinician.

But what is emotion? And what, if anything, do the emotions tell us? There is no one answer to these questions within modern mental health care. There are, instead, a host of different and sometimes conflicting answers, if the question is asked at all.

Historian Thomas Dixon argues that the term "emotion" is surprisingly new within the history of philosophy and psychology. There is no word in Greek or Latin that cleanly maps onto the modern English word "emotion," and the word "emotion" did not gain its current use as the name of a class of affective/feeling experiences, such as fear, joy, and delight, until the early nineteenth century. Ancient and medieval writers referred to what we now call "emotion" either as passions (derived from the Greek *pathos* and the Latin *passio*) or as "affections" (from the Latin *affectio*). Passions were understood as experiences of being moved, either by one's own appetites or by external objects and were often associated with lower emotions such as fear, anger, and sexual desire. Affections, never entirely distinct from passions, were often associated with higher emotions such as delight and joy and were often associated with the activity of the rational faculty of the soul, rather than the lower appetites. Dixon argues that this ancient and medieval language of passions and affections was broadly framed by Christian psychological and theological assumptions, which were themselves influenced by Greco-Roman

moral and philosophical traditions. Sometimes, as in certain texts of Augustine, the passions were seen to be at war with reason and needed to be coerced
into control by the reason and will. Sometimes (as we will see with Aquinas,
below) they could harmoniously participate in reason's judgments. But the
passions and affections were always related to reason and will, which found
their fulfillment and direction in God.[5]

All of that changed dramatically, Dixon argues, in the European Enlight-
enment of the seventeenth and eighteenth centuries. René Descartes, in *The
Passions of the Soul* (1649), argued that the passions were the result not of
the lower appetites impinging on reason but of the body mechanistically
impinging on the mind (see chapter 1). Operating within a dualistic understanding of mind and body, in which the body was understood as a machine,
the passions were mechanical for Descartes. Descartes occasionally used the
French term *émotion* for this eruption of bodily energy that impinged on
the mind, and Dixon argues that our modern English "emotion" may derive from Descartes's choice of this term. By situating the passions in the
activity of the body, Descartes was one of the first writers on the passions to
unlink the emotions from the activity of reason and will and to make the
emotions (feelings, passions, affections) into something like autonomous
agents in their own right—not following the dictates of reason and will but
rather complementing reason and will or, sometimes, directing them. David
Hume, writing a century after Descartes, famously stated in his *Treatise of
Human Nature* (1738-1740) that "reason is, and ought only to be the slave of
the passions, and can never pretend to any other office than to serve and obey
them."[6] For Hume, the passions were impressions of feelings produced by
the combination of a sensation with an idea, and both reason and will were
nothing but amalgamations of the passions.[7] Hume was one of the earliest
writers to use the term "emotion," possibly drawing it from Descartes. Other
writers, notably Adam Smith, began to use the language of "moral senti-
ments" to describe felt judgments about the rightness or wrongness of the

---

5. Thomas Dixon, *From Passions to Emotions: The Creation of a Secular Psychological
Category* (Cambridge: Cambridge University Press, 2003).

6. David Hume, *A Treatise of Human Nature* 3.3; quoted in Dixon, *From Passions to Emotions*, 106.

7. Dixon writes, "So the two pillars of a classically conceived Christian soul—will and
reason—vanished in Humean psychology, to be replaced by a multitude of passions, sen-
timents, affections, desires or emotions, each the product of the learned association of
certain impressions with other impressions of pleasure or pain in past experience"; *From
Passions to Emotions*, 106.

actions of others.[8] But Dixon credits the Scottish physician and philosopher Thomas Brown (1778–1820) with providing the language for the modern category of the emotions. In his widely read, posthumously published four-volume *Lectures on the Philosophy of the Human Mind* (1820), Brown wrote primarily not of "passions" or "affections" but rather of "emotions," treating them as freestanding psychological states that could be joined together, like atoms, in a "chemistry of the mind."[9] Brown's work anticipated and enabled a proliferation of nineteenth-century scientific writings, coinciding with the emergence of experimental psychology as an independent scientific discipline, that treated the emotions as mechanical, materialistic phenomena, often encompassing nonhuman animals (especially Charles Darwin's *Expressions of the Emotions in Man and Animals* [1872]). Though these physicalist accounts of emotion generated some resistance from Christian writers such as John Henry Newman, the physicalist account of emotion found its boldest expression in the writing of William James, who in an 1884 essay titled "What Is an Emotion?" famously posited that unlike the "standard account" of emotion, in which the mental experience of emotion follows on a particular perception that then gives rise to bodily manifestations, it is rather that "the bodily changes follow directly the PERCEPTION of the exciting fact, and that our feeling of the same changes as they occur is the emotion."[10] It is not, writes James, that "we lose our fortune, are sorry and weep; we meet a bear, are frightened and run; we are insulted by a rival, are angry and strike." Rather, "we feel sorry because we cry, angry because we strike, afraid because we tremble."[11]

Since James's time, psychologists, neuroscientists, and philosophers have offered a wide range of theories about the nature of emotion. While no simple categorization is possible, many of these responses can be considered according to two broad camps, each of which informs different practices and theories within modern mental health care.

Emotions as Feelings of the Body

First, building on nineteenth-century physicalist approaches, many theorists understand emotions as *feelings of the body*. William James's theory of

---

8. Dixon, *From Passions to Emotions*, 65.
9. Dixon, *From Passions to Emotions*, 118.
10. William James, "What Is an Emotion?," *Mind* 34 (1884): 189–90.
11. James, "What Is an Emotion?," 190.

emotion, generally known as the "James-Lange" theory because the Danish psychologist Carl J. Lange published nearly the same observation at the same time, was partially refuted in the 1920s by the experiments of physiologist Walter B. Cannon, who showed that there are too few visceral physiological responses to account for the vast range of human emotional experiences. But updated versions of the physicalist model of emotion continue to influence modern conversation about emotion.[12]

The physicalist model of emotion is deeply intertwined with the machine metaphor and runs deep within particular strains of modern mental health care. If emotions are primarily eruptions in bodily or brain activity, associated with events in the external world only through learned experience and through action-tendencies cultivated by evolutionary adaptation, then at best, emotions can teach us something about our learned experience—about the way that certain perceptions have accrued certain forms of value or disvalue for us over time—or about forms of response that were selected in evolution, or both. If, for instance, I am at the North Carolina State Fair and feel disgust and revulsion when I see corn dogs for sale, I can draw on that experience to think about previous negative experiences with corn dogs (in my case, too many soggy, greasy, lukewarm corn dogs on my elementary school lunch tray). But if emotions are considered *only* as evolved and learned movements of the body or brain, then they can be separated from broader frameworks of moral commitment. Furthermore, I can seek to modify my emotions as I wish. If I like the rush of fear that is associated with recreational activities that push the limit of safety, I can go rock climbing or skydiving. If, on the other hand, I am overwhelmed by anxiety, I can seek to change my emotional experience by changing the way that I think about the problems of my life, or by taking an antidepressant medication (not to mention other nonprescribed substances).

Because of its focus on emotion as the feeling of bodily processes, this phys-

12. Walter B. Cannon, "The James-Lange Theory of Emotions: A Critical Examination and an Alternative Theory," *American Journal of Psychology* 39 (1927): 106–24. Contemporary proponents of the view of emotions as feelings of the body include Robert Zajonc, Michael Gazzaniga, Joseph LeDoux, and Antonio Damasio; see, for example, LeDoux, *The Emotional Brain: The Mysterious Underpinnings of Emotional Life* (New York: Simon & Schuster, 1996), and Antonio Damasio, *The Feeling of What Happens: Body and Emotion in the Making of Consciousness* (San Diego: Harvest, 1999). Silvan Tomkins's affect theory, which we encountered in chapter 3, also generally fits this paradigm. See E. Virginia Demos, ed., *Exploring Affect: The Selected Writings of Silvan S. Tomkins* (Cambridge: Cambridge University Press, 1995).

icalist account of emotion coheres well with the machine metaphor and all five of the problematic presumptions of modern mental health care discussed in chapter 1. Because emotions are linked to the body of individual persons and are biological in nature, this account reinforces individual and self-body dualism. Because they are separable from the core commitments of the self, this account reinforces self-symptom dualism (understanding my emotional experience as something different from the self), technicism (seeking means by which to modify that experience), and commodification (assigning commercial value to those means). Modern mental health care, in its most commodified form, can become a craft for the manipulation and eradication of unwanted emotion. This is particularly true of my own field of psychiatry, which all too commonly displays a medication-first approach to treatment.

Emotions as Engagements with the World

Many psychologists and philosophers of emotion, however, do not agree that emotions are best understood in physicalist terms, as feelings of changes in the body. Emotions also involve judgments and tendencies to action. They have intentionality, in that they are *about* something.[13] They involve judgments, including judgments of salience. And they are associated with action-tendencies. If I am driving on an interstate highway at night and see in my rearview mirror a car following me at a safe distance, I feel little emotional response. But if that car suddenly activates flashing blue lights and a blaring siren, I feel a strong wave of emotion that is inextricably tied to the judgment that I may be in legal trouble and to action-tendencies to look at my speedometer and, unless the car quickly passes me, to pull to the side of the road. (For Black drivers in the United States, given the history of racial discrimination and violence associated with traffic stops, this wave of emotion may be even stronger and more complex.)

There are many variants of the view that emotions are more than bodily

---

13. Drawing on Anthony Kenny, Andrea Scarantino and Ronald de Sousa distinguish between the particular objects and the formal objects of emotion. Particular objects are persons or things to which an emotion is directed, and formal objects are the attributes or states of affairs of those things to which the emotion is a response. For example, if my wife is angry at me for coming home late without calling her to let her know that I would be delayed, I am the particular object of her anger, while my delinquency and poor communication are the formal object. See Andrea Scarantino and Ronald de Sousa, "Emotion," *Stanford Encyclopedia of Philosophy*, September 25, 2018, https://plato.stanford.edu/entries/emotion/.

happenings and that they also entail intentionality, judgments, and action-tendency.[14] Robert Solomon derides what he terms the "myth of the passions," associated in his view with the medieval and Christian tendency to understand emotion as misleading and nonrational, and defends the view that emotions are rational "engagements with the world."[15] Martha Nussbaum, quoting from Marcel Proust, draws on Stoicism to describe emotions as "upheavals of thought."[16] Robert C. Roberts describes emotions as "concern-based construals."[17] Science journalist Daniel Goleman echoed many of these developments in philosophy and psychology in his bestselling *Emotional Intelligence*, in which he argued that the traditional marker of intelligence, IQ, unfairly neglects the emotions and that recognizing, training, and properly deploying emotion constitutes its own form of intelligence.[18]

The view that emotions are (cognitive and rational) engagements with the world, as Solomon writes, is also represented in modern mental health care, especially in the psychotherapies. Early cognitive therapies such as Albert Ellis's rational emotive therapy and Aaron Beck's cognitive therapy (now referred to as cognitive behavioral therapy, or CBT) associated unwanted emotions with particular cognitive appraisals and demonstrated that lasting change in emotional reaction could come with different ways of thinking and acting.[19] Newer third-wave psychotherapies have their own ways of conceiving and formulating emotion. Emotion-focused therapy (EFT) leaders Leslie Greenberg and Jeanne Watson argue that emotions are "an adaptive form of information processing and action preparation that orient people to their environment and promote their well-being, disposing them to act on their behalf in a given situation."[20] They state that "emotions produce biologically based action tendencies that result from appraisals of the situation," both influencing and influenced by cognitive processes.[21] Marsha Linehan, the founder of

14. For a review, see Scarantino and de Sousa, "Emotion."

15. Robert C. Solomon, *The Passions: Emotions and the Meaning of Life*, 2nd ed. (Indianapolis: Hackett, 1993); Solomon, "The Logic of Emotion," *Nous* 11 (1977): 41–49.

16. Martha Nussbaum, *Upheavals of Thought: The Intelligence of Emotions* (New York: Cambridge University Press, 2001).

17. Robert C. Roberts, *Emotion: An Essay in Aid of Moral Psychology* (New York: Oxford University Press, 2003), 64.

18. Daniel Goleman, *Emotional Intelligence: Why It Can Matter More Than IQ* (New York: Bantam Books, 1995).

19. Aaron T. Beck et al., *Cognitive Therapy of Depression* (New York: Guilford, 1979).

20. Leslie S. Greenberg and Jeanne C. Watson, *Emotion-Focused Therapy for Depression* (Washington, DC: American Psychological Association, 2006), 17.

21. Greenberg and Watson, *Emotion-Focused Therapy*, 18.

dialectical behavior therapy (DBT), the most widely accepted psychotherapeutic treatment for borderline personality disorder (BPD), emphasizes that while emotional states are short-lived, lasting for minutes at most, longer-lasting emotional arousal (mood) results when emotional states affect cognitive processes by biasing the way that information is received and remembered and by affecting how we interpret situations in the light of this information. She argues that individuals with BPD tend to have high levels of emotional expression and reactivity but find themselves in "invalidating environments" in which these emotional experiences are met by "erratic, inappropriate, and extreme responses" and in which they are shamed and not taught how to make sense of these experiences and to use them for positive and constructive action. As a result, they lack self-confidence and self-worth, and they lack skills in regulating distressing affects and in navigating complex social situations and interpersonal relationships.[22]

Embodied Signs of Love: Aquinas on the Passions

In the *Summa theologiae*, Thomas Aquinas drew on over fifteen hundred years of philosophical and theological work on the passions to lay out what was, at the time, the most detailed and systematic account of emotion that had ever been written. His analysis of emotion, often referred to as the "Treatise on the Passions," became a benchmark in medieval philosophical thought.[23] Aquinas, like modern physicalists, agrees that the passions are embodied. He holds that passions involving sensory perceptions entail some sort of change in the body—a "corporeal transmutation" (*transmutatio corporalis*; see *STh* IaIIae q. 22 a. 3 *resp.*; *STh* IaIIae q. 22 a. 1 *resp.*)—though this may happen to a greater or lesser degree according to the nature of the passion (see *STh* IaIIae q. 22 a. 2 *ad1*). But he also strongly agrees that passions are forms of engagement with the world, and he notably anticipates the modern rediscovery of the intelligence of emotions. Aquinas also helps us to understand how the passions

22. Marsha Linehan, *Cognitive Behavioral Treatment for Borderline Personality Disorder* (New York: Guilford, 1993), 44–45, 49, 51–52.

23. In this section, I am drawing on three recently published studies of Aquinas's view of passion and emotion: Nicholas Lombardo, *The Logic of Desire: Aquinas on Emotion* (Washington, DC: Catholic University of America Press, 2011); Robert Miner, *Thomas Aquinas on the Passions: A Study of* Summa Theologiae 1a2ae 22–48 (New York: Cambridge University Press, 2009); Diana Fritz Cates, *Aquinas on the Emotions: A Religious-Ethical Inquiry* (Washington, DC: Georgetown University Press, 2009).

fit into the journey of the human wayfarer to God. He does this, specifically, by arguing that the passions hinge, above all else, on love.

Love, Desire, Delight: The Triad of Approach

As discussed above, Aquinas argues that we are by nature creatures who perceive what is good for us, who long to attain what we perceive to be good for us, and who then move toward that attainment. This is as natural to us as the fact that our lungs exchange oxygen and carbon dioxide, or that our kidneys filter electrolytes. The basic movement of this is as follows:

$$LOVE \; (amor) \rightarrow DESIRE \; (concupiscentia) \rightarrow$$
$$DELIGHT \; (delectatio) \; or \; JOY \; (gaudium)$$

First comes love, when we are inclined toward a person or a thing that we judge to be good for us. Love in this sense covers a wide ground. There is the kind of love that I feel for a ripe heirloom tomato that has just been picked off the vine in late summer in North Carolina. I do not love the tomato for its own sake—after all, I am going to eat it—but for the way that it will nourish my body and bring pleasure to me, as well as for the way that it manifests the care and skill of those who have grown it. Following Aristotle, Aquinas refers to this love—the love of something because of how it will serve us—as gratification-love (amor concupiscentiae; STh IaIIae q. 26 a. 4 resp.).[24] Sometimes we can love people in this way also—not for their own sake but because of how they can serve our own interests.

But love extends beyond the self. Beyond gratification-love, there is the kind of love that we feel toward other people to whom, because we love them, we wish that good will come. Aquinas refers to this as friendship-love. Friendship-love also covers a wide ground. There is a certain kind of love that I feel for colleagues at work, another that I feel for fellow church members, another that I feel for my wife, another that I feel for my children, another that I feel for extended family members whom I see once or twice a year at most. But the common thread in all of these forms of love, though they differ widely in intensity, is that I am in some way joined to those whom I love, so that their

---

24. While a more literal translation of amor concupiscentiae is "love of desire," I have chosen "gratification-love" because this term more clearly denotes that this form of love is specifically oriented to the pleasure or good of the self, not of the other.

good is somehow *my* good and their suffering *my* suffering. They have, in a real sense, become internal to me. Aquinas states that love is complacency in good (*complacentia boni*). I do not love my wife, my children, my work colleagues, or any true friends simply because of the benefit and pleasure that they can bring to me. I love them for their own sake; I desire benefit and pleasure for *them*, and because I have taken place with them and they are in me, their benefit and pleasure are, in a real sense, mine (see *STh* IaIIae q. 26 a. 4).[25]

For Aquinas, love is the fountainhead from which all our emotional life and all our action flows. Human beings are natural and inveterate lovers. As long as we are perceiving anything at all, we will perceive certain people or things as good for us, or as good in themselves and linked to us in relationship, and this apprehension of the other *as good* generates love. Our loves may, of course, be misguided. We may perceive that a certain person is good for us, when he is not, or that a certain community of friends is healthy for us, when they are not. But we are still lovers. The guiding question for all of us is not *whether* we love but *whom and what* we love.

Love is the fountainhead, but it quickly gives rise to desire (*concupiscentia*). Love and desire are often experienced together, and indeed they are two sides of the same coin. If love is the affective union sparked by the apprehension that a person or thing is good, desire is the longing to attain real union with that person or thing. If I love a summer heirloom tomato, I desire to taste it, or at least to look at and feel it. If I love my work colleagues, I desire to be with them (at least at certain times) and that good may come to them. If I love wisdom, I desire to attain it. Desire is the natural feeling of being drawn to someone whom or something that we love and that is not immediately present to us (*STh* IaIIae q. 30 a. 2 resp.). Some desires, such as for food and drink, are natural in that they relate to the basic needs of the body. Other desires—most of our desires, in fact—are acquired, in that we have learned, through teaching and practice, to value certain things or people as good for us (*STh* IaIIae q. 30 a. 3). These acquired desires are in principle unending, both because we can continue to desire more and more of a certain thing (e.g., money) and because we can desire an infinite number of things (*STh* IaIIae q. 30 a. 4).

Just as we can love people and things that are not good for us, so also we can desire people and things that are not good for us. Desire can get us into trouble. But desire is also a central building block of a healthy and whole life. Desire is an embodied response by which we are drawn to move toward what

25. Both gratification-love and friendship-love are examples of what in chapter 2 I called "ordinary love" (*amor*).

we love (*STh* IaIIae q. 30 a. 1). The key to a successful journey is not to ignore or to numb our desires but rather to learn to love and to desire life-giving people and life-giving things.

Aquinas distinguishes two forms of desire: simple desire (*concupiscentia*) and desire that has to do with a good that seems somehow difficult to attain. This latter form of desire comes in two varieties, hope (*spes*) and despair (*desperatio*). Let us consider, trivially, the example of the summer heirloom tomato. If I am at a picnic in July and there is a platter of freshly sliced North Carolina tomatoes in front of me on a serving table, then I am filled with simple desire to reach out for a slice. But let us say that I am driving to the picnic, thinking of ripe tomatoes, and am not sure whether anyone will be bringing them. If I desire tomatoes and think that after arriving I might find them, I feel not only desire but *hope* that the tomatoes will be present. Hope, for Aquinas, is desire for a good that seems possible, though somehow difficult, to attain (*STh* IaIIae q. 23 a. 2).[26] But let us imagine now that I arrive at the picnic and find, to my dismay, that no one has brought tomatoes. At least for the time, my desire is frustrated. Fresh summer tomatoes are unattainable, and I feel despair (*desperatio*), the passion associated with longing for something that seems impossible to attain.

Love is the fountainhead that gives rise to desire. Desire moves us to pursue what we love. When we attain what or whom we love, we feel pleasure or delight (*delectatio*). Delight is the passion associated with loving something, desiring it, and then attaining it; it is repose in the beloved (*STh* IaIIae q. 31 a. 1 ad2). Just as our loves and desires are highly diverse, so also our pleasures and delights are highly diverse. There are purely sensible delights that correspond to purely sensible loves, as when I enjoy the warmth of an extra sweatshirt on a cool autumn evening. There is delight that corresponds to good that comes to someone whom I love, as when I learn that a friend has received an attractive job offer. There is the delight of being with someone I love, as when I see my wife on returning home from work, or after one of us has been out of town. And then there is the less concrete but very real delight of viewing a sunset and contemplating the beauty of creation, or of grasping a difficult and elusive concept for the first time, or of seeing in someone an inner beauty that goes far beyond initial and outward appearances. This higher form of delight, which requires not only the senses but a deeper apprehension of truth and beauty, is joy (*gaudium*).

26. The passion of hope is distinct from the theological virtue of hope, which we will consider in chapter 8.

Like love and desire, we can take pleasure in the wrong things and the wrong people. Indeed, we all do just this, more often than we would like. But Aquinas is more focused on the *goodness* of our loves, desires, and pleasures— of the many, simple, everyday ways that we get it right. Our everyday lives are characterized by the rhythms of love, desire, and pleasure.

Revulsion, Aversion, Sadness: The Triad of Avoidance

The positive triad of love, desire, and delight or joy has a necessary negative counterpart. If we love those people or things that we judge to be good for us, or good in general, then what about those people or things that we judge to be *harmful* to us? For Aquinas, this inverse negative triad proceeds as follows:

REVULSION *(odium)* → AVERSION *(fuga or abominatio)* →
SADNESS *(tristitia)* or PAIN *(dolor)*

Revulsion *(odium)* is the negative counterpart to love. It is not the absence of love but rather the way that love positions itself with regard to a person or thing who is judged as harmful, just to the degree (and no more) that the object is judged as harmful.[27] Indeed, Aquinas describes love as the cause of revulsion: "nothing is [experienced as revulsive], save through being contrary to a suitable thing which is loved" (*STh* IaIIae q. 29 a. 2 *resp.*). Indeed, revulsion is always parasitic on love. We experience a person or thing as revulsive only because we first love the good that is threatened by the presence of that person or thing. The deeper the love that we feel for the good that is threatened, the deeper the revulsion that we will experience toward whatever threatens that good (*STh* IaIIae q. 29 a. 3 *resp.*). Revulsion, then, is a sign of love.

27. *Odium* is often translated as "hatred," but I offer "revulsion" instead. Hatred, in ordinary language, connotes not only a judgment that a person or thing is harmful but also a desire that the thing itself not exist, as when we speak of "hate crimes." But Aquinas's *odium* covers a broader ground. *Odium* is simply the judgment that a thing is harmful to a person's life: "love is a certain harmony of the appetite with that which is apprehended as suitable; while *odium* is dissonance of the appetite from that which is apprehended as repugnant and hurtful [*repugnans et corruptivum*]." It does not, for Aquinas, connote an overwhelming desire to destroy the harmful thing; one might choose to flee instead. Nor does it imply that the harmful thing is absolutely evil; one might be drawn in love toward and also repelled from the same object. So while a more literal translation would be "odiousness" or simply "odium," I have chosen the more familiar "revulsion" over "hatred." See *STh* IaIIae q. 29 a. 1 *resp.*

Having judged a person or a thing to be harmful for us or to be an obstacle to our good—having internalized it as a harm—we then naturally feel a desire to distance ourselves from that person or thing. This emotion, which is the converse of desire, Aquinas calls aversion (*fuga* or *abominatio*) (*STh* IaIIae q. 23 a. 4 *resp.*). It is the action-orientation that goes along with the apprehension of an evil. As with desire for a good, Aquinas holds that there can be simple aversion. Let us say that a faculty member with whom I work is known to be caustic and abrasive with colleagues. Though this colleague may be excellent in some aspects of his craft, in that moment I judge him to be evil *for me* (revulsion, *odium*). This is accompanied by an action-tendency to avoid contact with him (aversion, *fuga*). I am polite in our interactions, but I do not seek him out for conversation and generally try to stay out of his way.

But as with positive desire, there are more complex forms of aversion. Let us imagine, for example, that my immediate supervisor is promoted away from his or her position and that this caustic, abrasive colleague is named one of two finalists for the open position. As I think about the possibility that this colleague may move from being a distant coworker to my immediate supervisor, I appropriately feel the passion of fear (*timor*), which for Aquinas is the passion associated with an approaching evil (a difficult supervisor) that is not yet present but difficult to avoid. But let us imagine then that I am filled with resolve. I will speak to the search committee with my concerns. I will try to form a constructive working relationship with this person if he is named to the post. In the worst case, I will look for another job. In that case, fear (the passion associated with an approaching evil that seems impossible to avoid) gives way to daring (*audacia*), the passion associated with an approaching evil that can be overcome (*STh* IaIIae q. 23 a. 4 *resp.*).

But let us further imagine that, unfortunately, my worst fears are realized. This colleague is promoted to be my supervisor, and his abrasive nature soon leads to ugly interpersonal dynamics in the entire team. In this case, I no longer fear that this person might become my supervisor. He already is. Rather, I feel some combination of the passions of sorrow (*tristitia*) and pain (*dolor*)—the passions associated with the ongoing presence of an evil.

But for Aquinas, that is not the end. I leave work each day tired and embittered but also with the belief that the situation can be changed. I resolve to work within my organization's broader leadership structure to make my concerns heard. I speak with like-minded colleagues, and we agree to work together for common reforms. In this case, sensing that the evil (my supervisor's oppressive leadership) can be overcome with effort, I feel the passion of anger (*ira*), which for Aquinas is the passion associated with the sustained presence of an evil for which one has the hope of overcoming. But let us say, finally, that this comes to nothing. My pleas to superiors are rebuffed, and my work with colleagues fails. Things get worse and worse. I look for another job but do not find one, and I cannot afford simply to resign. In this case, I feel weighed down by intense sorrow—even to the point of what we might today call depression.

The full scope of Aquinas's treatment of the passions can be summarized in table 5.

Table 5. *Aquinas's Classification of the Passions*

Concupiscible (good or evil apprehended as such)		**Irascible** (apprehended as arduous or difficult to obtain or to avoid)
With respect to **intention** (the object as apprehended with relevance to the subject [Ia q. 78 a. 4]):	With respect to the **object itself**:	
Good Object appraised as good: **love (*amor*)**—"connaturality in respect of good," "complacency in good" (IaIIae q. 25 a. .2) "affective union" (IaIIae q. 25 a. 2 *ad2*)	Absent good: **desire (*concupiscentia*)**	Seems possible to obtain (approach [IaIIae q. 23 a. 2]): **hope (*spes*)** Seems impossible to obtain (withdrawal [IaIIae q. 23 a. 2]): **despair (*desperatio*)**
	Rest/repose in present good: **delight (*delectatio*) joy (*gaudium*)** "real union" (IaIIae q. 25 a. 2 *ad2*)	**n/a** (if present, the good is no longer arduous or difficult)

Evil Object appraised as evil: **revulsion (*odium*)**	Absent evil: **aversion (*fuga* or *abominatio*)**	Seems impossible to overcome (withdrawal [IaIIae q. 23 a. 2]): **fear (*timor*)** Seems possible to overcome (approach [IaIIae q. 23 a. 2]): **daring (*audacia*)**
	Suffering of present evil: **sadness (*tristitia*) or pain (*dolor*)**	Present evil with hope of overcoming (approach [23.3]): **anger (*ira*)** (no contrary, as present evil with no hope of overcoming would simply be intensified sorrow).

Emotions in the Context of the Journey

Though he wrote well before modern debates on the nature of emotion, Aquinas's account of the emotions resonates with both modern accounts of emotion—emotions as feelings of the body and emotions as engagements with the world—and places each in the context of a journey. First, the emotions (*passiones*) are always responses of being acted on by whomever or whatever is the object of the emotion, and Aquinas holds that this always involves a bodily change. Unlike Descartes, Aquinas did not believe that the mind was a separate substance from the body. Rather, for Aquinas, when the mind or soul loves, desires, abhors, and fears a person or thing—or experiences other emotions—this is inscribed in the body insofar as basic psychological faculties such as sensation, perception, and appraisal of danger are involved.[28]

28. Though Aquinas affirms in *STh* IaIIae q. 22 that "passion is properly to be found wherever there is corporeal transmutation," Nicholas Lombardo observes that Aquinas uses the broader term *affectus* (affection) to cover nonsensory movements of intellect and will that do not necessarily involve bodily change and that are not properly passions. God's love is one such example (*STh* Ia q. 20 a. 1 *ad1*), as perhaps are some human experiences of joy (*STh* IaIIae q. 31 aa. 3-4). Even in the case of joy, though, the body may be affected by a kind of overflow of the soul. Lombardo, *The Logic of Desire*, 75-93.

Consistent with physicalist accounts of emotion, Aquinas also implies that in some cases, when the body is not working properly, emotions may malfunction. We may have an emotional experience of love, desire, delight, hope, despair, revulsion, fear, daring, sadness, or anger that does not correspond to anything in the lived world. It comes from the body's dysfunction, not from the environment. Or we might have emotional experiences that are radically disproportionate to the lived world, in a way that cannot be accounted for by past or present experience. In these cases, our emotions are absurd, in that they do not mean anything other than that the body is not functioning properly.[29] There is room in Aquinas's thought for the view that sometimes emotions are just malfunctions of the body and should be understood and treated as such.

But for Aquinas, the emotions are generally not absurd, nor are they only bodily disturbances to which we secondarily assign meaning. Rather, most of the time, emotions are signs of whom and what we love. If I feel drawn toward a person or thing—if, that is, I feel desire, *concupiscentia*—then love of some sort stands behind that desire. If I fear a person or thing, then I can infer that I judge something or someone I love to be threatened by the approaching evil. If I am angry, Aquinas encourages me to consider not only the perceived evil that is currently smothering me but also the relationships with those people and things that I love—including me—that are left unfulfilled as long as the evil is present. In short, in most cases, emotions are signposts for the journey that help to orient us to whom and what we love.

Understanding emotions as signs of whom and what we love is the first step toward refusing the sort of focus on symptoms that leads to technicism and commodification in modern mental health care. Let us think, for example, about the experience of major depression. If I am depressed, then certain strains of modern psychiatry would encourage me to understand my experience as a collection of symptoms—poor sleep, poor energy, thoughts of suicide, and so on—and to seek any treatment that would effectively reduce these symptoms. This technical approach to mental health treatment may well be helpful in reducing certain symptoms, but it has little to contribute to what I am to do with my life once these symptoms have become less intense.

---

29. This follows from Aquinas's affirmation in *STh* Ia q. 84 aa. 7–8 that the use of reason can be hindered through indisposition of the body, as well as his affirmation that individuals with certain forms of cognitive impairment and mental illness are not morally culpable for their behavior—for example, *STh* IIaIIae q. 45 a. 5 *ad3*; IIIa q. 68 a. 12 *ad2*.

On the other hand, a wayfaring perspective would encourage someone who is depressed to discern *from his or her experience* what loves are being blocked by a perceived evil. Perhaps a root of depression is painful childhood trauma: what is loved is one's own childhood self, wounded and defiled by another who remains present in experience and memory. Perhaps a root of depression is chronic homelessness: what is loved is the seemingly distant experience of a safe and secure home of one's own. Perhaps a root of depression is rejection by one's family on the basis of religious conversion or sexual identity: what is loved is one's own kin, now distant and unapproachable. Perhaps a root of depression is loneliness on a college campus: what is loved is the simple experience of being known and treasured, not for performance but simply for one's own sake. Or, more likely, perhaps depression has multiple roots, spanning multiple periods of life, that point to an intertwined tree of loves. Discerning these loves is the good and ordinary work of psychotherapy, properly done. It is also the good and ordinary work of spiritual direction, pastoral counseling, and Christian formation in the church.

There are two important qualifications for this view that emotions are signs of love. First, Aquinas was clear that even when emotions are signs of love—even when they make sense and are not absurd—they can still overwhelm normal human capacities for psychological function. In his discussion of the passions of pain and sorrow, he comes close to describing what would today be described as catatonia:

> If, on the other hand, the strength of the evil be such as to exclude the hope of evasion, then even the interior movement of the afflicted soul is absolutely hindered, so that it cannot turn aside either this way or that. Sometimes even the external movement of the body is paralyzed, so that a man becomes completely stupefied. (*STh* IaIIae q. 37 a. 2 *resp.*)

In cases such as this, when the psychological and physical functions that would normally orient the life of the wayfarer are frozen, then practices of care for the body—including medication, in many cases—play an important role. In an intriguing part of the "Treatise on the Passions," Aquinas considers various remedies for sorrow and pain—which, as discussed above, resemble our modern conception of depression, not least in the way that Aquinas so closely links together the experiences of psychological and physical pain. Aquinas offers a remarkably holistic description of remedies that could serve as a model for many modern-day treatment plans for depression. Two of his remedies are what we would now consider cognitive or psychological: he argues that sorrow and pain are assuaged by pleasure of any sort and by the contemplation of truth, especially of future happiness (*STh* IaIIae q. 38 aa. 1, 4). With these remedies, Aquinas anticipates modern cognitive-behavioral approaches that focus on engaging in pleasurable activities (behavioral activation) and altering one's structure of belief (cognitive reframing). One of his remedies is clearly relational: he argues that pain and sorrow are assuaged by the sympathy of friends, because "when one is in pain, it is natural that the sympathy of a friend should afford consolation." Following Aristotle, he gives two reasons for this:

> The first is because, since sorrow has a depressing effect, it is like a weight whereof we strive to unburden ourselves: so that when a man sees others saddened by his own sorrow, it seems as though others were bearing the burden with him, striving, as it were, to lessen its weight; wherefore the load of sorrow becomes lighter for him: something like what occurs in the carrying of bodily burdens. The second and better reason is because when a man's friends condole with him, he sees that he is loved by them, and this affords him pleasure. (*STh* IaIIae q. 38 a. 3 *resp.*)

Finally, Aquinas offers two remedies for pain and sorrow that clearly lodge in the body. First, he argues that pain and sorrow can be assuaged by tears and groans (*lacrimae et gemitus*), "because a hurtful thing hurts yet more if we keep it shut up, because the soul is more intent on it: whereas if it be allowed to escape, the soul's intention is dispersed as it were on outward things, so that the inward sorrow is lessened" (*STh* IaIIae q. 38 a. 2 *resp.*). Second, he argues that pain and sorrow can be assuaged by "sleep and baths" because "sorrow, by reason of its specific nature, is repugnant to the vital movement of the body; and consequently whatever restores the bodily nature to its due state of vital movement, is opposed to sorrow and assuages it" (*STh* IaIIae q. 39 a. 5 *resp.*). Throughout this discussion, Aquinas presupposes that sorrow and pain are serving their proper functions of reflecting the ongoing, sustained presence of an evil that thwarts love; sorrow and pain are meaningful and not absurd. But the *response* to sorrow and pain must be holistic and, in modern terms, biopsychosocial.

The second qualification is that the fact that emotions are usually signs of love, in that they are not meaningless or absurd, does not mean that for that reason alone they are trustworthy guides to a well-lived life. Emotions may be truthful signs of whom or what we love, but, of course, our loves may themselves be disordered. Right this minute, not to mention many thousands of previous times while writing this book, I feel a strong desire to click on my internet browser to a website that would take me away from the work of writing—likely to a news site like the *Washington Post* or the *New York Times* but possibly to a social media site or my email application. In Aquinas's framework, this desire is a truthful sign of my loves in this moment and is most likely a compound of desire and aversion: desire to be passively carried away with someone else's thinking, to be in the know, or to be entertained; and aversion to the hard work of writing that requires me to sit with myself and with my thoughts and to confront the limits of my ability as a writer and scholar. The former is easy and pleasurable, the latter uncomfortable and exposing. But I have learned from hard experience that the pleasures afforded by these internet sites, including my email, are fleeting and that ordering my life toward being ever connected and in the know leaves me in a hyperalert, distracted haze, unable to focus attention on hard intellectual work or even to sit comfortably in silence without reaching for my iPhone. My own journey requires attending to *all* of my loves and learning to foster and to nurture those loves that are more life-giving. For me that entails the ability to say no to news sites in order to stay focused on this project. It also entails the ability to say no to this project at times so that I can focus on other commitments that require my full attention, such as commitments to my family and to my patients.

We see, in summary, that Aquinas offers a rich account of emotion that encourages us to interpret our emotions in the context of a journey. In some cases, when there is a malfunction of the body's emotion-generating function, emotions can be absurd or disproportionate to context. In these cases—as, for example, in the context of many forms of delirium or bipolar mania—the emotions do not signify anything other than that the body is not working properly. Aquinas's approach would support somatic or pharmacological treatment approaches that are focused on restoring the body's ability to maintain these psychological functions. But the default approach for Aquinas is not to assume that emotions are absurd and that unwanted emotions are simply objects to be technologically manipulated. Rather, he encourages us to interpret emotions as signs of whom or what we love—*not only* bodily feelings *but also* engagements with the world. Anxiety, depression, PTSD, cravings for addicting substances, cravings and aversions associated with disordered eating—all of these experiences are at least in part reflections of what, in the present, is loved, and there is much to learn from the exercise of tracing these loves to their source.

But beyond simply treating the emotions diagnostically, as ways to understand the structure of our loves, emotions can be a powerful resource for a full and well-lived life—depending on the loves to which they are ordered. It is here that the image of the journey is centrally important. If our loves are ordered to goods and goals that, however appropriate in their own right, distract us from what leads to our participation in blessing—such as my penchant for seeking distraction in social media and the *Washington Post* when I am writing—then we will experience emotion as in some way an enemy to be conquered, an unreliable guide. But if our loves are ordered to what is life-giving, then we can lean into our emotions as reliable guides to what is life-giving for us. Aquinas closely follows Augustine's dictum that

> the right will is, therefore, well-directed love, and the wrong will is ill-directed love. Love, then, yearning to have what is loved, is desire; and having and enjoying it, is joy; feeling what is opposed to it, is fear; and feeling what is opposed to it, when it has befallen it, it is sadness. Now these motions are evil if the love is evil; good if the love is good.[30]

For Aquinas, as for Augustine, the goal of the journey is not elimination of emotions or technological mastery of the emotions but rather training the emotions so that they can be faithful signs of what is good and life-giving for us as we pursue participation in blessing.

30. Augustine, *City of God* 4.7.

CHAPTER 8

From Constraint to Freedom

....

We Are Guided and Helped on the Journey

> For it was you who formed my inward parts;
>   you knit me together in my mother's womb.
> I praise you, for I am fearfully and wonderfully made.
>   Wonderful are your works;
>   that I know very well.
>
> *—Psalm 139:13–14*

So far in this exploration of the process of the journey, following Aquinas's order of presentation in the *Summa theologiae*, I have discussed intellect and will as the enabling capacities of action, and emotions as embodied signs of whom and what we love. We journey as wayfarers not simply as thinking and choosing beings but also as passionate, feeling animals, guided by the constant cycles of love-desire-pleasure and, its inverse, revulsion-aversion-sadness.

Developing his argument, Aquinas then clarifies that the powers of intellect and will and the associated passions do not operate arbitrarily or randomly over time. As humans, we do not operate like computers that may at any point be reset to factory default settings, erasing all traces of previous use. Rather, as embodied creatures, there is a pattern and continuity to our thinking, acting, and feeling. These patterns of continuity both facilitate our freedom in the journey toward participation in blessing and undergird many of our frustrations and challenges. Following Aristotle, Aquinas refers to these patterns of thinking, acting, and feeling as habit (*habitus*).[1]

---

1. Following Aristotle, Aquinas holds that habits are qualities of lasting disposition and distinguishes two species of habit: habits that dispose something well or ill according to its nature, and habits that dispose something well or ill according to its end. The former

Embodied Dispositions to Action: Aquinas on Habit

Habits for Aquinas are stable dispositions to act in certain ways in response to certain contexts, and it is important to note that for Aquinas, "habit" encompasses a broader range of human life than our modern ordinary English term "habit" often connotes. We often speak of habits in a negative sense: a habit of smoking, or a habit of cursing, or my own habit of checking websites for distraction when I am writing. Indeed, these are habits in Aquinas's sense. But so is any pattern of thought, feeling, or behavior that disposes us to respond consistently to particular contexts. To borrow a well-known example from philosopher Anthony Kenny, when I walk into a room of people speaking English, I am easily able to join in the conversation. I have acquired, through training and practice, the disposition to speak English when others are speaking English.[2] I have the habit of English-speaking. But to my dismay, when I walk into a room where people are speaking to each other in Spanish, I can catch only fragments of words and phrases. I have not acquired the habit of Spanish-speaking. Similarly, riding a bicycle, swimming freestyle, and driving a car all come easily for me, because I have acquired the habits that dispose me to be able to perform these activities. I am conspicuously *lacking* in other habits, such as swinging a golf club, hitting jump shots, and dancing. Habits properly reside in the life (soul) of the person and involve the body insofar as the soul forms the body.[3]

---

have become known as *entitative* habits, the latter as *operative* habits. Health (*sanitas*), for Aquinas, is an entitative habit, in that it names the disposition of something to its nature. In theory, using Aquinas's Aristotelian distinction, it would be possible to pursue a lasting disposition to health without reference to the end (participation in blessing) toward which humans are directed. But as I have argued in more detail elsewhere, Aquinas makes little use of this distinction in the *Summa* and is far more focused on the operative habits, which dispose us to act in particular ways for good or for ill. In fact, it is not clear in Aquinas's account how one would ever recognize an entitative habit of health apart from reference to the operation of the creature: a healthy human, especially a mentally healthy human, is one who does what healthy humans do, which is to act in a way that is consistent with the pursuit of *beatitudo*. See Warren Kinghorn, "Medicating the Eschatological Body: Psychiatric Technology for Christian Wayfarers," ThD diss., Duke University, 2011, 361-66. For discussion of entitative and operative habits, see Robert Edward Brennan, *Thomistic Psychology: A Philosophic Analysis of the Nature of Man* (New York: Macmillan, 1941), 29-31, 262-63.

2. Anthony Kenny, introduction to volume 22 of Blackfriars edition of the *Summa theologiae*; quoted in introduction to Brian Davies, ed., *Thomas Aquinas: Contemporary Philosophical Perspectives* (New York: Oxford University Press, 2002), 15-16.

3. Aquinas argues that operative habits are properly in the soul—that is, the life of the acting person—but that "they can be secondarily in the body: to wit, in so far as the body

Habits are the grooves inscribed in our patterns of thinking and acting, through a combination of innate capacity and repeated practice.[4] Nearly all humans are born with the capacity to acquire any language, but no human who is alive can speak every human language. We are born, instead, into a community of speakers of a particular language (or, in some cases, a handful of languages), and we develop habits of speaking the particular languages into which we are formed. Habit in this sense stands between natural capacity and act. Language-speaking is a natural capacity of human beings as a whole, unlike in dogs and horses, even though infants are born unable to form words, and some humans, often in the context of intellectual disability or neuro-cognitive disorders, do not display speech. But learning to speak a language requires training, modeling, and extensive practice, and this disposition to speak a particular language (habit) is required for the practice of *speaking* the language fluently (act). Our personalities and characters take shape through the habits that form within us.

Habits for Aquinas involve every aspect of who we are and are key to journeying well. Aquinas taught that God has created humans with the innate capacities for intellect and will and the capacity for purposeful and intentional action. He also taught that as embodied beings who know first through the senses, we are *passionate* beings who are drawn to others in love and who participate in a rich emotional life that stands as a sign of whom, or what, we love. But placing these rich capacities in the context of a journey requires the formation of habit. I may have (as I do) the physical and psychological capacity to fly a twin-engine airplane from North Carolina to Mexico and even may have a well-maintained, fueled airplane at the ready, but if I have not acquired the skill of flying, through long study and practice (which I have not), all of my innate capacity and access to aviation will be useless. I need to develop the *habit* of flying in order to be able to do so. Otherwise, I cannot make the journey. In the same way, the capacities for intellect, will, and emotion must be formed into grooves of knowing and acting that will enable us to pursue our journey toward *beatitudo*. The key to mental health, in Aquinas's account, is not innate capacity (though that is important), or even behavior alone (though that is important also), but rather the habits that form in us over the course of a lifetime.[5]

---

is disposed and enabled with promptitude to help in the operations of the soul" (*STh* IaIIae q. 50 a. 1 *resp.*).

4. See *STh* IaIIae q. 51.

5. Ezra Sullivan analyzes Aquinas's treatment of habit in considerably more detail than I have provided here, distinguishing among eight ways that Aquinas deploys the term *habitus*. *Habitus* may connote, for Aquinas, "a stable disposition toward action that comes from

Ann and Dave, whose story we encountered in the introduction to this book, spoke of the importance of developing these habitual grooves of thinking and acting in their own family's experience with depression. Dave, reflecting not only on his family but on his work as a pastor, speaks of working with a group of congregants in their mideighties, for whom "the threat of disease and death is more real than for most of us." The group recites Psalm 23, "The LORD is my shepherd," often. Dave says that a pastor colleague once taught him that "it's important to rehearse the truth and promises of God 'in the daylight' so that we might remember some of them in the darkness." Repeatedly reciting as a group "even though I walk through the darkest valley, I fear no evil" (Ps. 23:4) forms those facing their own death to remember that "the Shepherd is with the psalmist 'in the valley,' not waiting for him on the other side."[6]

Aquinas goes to great length to describe habits that help the wayfarer toward *beatitudo*, which he calls virtue (*virtus*), and habits that detract from the wayfarer's journey toward *beatitudo*, which he calls vice (*vitium*). Aquinas defines virtue, following his predecessors, as "a good quality of the mind, by which we live righteously, of which no one can make bad use, which God works in us, without us" (*STh* IaIIae q. 55 a. 4 *obj1*). He clarifies that virtue, as a perfection of the human powers of action and choice, is a perfection of habit. For Aquinas, virtues are embodied dispositions to action that are consistent with the journey to *beatitudo*, and vices are habits that get in the way of this journey.

The Virtues as Helps for the Journey

In ordinary language, "virtue" is often associated with moral scrupulosity and with purity. To call an activity "virtuous" is, more often than not, to damn it with praise: it is a good act, but *too* good, perhaps done for show or to prove the

---

possessing something entirely extrinsic to oneself," such as clothing; "a stable disposition derived from 'general nature,'" such as health; "a stable disposition derived from individual nature," such as individual dispositions due to genetic variation; "a stable disposition acquired in a nonvolitional way," such as language acquisition and accent; "an acquired and stable disposition of one's soul" directed to properly human acts, such as intellectual and moral virtue; "the supernatural entitative habit of grace"; the "non-acquired, stable, supernatural, voluntary dispositions" of the theological and infused moral virtues; and the gifts of the Holy Spirit, which are dispositions "primarily activated by God moving man freely." See Ezra Sullivan, *Habits and Holiness: Ethics, Theology, and Biopsychology* (Washington, DC: Catholic University of America Press, 2021), 28–34.

6. Comments delivered at a congregational gathering, May 1, 2016.

goodness of the actor. "Virtue signaling" is to portray oneself as good and pure, even if that is not the case. The term evokes judgmentalism, Victorian sexual morals, and holier-than-thou purity. For that reason, with rare exceptions, modern mental health clinicians often avoid the language of virtue in their work.[7]

To interpret virtue in this way, however, is to misunderstand what Aquinas meant by virtue and also to disregard the power of virtue for thinking about the wayfarer's journey toward God. Indeed, Aquinas would not have understood these modern uses of "virtue" to represent virtue at all. "Virtue signaling," insofar as it connotes a desire to convince others of one's virtue and makes the perception of others a primary goal, is not virtue at all but rather an example of the vices of dissimulation (*simulatio*), hypocrisy (*hypocrisis*), and boasting (*iactantia*), which are contrary to the virtue of justice.[8] In the same way, someone who is fixated on purity (e.g., in a sexual sense) so as to avoid disgraceful action is not fully virtuous but rather is feeling the passion of shame (*verecundia*) in an effort to maintain continence (*continentia*). The word "virtue" has been poisoned for modern mental health conversations, because it is often used to signify what Aquinas would have called vice.

The virtues, for Aquinas, are the grooves of thinking, feeling, and acting that enable us to move toward what is good and freeing for us—to move, that is, toward God and toward *beatitudo*—with ease and pleasure. While rules remain important, the virtues are not fundamentally about following rules. They are about becoming the kind of people who think, feel, and act in life-giving

7. Christopher Peterson and Martin Seligman (*Character Strengths and Virtues: A Handbook and Classification* [New York: Oxford University Press, 2004]) engage the concept of virtue, but only as a metalevel way to classify character strengths, which are the primary focus of their project to assemble a "manual of the sanities." Blaine Fowers (*Virtue and Psychology: Pursuing Excellence in Ordinary Practices* [Washington, DC: American Psychological Association, 2005]), following Aristotle, argues for virtue as a central organizing principle for psychology. Unfortunately, most uses of virtue in the psychology and psychiatry literature in the past two decades have followed Peterson's and Seligman's approach, which makes very little use of classical virtue theory, and few have followed Fowers's model. I have critiqued the philosophical and political basis of Peterson's and Seligman's approach in Warren Kinghorn, "The Politics of Virtue: An Aristotelian-Thomistic engagement with the VIA Classification of Character Strengths," *Journal of Positive Psychology* 12 (2017): 436-46.

8. *STh* IaIIae qq. 111-12. Aquinas, for example, argues that "the hypocrite in simulating a virtue regards it as his end, not in respect of its existence, as though he wished to have it, but in respect of appearance, since he wishes to seem to have it. Hence his hypocrisy is not opposed to that virtue [that he is portraying], but to truth, inasmuch as he wishes to deceive men with regard to that virtue. And he performs acts of that virtue, not as intending them for their own sake, but instrumentally, as signs of that virtue, wherefore his hypocrisy has not, on that account, a direct opposition to that virtue." See *STh* IaIIae q. 111 a. 3 *ad1*.

ways even *without* rules, because it is in our nature to do so. The virtues enable freedom; they allow us to journey wholeheartedly and well.[9]

Aquinas names three broad types of virtue, which overlap with one another to some degree. There are, first, the virtues of knowing, or intellectual virtues, which are oriented to what is true. Second, there are the virtues of acting, or moral virtues, which are oriented to what is good. Third, there are virtues of knowing and acting that cannot be acquired by human effort alone and must be infused directly by God; these are the theological virtues. All are necessary for the wayfarer's journey to God.

Virtues of Knowing

Aquinas first described several dispositions that have to do with knowing what is true. Though we will not engage this discussion in detail (see table 6), he describes several different types of knowing. There are two forms of knowing, he taught, that are basic to the others and that are difficult if not impossible to corrupt: understanding of first principles of logic, such as the principle of noncontradiction (*intellectus*), and understanding of first principles of ethics, such that good is to be done and evil is to be avoided (*synderesis*). But every other form of knowing requires practice and discipline to get right. As every first-year college student knows, it takes practice and experience to learn deductive reasoning (*scientia*). As everyone who has learned an art or craft knows, it takes practice and experience to learn how to make something good and beautiful (*ars*).

One of Aquinas's virtues of knowing is closely associated with feeling and acting and is so important to human life that Aquinas, following longstanding tradition, classified it as a cardinal virtue (a core virtue from which other virtues spring). This is the virtue of prudence (*prudentia*), the wisdom to know in any given situation what is to be done. Prudence in Aquinas's use is not, as in our modern use of the term, to act hesitantly and with caution or to rigidly follow a code of propriety. Rather, prudence is the ability to navigate complex

9. Herbert McCabe aptly states that "virtues are dispositions to make choices which make you better able to make choices." See Herbert McCabe, *The Good Life: Ethics and the Pursuit of Happiness* (New York: Continuum, 2005), 29. Servais Pinckaers appropriately remarks that "virtue is not a habitual way of acting, formed by the repetition of material acts and engendering in us a psychological mechanism. It is a personal capacity for action, the fruit of a series of fine actions, a power for progress and perfection." See Servais Pinckaers, *The Sources of Christian Ethics*, trans. Mary Thomas Noble (Washington, DC: Catholic University of America Press, 1995), 364.

relationships, challenges, and situations and to know within oneself what needs to be done. It is the ability to know what to say in a conversation that will bring out the best in someone else. It is the ability to understand what is happening in a group experiencing conflict and to know what needs to be said or done next. Aquinas emphasizes that prudence requires a wholehearted and open stance toward life as it is.[10] Prudence, for example, entails the ability to remember the past while also being open to the present and attentive to the future; an openness to being taught; the ability to grasp subtle connections; and mindful awareness of one's present context (see *STh* IIaIIae q. 49). Much of what modern mental health clinicians hope to cultivate by practicing and recommending mindfulness is contained in Aquinas's account of prudence.[11]

Table 6. *Aquinas's Virtues of Knowing*

Domain	Virtue	Associated Virtues	Associated Vices
Apprehension of truth in itself	Understanding of principles (*intellectus*) (*STh* IaIIae q. 57 a. 2)		
Apprehension of truth as known through a chain of causes	Wisdom (*sapientia*)—understanding of the nature and first cause of things (*STh* IaIIae q. 57 a. 2) Deductive reasoning (*scientia*)—understanding what is last in the genus of knowable matter (*STh* IaIIae q. 57 a. 2)		

10. Josef Pieper, "Prudence," in *The Four Cardinal Virtues: Prudence, Justice, Fortitude, Temperance* (Notre Dame: University of Notre Dame Press, 1966), 1–40
11. Warren Kinghorn, "Presence of Mind: Thomistic Prudence and Contemporary Mindfulness Practices," *Journal for the Society of Christian Ethics* 35 (2015): 83–102.

Domain	Virtue	Associated Virtues	Associated Vices
Right reason about what is to be made (*recta ratio factibilium*)	Craftsmanship (*ars*) (*STh* IaIIae q. 57 a. 3)		
Right reason about what is to be done (*recta ratio agibilium*)	Prudence (*prudentia*)—overlaps with the virtues of acting (*STh* IaIIae q. 57 a. 4)	*Euboulia* (the disposition to take good counsel) (*STh* IIaIIae q. 51 aa. 1–2) *Synesis* (good judgment about practical matters) (*STh* IIaIIae q. 51 a. 3) *Gnome* (wisdom to know when to set rules aside for a higher good) (*STh* IIaIIae q. 51 a. 4)	Imprudence (*imprudentia*) (*STh* IaIIae q. 53) Negligence (*negligentia*)—lack of due solicitude, carelessness (*STh* IIaIIae q. 54) Excessive concern for one's body (*prudentia carnis*) (*STh* IIaIIae 1. 55 a. 1) Craftiness (*astutia*), guile (*dolus*), and fraud (*fraus*)—invoking fabricated means to reach an end (*STh* IIaIIae q. 55 aa. 3–5)

Virtues of Acting

The virtues of knowing, however, cannot stand alone. They are associated with virtues of acting, oriented toward what is good, often referred to as the "moral virtues." Aquinas distinguishes the virtues of acting into three broad categories: virtues of relationship, of which the overarching virtue is justice; virtues of pursuit, of which the overarching virtue is courage; and virtues of self-regulation, of which the overarching virtue is temperance.

Virtues of Relationship

Aquinas gives primacy of place among the virtues of acting to justice, the virtue of establishing and maintaining right relationships among people and between people and God. His treatment of the acts and habits associate with justice is remarkably detailed, focusing on judicial proceedings—justice under the law—but also engaging at length other relationships among people and between people and God (see table 7). Aquinas understood that journeying well toward *beatitudo* means journeying well *together* with other travelers and also orienting one's life rightly to God.[12] Absent the virtues of relationship, all of the other virtues will easily corrode.[13] As discussed throughout this book, the pursuit of justice is a requirement for any community or any health care system that seeks to promote and to protect the flourishing of its members.[14]

Table 7. *Aquinas's Virtues of Relationship*

Justice (*iustitia*)—the perpetual and constant will to render to each one their right (*ius*). Opposed to injustice (*iniustitia*) (*STh* IIaIIae qq. 58–59)

---

12. Jean Porter argues that contrary to many modern accounts of justice that focus on "abstract principles and the social and institutional arrangements expressing and safeguarding them," Aquinas consistently holds that justice is a personal virtue of the will, "a stable disposition to care about and to pursue just relations, informed by some sense of the point or the worth of just actions and the kinds of relationships that they generate." See Jean Porter, *Justice as a Virtue: A Thomistic Perspective* (Grand Rapids: Eerdmans, 2016), 7–8.

13. Alasdair MacIntyre argues that as dependent rational animals, human practical reason emerges from social interactions and relationships and that the "virtues of acknowledged dependence," which contribute to the flourishing not only of the agent but of the vulnerable and disabled in his or her community, are essential for collective flourishing. See Alasdair MacIntyre, *Dependent Rational Animals: Why Human Beings Need the Virtues* (Chicago: Open Court, 1999), 81–146.

14. For a feminist account that critiques Aquinas's Aristotelian anthropology while defending a broad vision of justice as a virtue of upholding the common good in relation to health care, see Susanne M. DeCrane, *Aquinas, Feminism, and the Common Good* (Washington, DC: Georgetown University Press, 1994).

Domain of relationship	Associated virtues	Opposing vices
Interpersonal, in judicial proceedings	Distributive justice—justice related to the order of what belongs to the community in relation to each single person (*STh* IIaIIae q. 61 a. 1) Commutative justice—justice related to the order of one private individual to another (*STh* IIaIIae q. 61 a. 1) (pertains to restitution of what has been taken [*STh* IIaIIae q. 62])	Respect of persons (*personarum acceptio*)—according unfair privilege to persons because of who they are and not what they have done or deserved Unjust imprisonment, torture, and execution Judicial injustice False accusation Lying False witness Weak representation Perjury
Interpersonal, apart from judicial proceedings		Murder Bodily harm (mutilation, blows, imprisonment) Theft and robbery Reviling Backbiting Talebearing Derision Cursing Cheating Usury
	Just punishment of wrongdoers	
	Truth	Lying Dissimulation and hypocrisy Boasting Irony
	Friendliness	Flattery Quarreling

Domain of relationship	Associated virtues	Opposing vices
	Liberality	Covetousness
		Prodigality
	Epikeia (equity)	
Between people and God	Religion and piety (devotion, prayer, adoration, sacrifice, offerings, vows, and oaths)	Superstition
		Undue worship
		Idolatry
		Divination
		Vain observance
		Temptation of God
		Perjury
		Sacrilege
		Simony
		Disobedience
	Gratitude	Ingratitude

Virtues of Pursuit

In his discussion of the virtues of acting, Aquinas second considers dispositions to pursue what is difficult and not to shrink back from pursuing what is good in the face of danger. The cardinal virtue of pursuit is *courage*. To live courageously is to be able to journey toward God with full awareness of the many challenges to doing so, and with full awareness of danger and evil—but not to turn away.

Aquinas's account of courage is deeply relevant to those who live with mental illness. Survivors of trauma, for example, live constantly with the awareness that the world is a potentially dangerous place and have often been deeply betrayed by others whom they previously trusted. Many of the characteristic behaviors of PTSD can be understood as ways to protect oneself and one's loved ones against exposure to the dangers that lie all around. Constant awareness of danger, brought constantly to consciousness by intrusive memories and dreams of traumatic events, gives way to behaviors of avoidance of danger: limiting relationships, avoiding crowds, cutting oneself off from the world. This attempt to control one's external world is then often associated with attempts to control one's experience of the self, through dissociation, numbing, and the use of external means (such as alcohol) to blunt negative emotion.

Survivors and clinicians alike recognize the avoidance behaviors associated with PTSD as understandable solutions to the reality of post-traumatic experience—but as solutions that, however understandable, cause further problems of their own and do not lead to healing. Using the language of this chapter, we would say that these solutions distract, rather than facilitate, the journey of the wayfarer toward *beatitudo*. Rather, as survivors and trauma therapists know, the only way out of PTSD is to navigate *through* the post-traumatic memories, through some version of establishing safe ways to cope with intensely negative emotions, remembering the felt experience of trauma, processing these experiences, and then finding new sources of life and connection.[15] The ability to live on in the face of trauma is enabled by the virtue of pursuit that Aquinas describes as courage.

Beyond courage itself, other virtues of pursuit are relevant to mental health and mental illness (see table 8). Following tradition, Aquinas considers the disposition to engage in great works and tasks and to build institutions of significance, which he calls magnanimity and magnificence, and which are opposed on each side by the vices of thinking of ourselves more highly than we ought (presumption, ambition, vainglory) and thinking of ourselves less highly than we ought and shrinking back into a safe zone of irrelevance (pusillanimity). And he considers two virtues of pursuit that each require God's grace and yet are central for living with mental health challenges: patience, the virtue of holding to what is good even in the face of sorrow caused especially by evils perpetrated on us; and perseverance, the virtue of staying with a difficult, good task even when it is hard and we want to give up (*STh* IIaIIae qq. 136-137).

Table 8. *Aquinas's Virtues of Pursuit*

Domain of Pursuit	Associated Virtues	Opposing Vices
Pursuit in general, in the face of danger and obstacle	Courage	Fear Fearlessness Daring

15. Judith Herman, *Trauma and Recovery: The Aftermath of Violence—from Domestic Abuse to Political Terror* (New York: Basic Books, 1997). The principle of navigating through traumatic memories is central to cognitive processing therapy and prolonged exposure therapy, two evidence-based trauma therapies widely used within the Veterans Affairs health system.

Domain of Pursuit	Associated Virtues	Opposing Vices
Pursuit of establishing and building great things	Magnanimity	Presumption Ambition Vainglory Pusillanimity
	Magnificence	Meanness
Pursuit of what is good even in the face of sorrow, especially regarding interpersonal evils	Patience (requires grace [STh IIaIIae q. 136 a. 3])	
Pursuit of what is good even when the act itself is difficult	Perseverance (requires grace [STh IIaIIae q. 137 a. 4])	Softness (withdrawing because of the lack of pleasure associated with the difficulty of the act) (STh IIaIIae q. 138 a. 1) Pertinacity (pushing forward from pride, to an excess) (STh IIaIIae q. 138 a. 3)

Virtues of Self-Regulation

Aquinas recognized that for a successful journey, a wayfarer needs the ability to press forward toward the good even in the face of danger and trial. These are the virtues of pursuit. But he also recognized that the wayfarer needs the ability to regulate desire and other emotions in ways that allow the wayfarer not to be distracted and derailed by desires that, however understandable in context, do not lead to a successful journey. These are the virtues of self-regulation, of which the cardinal virtue is temperance (*temperantia*).

As discussed above, emotions are usually truthful signs of whom and what we love, but insofar as our loves may be misdirected, our emotions may be misdirecting, leading us to distraction and even ruin rather than to *beatitudo*. Our love for ourselves, and for our bodies, may lead us to desire chemical substances that will make us *feel* that all is well with us, even when that is not the case, and so we may become dependent on comfort eating or on the use of alcohol, opioids, or other substances to maintain a certain feeling that is elusive when we are not using these substances (*STh* IIaIIae qq. 148, 150). Our natural desire to be known and loved, which stems from love for ourselves and for others, may lead us to seek intimacy in relationships, especially in sexual relationships, that are destructive and not life-giving for us (*STh* IIaIIae q. 141 a. 4; qq. 153-154). Aquinas held that the virtues of self-regulation apply particularly to food and drink (the substances by which life is maintained) and sexual behavior (by which life of the species is continued), both of which are mediated by touch. Self-regulation, then, is primarily about regulating our need for touch, and secondarily regulating other senses like taste and sight (*STh* IIaIIae q. 141 aa. 4-6). Insofar as food, drink, and sex are important human practices that meet bodily desires and needs, the virtues of self-regulation might be understood as dispositions to care rightly for the body. To display the virtue of temperance is to desire and to choose things that serve the body well, rather than desired things that *seem* to care for the body but that cause greater pain and trouble in the long run.

The virtues of self-regulation apply to more than food, drink, and sex, however (see table 9). Our natural desire for retribution against someone who has wronged us, which stems from our love for ourselves and our natural abhorrence of this perceived enemy, may lead to a life consumed by anger and characterized by increasingly dehumanizing acts that seem justified by the wrong done to us (*STh* IIaIIae q. 159). Even our natural desire to know the world around us, if engaged primarily as a mode of control or self-satisfaction, can lead us away from what is true.[16]

It is common to imagine self-regulation as a constant battle between reason and desire (Dialectical Behavior Therapy therapists may refer to this as a conflict between "reasonable mind" and "emotion mind").[17] Aquinas recognizes that sometimes this describes everyday life: when one is overcome by a desire to pursue something unhealthy or to avoid something healthy, then the right course is to fight to act against that desire. Aquinas refers to the disposition

---

16. This is for Aquinas the vice of curiosity (*STh* IIaIIae q. 167).

17. Marsha Linehan, *Cognitive Behavioral Treatment of Borderline Personality Disorder* (New York: Guilford, 1993), 214.

to stand firm against unhealthy desires as continence. But continence is a halfway virtue. The virtues, we may recall, are habits that enable us to journey toward participation in blessing with ease and pleasure; but continence by definition is not easy. Better, Aquinas argues, is the virtue of temperance (*temperantia*), in which we are able to focus on what is truly good, rather than what is pleasurable but distracting, so that we no longer even desire that which distracts us.

The virtues of self-regulation are broadly relevant to modern mental health care, because many approaches to recovery and treatment (e.g., treatment of anxiety, depression, eating disorders, and obsessive-compulsive disorder) focus on the capacity to focus on one's central goals for recovery and to ignore or reject alternative pathways that will lead to a perpetuation of behavioral cycles that lead to suffering. But Aquinas's description of the virtues of self-regulation applies in particular ways to substance use issues, as Aquinas himself was well aware.

Aquinas's analysis of the vice of problematic alcohol use (*inebrietas*) provides a helpful case study for how his work can inform mental health care more broadly. He describes sobriety (*ebrietas*) as the disposition to drink alcohol and other intoxicating drinks in a healthy way and makes clear that drinking alcohol is not inappropriate in itself. But it may become inappropriate

> owing to a circumstance on the part of the drinker, either because he is easily the worse for taking wine, or because he is bound by a vow not to drink wine: sometimes it results from the mode of drinking, because to wit he exceeds the measure in drinking: and sometimes it is on account of others who would be scandalized thereby. (*STh* IIaIIae q. 149 a. 3 *resp.*)

He then turns to the opposing vice of drunkenness (*inebrietas*) and displays a nuanced and compassionate stance. Considering whether drunkenness is a sin, he argues that it depends on the context. If drunkenness is understood simply as the state of *being intoxicated*, then it is not a sin. Similarly, if one is mistaken or deceived about the alcohol content of a drink and accidentally consumes too much, then the resulting intoxication is not a sin. But if one drinks too much because of unhealthy desire, then drunkenness is sinful (*STh* IIaIIae q. 150 a. 1 *resp.*). Even in this case, though, Aquinas argues that the person should be treated with compassion rather than with stigma and shame. Following the examples of Saint Gregory the Great and Saint Augustine, he argues that sometimes the correction of a sinner is to be foregone. . . . Hence Augustine says in a letter, "Meseems, such things are cured not by bitterness, severity, harshness, but by teaching rather than commanding, by advice rather than threats. Such is the course to be followed with the majority of sinners: few are they whose sins should be treated with severity." (*STh* IIaIIae q. 150 a. 1 *ad4*)

Furthermore, he argues that harmful actions done while intoxicated may or may not be sinful. If one became intoxicated without sin—say, one was deceived into drinking too much—then actions done while impaired are not sinful. If, however, one voluntarily chose to become intoxicated and then did something unhealthy, then that action "is rendered voluntary through the voluntariness of the preceding act. . . . Nevertheless, the resulting sin is diminished, even as the character of voluntariness is diminished" (*STh* IIaIIae q. 150 a. 4 *resp.*).

Table 9. *Aquinas's Virtues of Self-Regulation*

Domain of Self-Regulation	Associated Virtues	Opposing Vices
Self-regulation in general	Temperance	Intemperance Timidity
Self-regulation concerning food and drink	Abstinence Fasting Sobriety	Gluttony Drunkenness
Self-regulation concerning sex	Chastity Virginity	Lust
Self-regulation against unwanted desire	Continence	Incontinence
Self-regulation in seeking vengeance	Clemency and meekness	Anger Cruelty
Self-regulation in seeking excellence, in desiring knowledge, in bodily movement and actions, and in dress	Modesty Humility Studiousness	Pride Curiosity

Virtues That God Alone Can Give

In his account of the virtues, Aquinas draws deeply on the tradition handed on to him by Christian, Jewish, and Muslim commentators that flows from Aristotle primarily, and also from Plato, Cicero, Seneca, and other prominent classical moral thinkers. With Aristotle, he holds that the virtues of knowing and acting can be cultivated to a significant degree by learning and practice under the guidance of capable and wise teachers. But as a Christian, he believes that there are limits to this. Humans, even in our created goodness, are not able to attain union with God by our efforts alone. The special assistance of grace is required. Sin, and the destructive effects of sin on our capacity to know what is true and to do what is good, then compounds this problem. We require God to do for us what we are unable to do for ourselves.

Following Scripture and Christian tradition, Aquinas holds that faith, hope, and love are virtues that God alone can give.[18] For this reason, he separates them from other virtues of knowing and acting and describes them as *theological* virtues that have a certain sequence. Faith is the first of the theological virtues and is the disposition for the intellect to assent to truths of God's being and God's activity that are not apprehended by the senses and not able to be grasped through natural reason. Faith is "a habit of the mind, whereby eternal life is begun in us, making the intellect assent to what is non-apparent" (*STh* IIaIIae q. 4 a. 1 *resp.*). It is a virtue of knowing that requires not only a healthy will and the corresponding virtues of acting but also the direct work of God (*STh* IIaIIae q. 4 a. 2; q. 6 a. 1). It is through faith that God enables humans to *know* God and God's work.

The second virtue that God alone can give is hope. Hope as a virtue, for Aquinas, is distinct from hope as a passion. Whereas the *passion* of hope is the form that desire takes when we perceive a loved person or thing to be difficult and yet possible to attain, the *virtue* of hope has more to do with the capacity to rest not in our own effort but in the assistance and activity of God (*STh* IIaIIae q. 17 a. 1 *resp.*). The passion of hope says, "With effort, I can attain what I long for." The virtue of hope, in contrast, says, "I can align my activity with God, trusting that God will make a way out of no way, and will rest in that." Hope is the capacity to rest in the good future that God alone will bring forth, including our own enjoyment of God (*STh* IIaIIae q. 17 a. 2). It is opposed to

18. While God alone can give these virtues, Aquinas holds that human interactions and relationships may be means that God uses. God may give faith, for example, by sending preachers (*STh* IIaIIae q. 6 a. 1 *resp.*).

the vices of despair, the inability to rest in God's promises due to the belief that God cannot or will not bring them about (*STh* IIaIIae q. 20 a. 1),[19] and presumption, the belief that we can attain God's promises through our power alone (*STh* IIaIIae q. 21).

Both faith and hope point to the third and highest of the theological virtues, love (*caritas*, charity). As we have already examined in chapters 2 and 5, Aquinas understands love as the form of all of the other virtues—the virtue that undergirds all of the other virtues, and to which all other virtues point. Its animating force is God's love, given freely in creation and in grace to us. God's love then forms in us a corresponding love that is possible only because of the work of God in us. Aquinas describes this disposition to love in a way that resonates with God's love as friendship with God:

> since there is a communication between man and God, inasmuch as he communicates His happiness to us, some kind of friendship must needs be

---

19. Aquinas refers to despair not only as a vice and a mortal sin but as the most dangerous of sins, because "since hope withdraws us from evils and induces us to seek for good things, so . . . when hope is given up, men rush headlong into sin, and are drawn away from good works" (*STh* IIaIIae q. 20 a. 3). He then offers two common causes of despair. The first is lust (*luxuria*), since "the fact that spiritual goods taste good to us no more, or seem to be goods of no great account, is chiefly due to our affections being affected with the love of bodily pleasures, among which, sexual pleasures hold the first place: for the love of these pleasures leads man to have a distaste for spiritual things, and not to hope for them as arduous goods" (*STh* IIaIIae q. 20 a. 4 *resp.*). But a second cause is *acedia*, when "a man deems an arduous good impossible to attain . . . due to his being over downcast, because when this state of mind dominates his affections, it seems to him that he will never be able to rise to any good" (*STh* IIaIIae q. 20 a. 4 *resp.*). Despair is also caused by sorrow (2 Cor. 2:7), "for when a man is influenced by a certain passion he considers chiefly the things which pertain to that passion: so that a man who is full of sorrow does not easily think of great and joyful things, but only of sad things, unless by a great effort he turns his thoughts away from sadness" (*STh* IIaIIae q. 20 a. 4 *ad3*). This formulation provides challenging and yet insightful ways to consider the experience of depression in modern times. For many people, depression is not the same as despair. Many people who are depressed are still able, in the midst of depression, to rest in God's good future beyond depression. But some who are depressed find that hope is gone. In this case, Aquinas would caution against pursuing short-term pleasures—whether academic or professional success, alcohol, exercise, sex, or relationships—that may be distracting from what is truly life-giving (*luxuria*). Second, Aquinas would encourage those with depression to examine their lives, preferably in relationship with wise counselors, to discern whether they might be stuck in ruts of joyless daily practice (*acedia*) and how to persevere in pursuit of what is good. Third, Aquinas would want clinicians and patients alike to be realistic about the external evils that are causing sorrow that leads to the experience of hopelessness.

based on this same communication, of which it is written, *God is faithful: by Whom you are called into the fellowship of His Son.* The love which is based on this communication, is charity: wherefore it is evident that charity is the friendship of man for God. (*STh* IIaIIae q. 23 a. 1 *resp.*)

This is not love that we concoct out of our own effort. It is God's love, given to humans, by which we are enabled to love God in return. And we are enabled not just to love God but *in God* to love ourselves, our bodies, our friends, the nonhuman creation, and even our enemies (*STh* IIaIIae q. 25 aa. 1, 3, 4, 5–9). The effect of God's love is to make us deeper and better lovers—the kind of lover that God is.

The Gifts of the Holy Spirit

The virtues that God alone can give are not simply supplements for the life of the wayfarer, tacked on at the end to allow those on a journey to bridge the last remaining distance between God and us. Rather, they make the rest of the journey possible in ways that would not be possible otherwise. Aquinas speaks in several registers about the difference that God's love makes for our journey beyond the theological virtues of faith, hope, and love. First, he speaks of virtues of acting that cannot be acquired through practice alone but are infused directly by God, just as the theological virtues are, and that enable us to live into the life that God alone can make possible (*STh* IaIIae q. 63 a. 3 *resp.*). These divinely infused virtues of acting are often referred to as the infused, rather than acquired, moral virtues. Aquinas illustrates the difference between the infused and acquired moral virtues by the example of the virtue of self-control with respect to eating. Acquired self-control, as a virtue of self-regulation, provides "that food should not harm the health of the body, nor hinder the use of reason" (*STh* IaIIae q. 63 a. 4 *resp.*). The self-control that God alone gives, by contrast, allows someone to engage in practices of fasting and self-discipline that lead to deeper union with God. The point of Aquinas's nonsystematic and sometimes confusing account of the infused moral virtues is that having loved us first and having infused the dispositions of faith, hope, and love within us, God also provides the capacity to live in a way that leads to union with God, that enables us to be "fellow-citizens with the saints, and of the household of God" (Eph. 2:19) (*STh* IaIIae q. 63 a. 4 *resp.*).

The scriptural and traditional account of the seven gifts of the Holy Spirit, drawn from Isaiah 11:2–3, is another way that Aquinas describes the ways that God helps wayfarers toward the goal of the journey. The seven gifts of the Spirit—understanding, counsel, wisdom, knowledge, piety, fortitude, and fear—are dispositions given by God and infused by God into the soul that enable the soul to respond to the prompting of the Holy Spirit. Like polarized sunglasses on a bright, hazy day, the gifts bring God's operation in the world into sharper relief, enabling us to respond to the ways that God is moving and acting. The gifts of wisdom and understanding sharpen, perfect, and aid our ability to apprehend what is true, while the gifts of knowledge and counsel perfect and aid our reasoning about what to do. Our longings and desires related to relationship are perfected by the gift of piety, our aversion to danger by the gift of fortitude, and our longing for pleasure by the gift of fear (*STh* IaIIae q. 68 a. 4).[20]

Blessings along the Way: The Beatitudes and the Fruits of the Spirit

I have described Aquinas's account of *beatitudo* or participation in blessing as the elusive goal of the journey of the wayfarer, and then of Aquinas's account of the journey's process. Through practice, habit, and God's grace and gift, our natural capacities for knowing, feeling, and acting can be shaped and transformed to reliably direct us to *beatitudo*. The virtues of knowing, the virtues of acting, the virtues that God alone can give, and the gifts of the Holy Spirit are helps for the journey that also show that the journey is going well. Along with this, drawing on tradition, Aquinas offers two additional descriptions of blessings along the way: the fruits of the Spirit and the beatitudes.

If the gifts of the Spirit enable us to respond with promptness to the movement of the Holy Spirit, the fruits emerge and proceed when we successfully align with this movement. Aquinas follows a tradition that began with the apostle Paul's list in Galatians 5:22–23 and was continued by many who came after him.[21] He divides the fruits of the Spirit into three groups: those that

20. Servais Pinckaers emphasizes that while these infused virtues and gifts are from God, they are nonetheless perfections of our own natural inclinations. They operate *within* our nature, not outside of it. "The natural inclination toward truth and goodness is the work of God. God conforms the human person to the likeness of his wisdom and goodness and, as an interior master, calls him to participate more deeply in his creative freedom. This bond with God is intimate and from birth. It touches the essence of our personality in our longing for happiness and love. It does not limit human freedom, but grounds it." See Servais Pinckaers, *Morality: The Catholic View* (South Bend: Saint Augustine's, 2001), 70-71.

21. Galatians 5:22 begins, "The fruit of the Spirit is" (singular noun and verb), but Aqui-

pertain to our response to God's indwelling presence; those that pertain to relationship with others; and those that pertain to relationship with pleasure.

Love comes first—not only as the root of all of the emotions and the form
of all the virtues but as the first fruit of the Spirit. Love is not just a fruit of the
Spirit but the Spirit in actuality: "the Holy Ghost is given in a special manner,
as in His own likeness, since He himself is love. Hence it is written (Rom. 5:5):
'The charity of God is poured forth in our hearts by the Holy Ghost, Who is
given to us'" (STh IaIIae q. 70 a. 3 resp.). Love is the fruit of God's presence in us.
But love leads to other fruits also: the experience of being united to God in love
brings forth joy, "because every lover rejoices in being united to the beloved"
(STh IaIIae q. 70 a. 3 resp.). This joy at being united to God gives rise to peace,
the capacity to rest content in the presence of God, and the corresponding
fruits of patience and longsuffering, which enable us not to be disturbed when
evil threatens us or when what is good is delayed.

Other fruits, Aquinas holds, have to do with our relationship with other
humans. The will to do good to those around us bears the fruits of goodness
and benevolence (benignity), the capacity to bear with others even when they
have wronged us bears the fruit of meekness, and the commitment not to
abuse or exploit those around us bears the fruit of fidelity. Third, modesty,
continence, and chastity are the fruits of not being led astray by unlawful or
by lawful desires (STh IaIIae q. 70 a. 3 resp.).

Exceeding the fruits of the Spirit, though, are the beatitudes. Aquinas comments that whereas fruits must be "ultimate and delightful," the beatitudes
are in addition "perfect and excellent." For the closest approximation of what
participation in blessing can look like in this life, therefore, we may look to
how Jesus himself described blessing (Matt. 5:1-12). Unlike the virtues and
gifts, the beatitudes mark not just the *disposition* to journey well but journeying well itself (STh IaIIae q. 69 a. 1). The beatitudes are an inbreaking of the
life to come, the life of perfect happiness in union with God, in this life (STh
IaIIae q. 69 a. 2 resp.).

The first of the beatitudes, Aquinas argues, display participation in blessing with regard to the senses, and especially with regard to pleasures. To be
poor in spirit, Aquinas holds, is to display humility and contempt for riches
and honors, but in place of the "excellence and abundance" of riches, the one

---

nas speaks of the "fruits" (plural) of the Spirit. Also, following the Latin manuscript tradition of his day, Aquinas lists two fruits (long-suffering and modesty) that are not found
in the earliest Greek manuscripts or modern biblical translations and divides the fruit of
self-control into two fruits, continence and chastity.

who is poor in spirit is granted the excellence and abundance of the kingdom of heaven (*STh* IaIIae q. 69 aa. 3–4). Those who are able to bring desires for pleasure and domination of others under control—the meek—find as a reward "a secure and peaceful possession of the land of the living, whereby the solid reality of eternal goods is denoted" (*STh* IaIIae q. 69 aa. 3–4). Those who are able to look beyond their own desires and to mourn the world's brokenness will find comfort.

The next set of beatitudes, in Aquinas's interpretation, deals with engaged life in the world—the active life. Aquinas describes these beatitudes in contrast with patterns of living and thinking that are all too common in human life. People exploit others and create situations of inequity and injustice so that they can enjoy the material goods gained by way of exploitation, but in God's life, those who not only accede to the demands of justice but who "hunger and thirst for justice" will have their fill (*STh* IaIIae q. 69 a. 3 *resp.*). The life of God is marked by joyful justice-seeking, the pursuit of justice with an "ardent desire, even as a hungry and thirsty man eats and drinks with eager appetite." Similarly, many people retreat from the misery of others in order to limit their own misery. But the life of God turns this around: it is those who show mercy, even when it means opening themselves to the pain of others, who will be comforted. Aquinas reminds readers that Jesus told his followers, "When thou makest a dinner or supper, call not thy friends, nor thy brethren, etc. . . . but . . . call the poor, the maimed" (Luke 4:12-13) (*STh* IaIIae q. 69 a. 3 *resp.*). Mercy is the way of God and a mark of participation in blessing.

Finally, there are beatitudes that deal with the contemplative life, which is already (as we will see in chapter 9) a participation in the life of God. The person who is not clouded by distracting passions but able to be "clean of heart" is promised fellowship with God. And the person who seeks peace with others shows himself or herself to be a true "follower of God, who is the God of unity and peace." As a reward, the peacemaker is promised "the glory of the Divine sonship, consisting in perfect union with God through consummate wisdom" (*STh* IaIIae q. 69 a. 4 *resp.*).

Challenges of Wayfarers: Understanding Mental Health Problems in the Light of the Journey

The details of Aquinas's understanding of how humans think, act, feel, and live, which I have presented here only briefly and in overview form, are complex. But the picture that he paints—viewed from thirty thousand feet rather than at ground level—is breathtakingly beautiful. For Aquinas, humans are God's good, beloved creatures, embodied manifestations of God's love, formed in a way that we are able to know God and the things of God, and to conform our lives to God's *ratio*, God's good ordering of the world. As creatures formed for God, we seek *beatitudo* in all of our actions—and perfect *beatitudo* is found only in pursuing God as our highest end. We are wayfarers on a journey from God to God—a journey made possible not only by our activity but by God's gracious action toward us, in the person and work of Christ. We are *on* the way; Christ *is* the way; and all of our lives are those of wayfarers on a journey (*STh* Ia q. 2 *proem.*).

The image of human beings as wayfarers provides a sharp contrast to the machine metaphor. The goal of human life is not the optimal functioning of a machine but rather the wayfarer's active participation in blessing. The human capacities to know and to act are best understood not as evolved products of neural circuits, to be directed toward whatever ends are chosen for them, but rather as powers that reflect our status as creatures who are fitted for life with and in God. Emotions are not simply feelings of the body, to be adjusted at will, but are embodied signs of the wayfarer's love. Stable dispositions of thinking and acting are not simply products of genes and learning but are the cognitive and conative grooves that either aid or hinder the wayfarer's journey. God's grace is not an outside intervention from God in the body-machine but the perfection of the wayfarer's nature and the inner prompting that allows the wayfarer to move toward God and to realize his or her participation in blessing.[22] The human is not a machine to be fixed but a wayfarer to be attended and accompanied.

How does Aquinas's image of the human as wayfarer inform our understanding of mental health and mental illness? Though we have been engaging this question throughout this chapter and book, I conclude with several ways that the wayfarer image helps us to understand mental health problems. In chapter 10, we will return to how the wayfarer image informs Christian engagement with mental health care.

In brief, the wayfarer image helps us understand mental health problems not as technical problems to be fixed but as challenges to be navigated. To be sure, mental health problems can feel simply like problems that need fixing. Someone who is depressed may feel cut off from God and from happiness. Someone struggling with substance use may feel unable to move consistently toward what she knows is most life-giving. It may seem like the only reasonable approach to such conditions is to seek a fix that would banish them entirely.

22. Pinckaers, *Sources of Christian Ethics*, 48–74.

But viewed in the light of Aquinas's understanding of the human as way-farer, mental health problems are more nuanced than that. In my clinical work as well as in my broader life, I have observed that people (including me) will do the best they can with what they have learned in order to get what they think they need in any given situation. Viewed in this perspective, mental health problems are often best understood not as states or conditions that descend on a person (or that arise only from some internal dysfunction; see chapter 3) but rather as complex emotional, cognitive, and behavioral patterns in which people with particular life experiences and bodily dispositions encounter challenges and respond to them as best they can, in ways that might or might not successfully overcome the challenges and might or might not lead to growth in freedom. In any given situation, it is useful to ask: What past experiences has a person lived through, and what have they learned from these experiences? What do they think they need in the present? In what concrete situations do they find themselves? Are their responses to these situations fostering growth in agency and freedom? If not, what kind of responses might the person identify that would do so?

Mental health problems, that is, are best understood not as obstacles per se but rather as particular ways that people encounter perceived obstacles and respond to them. Sometimes people experience themselves as stuck. But over time, as someone learns to navigate obstacles in life-giving ways—perhaps with the aid of a mental health practitioner, counselor, or pastor—the experience of living with mental health challenges can allow a person to find and develop wise ways of seeing, knowing, and acting (that is, virtues). These virtues not only can aid the journey to *beatitudo* but can help other wayfarers also. Mental health problems can be sites of blessing as well as challenge, fertile soil from which tenacious and deeply rooted virtues can grow. They are not so much *constraints* on the journey as possible *conditions* of the journey.

That said, living with mental health challenges does require coming face-to-face with various kinds of obstacles and learning to navigate them. What does the image of the wayfarer teach us about the nature of the obstacles that people with mental health challenges face? While no list can be comprehensive, several such obstacles are worth considering in detail.

Trauma. Trauma names any experience or set of experiences that, in the words of Judith Herman, "overwhelm the ordinary systems of care that give people a sense of control, connection, and meaning."[23] While the precise boundaries of trauma are fuzzy and depend not only on what is experienced

---

23. Herman, *Trauma and Recovery*, 33.

but also on how,[24] it is clear that trauma associated with childhood sexual and physical abuse, childhood emotional abuse, intimate-partner violence, sexual assault, and other violent experiences are all too common (see chapter 1). It is also clear that such experiences can either prevent the healthy formation or disrupt the integrity of the psychological infrastructure that, for Aquinas, aids the wayfarer's journey. Childhood sexual abuse, for example, is a common antecedent of borderline personality disorder, which is characterized among other things by difficulty naming and regulating emotions, chronic feelings of emptiness, an unstable sense of self, and challenges in interpreting and navigating interpersonal relationships.[25] Combat experiences leave many veterans with challenges in appraising and responding to the actual threat of everyday situations upon return to civilian life.

Like the man on the way from Jerusalem to Jericho who was assaulted and left for dead (Luke 10:30), trauma can profoundly disrupt the wayfarer's journey. In Thomistic terms, trauma leads to an overvaluation of threat and danger, which in turn hyperactivates the emotional triad of avoidance (causing a wider range of things to be judged harmful and avoided) and directs the emotional triad of approach toward those things that promise safety and control (one loves what allows a world experienced as uncontrollable to come

24. Though it is clear that "trauma" is increasingly being used to describe a broader range of experiences than the "actual or threatened death, serious injury, or sexual violence" specified in Criterion A of the diagnostic criteria for post-traumatic stress disorder in *DSM-5-TR*, I prefer not to set limits on the kinds of experiences that can be traumatic because (a) the use of any clinical term is ultimately a matter of social convention and (b) rejecting certain events (e.g., racial microaggressions) as potential sites of trauma makes it harder to hear and understand the perspectives of those who have experienced these events. When I hear someone describe an event as "traumatic" that is not generally associated with trauma, I find it best not to police the boundary of the term but rather to ask, "What was it about that experience that makes the concept of trauma resonate for you?" Answers to these questions help to illuminate how events that are often dismissed can indeed be associated with a loss of control, connection, and meaning. I also follow Catherine Dulmus, Carolyn Hilarski, and other trauma theorists in observing that traumatic events fall on a "stress-trauma-crisis continuum" and that it is unhelpful to draw a precise boundary between traumatic events and stressors. See Catherine Dulmus and Carolyn Hilarski, "When Stress Constitutes Trauma and Trauma Constitutes Crisis: The Stress-Trauma-Crisis Continuum," *Brief Treatment and Crisis Intervention* 3 (2003): 27–35.

25. Lucas Fortaleza de Aquino Ferreira et al., "Borderline Personality Disorder and Sexual Abuse: A Systematic Review," *Psychiatry Research* 262 (2018): 70–77; for the borderline personality disorder diagnostic criteria, see American Psychiatric Association, *Diagnostic and Statistical Manual of Mental Disorders*, 5th ed. rev. [*DSM-5-TR*] (Washington, DC: American Psychiatric Association, 2013), 752–53.

under control). Because of this overactivation of threat responses, it also disrupts the virtues of knowing and acting, particularly the virtues of prudence and *synesis*, which have to do with making intuitive judgments about what needs to be done in challenging particular situations.[26]

Stress. More broad than traumatic events that threaten the wayfarer's capacities for control, connection, and meaning, it is clear that stress can affect the wayfarer's journey. A friend who recently completed part of the *Camino de Santiago* in Spain, a noted medieval pilgrimage route, shared that even for well-prepared pilgrims, the journey can be arduous. He described hostels with bedbugs, challenges maintaining hydration in the baking sun, and unpredictable weather. Stresses like these can make any journey more difficult and are trivial compared to the stress experienced by many people diagnosed with mental illness. Food and housing insecurity are associated with depression and anxiety, in likely a bidirectional causal relationship.[27] Living in a violent neighborhood is associated with depression and psychological distress.[28]

Lack of traveling companions or challenges with traveling companions. Wayfaring is a corporate activity. Pilgrims usually travel in groups. My *caminante* friend described how important it was to have fellow pilgrims around him on the journey. In some villages, the path of the *camino* would not be clear, and others would help him find the way. At other times, fellow pilgrims were a deep source of delight and encouragement. And at other times, conflicts among pilgrims would emerge and would make the journey more unpleasant and difficult. In the same way, all human wayfarers need good traveling

---

26. Lisa Tessman argues that traumatic experience fosters the development of "burdened virtues," engrained patterns of responding and acting to traumatic situations that foster survival and resistance in traumatic situations but that create challenges when generalized to the whole of one's life. For an American soldier guarding a perimeter of a base camp in Vietnam, monitoring one's environment for threat and responding with violence if necessary is (arguably) adaptive, but those action tendencies might not work well when soldiers return home to their families and to civilian life. While Tessman's insight is important and while I agree with her argument that virtue always corresponds to a particular context and community, from a Thomistic perspective, burdened virtues are not complete virtues insofar as they hinder, rather than facilitate, a person's flourishing. See Lisa Tessman, *Burdened Virtues: Virtue Ethics for Liberatory Struggles* (New York: Oxford University Press, 2005).

27. Merryn Maynard et al., "Food Insecurity and Mental Health among Females in High-Income Countries," *International Journal of Environmental Research in Public Health* 15 (2018): 1424–60.

28. Gergő Baranyi et al., "The Impact of Neighbourhood Crime on Mental Health: A Systematic Review and Meta-analysis," *Social Science and Medicine* 282 (2021): https://doi.org/10.1016/j.socscimed.2021.114106.

companions. Loneliness is prominently associated with depression and other adverse mental health outcomes.[29] Beyond that, the outside-in model of mental health challenges makes clear that relational challenges can be the burner under the pot of depression, anxiety, and other mental health challenges.

Limitations of the body. For my friend on the *Camino de Santiago*, it was not just external stressors and relational challenges that created problems for the journey. He also described unexpected and uncomfortable blisters and aches that made it hard to go on. Though humans are not machines, our journeys are embodied. Similarly, as made clear in chapters 2 and 3, Aquinas understood that challenges in the body can create obstacles in the wayfarer's journey to God. Sometimes, as in the case of my pilgrim friend's blisters, these are problems that do not directly affect a person's capacity for thinking and acting. But sometimes bodily problems can impair appropriate cognition and action and so can be the primary cause of mental health problems. Aquinas held that there were instances, for example, in which the body impairs the operation of the sensitive faculty of the soul so that sensory and perceptual information is not delivered correctly to the intellect (*STh* Ia q. 84 aa. 7–8; *STh* IIIa q. 68 a. 12 *ad2*). In this case, as discussed in chapters 2, 3, and 7, there is still room in Aquinas's thought for mental health challenges to be caused primarily by problems in the body; though in the absence of physiological evidence, this will generally be a diagnosis of exclusion, applied only when one is unable to make sense of mental health challenges as embodied responses to context.

Habits that get in the way. The most common forms of mental health challenges, such as anxiety, depression, and substance use disorders, are frequently rooted in trauma and stress that come to a person from without. But how we respond to trauma and stress can either lead to healing or lead to more problems, and at worst lead to cycles that can be hard to escape. When these responses are ingrained and lead to dispositions to think and to respond to stress in a way that leads not to flourishing but to further pain, this is not virtue but vice. As detailed above, it is important to remember that for Aquinas, all vices *begin* in behavior that seeks *beatitudo*, as people do their best in particular situations to do what is good for them. Problematic substance use, for example, often begins when someone who is suffering finds that a particular drug takes their suffering away. Using the substance is a way of caring for the body and its needs. In this case, the problem is not the original intention to alleviate suffering but

29. Stephanie Cacioppo et al., "Loneliness: Clinical Import and Interventions," *Perspectives on Psychological Science* 10 (2015): 238–49.

rather the fact that substances like heroin, fentanyl, and cocaine don't deliver what they promise for long. They wear off quickly and demand frequent and repeated patterns of use that, before long, can severely derail a person's journey. The response to stress gets in the way and becomes an obstacle in its own right. While it may seem stigmatizing to refer to such patterns as "vice," it is no different from the way that modern therapists might refer to "maladaptive coping strategies." When habits get in the way, as they do for all of us, it is important not to get locked in self-condemnation or shame (chapter 4). Rather, as we will consider in chapter 10, we are invited to name the problem honestly, to carefully and creatively ask what we really need, and to discern how to meet these needs—such as the needs to care well for the body, to seek relationship, and to face suffering—in life-giving and sustainable ways.

CHAPTER 9

From Control to Wonder

....

We Are Called to Love, Wonder, Praise, and Rest

> How weighty to me are your thoughts, O God!
>> How vast is the sum of them!
> I try to count them—they are more than the sand;
>> I come to the end—I am still with you.
>
> —*Psalm 139:17-18*

He is known to us as "the man in the tombs," or as "the Gerasene demoniac."
We do not know his given name. But let's hear his story:

> They came to the other side of the sea, to the region of the Gerasenes. And
> when [Jesus] had stepped out of the boat, immediately a man from the
> tombs with an unclean spirit met him. He lived among the tombs, and no
> one could restrain him any more, even with a chain, for he had often been
> restrained with shackles and chains, but the chains he wrenched apart,
> and the shackles he broke in pieces, and no one had the strength to subdue
> him. Night and day among the tombs and on the mountains he was always
> howling and bruising himself with stones.
>
> When he saw Jesus from a distance, he ran and bowed down before
> him, and he shouted at the top of his voice, "What have you to do with
> me, Jesus, Son of the Most High God? I adjure you by God, do not torment
> me." For he had said to him, "Come out of the man, you unclean spirit!"
> Then Jesus asked him, "What is your name?"
> He replied, "My name is Legion, for we are many." He begged him ear-
> nestly not to send them out of the region.
> Now there on the hillside a great herd of swine was feeding, and the
> unclean spirits begged him, "Send us into the swine; let us enter them." So

he gave them permission. And the unclean spirits came out and entered the swine, and the herd, numbering about two thousand, stampeded down the steep bank into the sea and were drowned in the sea.

The swineherds ran off and told it in the city and in the country. Then people came to see what it was that had happened. They came to Jesus and saw the man possessed by demons sitting there, clothed and in his right mind, the very man who had had the legion, and they became frightened. Those who had seen what had happened to the man possessed by demons and to the swine reported it. Then they began to beg Jesus to leave their neighborhood. As he was getting into the boat, the man who had been possessed by demons begged him that he might be with him. But Jesus refused and said to him, "Go home to your own people, and tell them how much the Lord has done for you and what mercy he has shown you." And he went away and began to proclaim in the Decapolis how much Jesus had done for him, and everyone was amazed. (Mark 5:1–20 NRSVue)

The story of the man in the tombs is frequently interpreted as a paradigmatic instance of the healing of mental illness in the Bible. But how might we interpret this passage? Four dimensions of interpretation reveal themselves.

First, it is possible to understand Jesus's healing of the man as a kind of *medical healing*. Perhaps, indeed, he lived with what we would now consider a serious and persistent mental illness. Using modern psychiatric language, we can confidently say, at the least, that he displayed persistent self-harming behavior and appeared to be emotionally dysregulated. Similar to the way that people with mental illness used to be (and sometimes still are) forcibly restrained, we are told that he had "often been restrained with shackles and chains," perhaps for his own safety or the safety of others. Ostracized from his community, living among the dead, he certainly bore stigma. Though the text gives little information beyond this that resonates with the modern *DSM* diagnostic criteria, we can speculate that perhaps he lived with a psychotic disorder like schizophrenia, or perhaps even post-traumatic stress disorder.[1]

---

1. Michael Yandell, agreeing that the text is open to interpretation, suggests that the man may have been a military veteran tormented by memories of violence associated with military service. The man's choice of the Latin term translated "legion" for a name may not be a metaphor, Yandell argues, but rather an example of the fused identity of those "who cannot distill their own being and actions from those of the institution" of the military. See Michael Yandell, "'Do Not Torment Me': The Morally Injured Gerasene Demoniac,"

While interpreting this text as a medical healing is most consistent with modern ways of understanding mental health and mental illness, however, it is not the plain sense of the text. The Gospel of Mark (along with Matthew and Luke, in slightly different versions) describes the Gerasene man's healing as a *spiritual healing*, an exorcism of "unclean spirits." The individualistic and materialistic machine metaphor cannot account for the reality of unclean spirits, how they might affect people, and what response might be necessary. But the existence of pervasive spiritual agents and forces—what this text refers to as unclean spirits and demons—was widely assumed in the first century. While unclean spirits and demons were more likely to cause what would now be called "physical" symptoms rather than "psychological" symptoms, the text asks us to see unclean spirits as the proximate cause of this man's distress.[2] Jesus's exorcism of the unclean spirits tormenting this man was a sign of his authority over heaven as well as earth.

The man's (or, more precisely, the unclean spirits') self-identification as "Legion," however, points to a third possible way of interpreting the nature of Jesus's healing, specifically as a *political* or *liberatory* healing. Though the Gospel of Mark was written in Greek, the term "Legion" is a transliterated Latin term that in the first century referred only to the legions of the Roman military—military units of several thousand soldiers, approximately the same size as brigades in the US Army and British Army.[3] If a similarly disturbed person in the United States or United Kingdom today were to state, "my name is Brigade, for we are many," listeners would immediately notice the word choice and would wonder about his relationship, if any, with the military. Perhaps, as Michael Yandell has suggested, the man was a military veteran tormented by participation in violence.[4] Or, perhaps, the name "Legion" in the story would simply have evoked comparison of the unclean spirits that were controlling and oppressing the man and the Roman imperial powers that were controlling and oppressing the people of Israel in first-century Palestine. Either way, Jesus's public exorcism of the legion of unclean spirits, and the

---

in *Exploring Moral Injury in Sacred Texts*, ed. Joseph McDonald (London: Kingsley, 2017), 135–49, quotation from 138.

2. John Swinton, *Finding Jesus in the Storm: The Spiritual Lives of Christians with Mental Health Challenges* (Grand Rapids: Eerdmans, 2020), 193–94; Christopher C. H. Cook, "The Gerasene Demoniac," in *The Bible and Mental Health: Towards a Biblical Theology of Mental Health*, ed. Christopher C. H. Cook and Isabelle Hamley (London: SCM, 2020), 141–56.

3. Joel Marcus, *Mark 1–8: A New Translation with Introduction and Commentary* (New York: Doubleday, 2000), 344–45.

4. Yandell, "'Do Not Torment Me.'"

subsequent humiliating fate of the legion in the drowning of the swine (an echo, perhaps, of the closing in of the sea over the pursuing Egyptians), might be interpreted as Jesus's assertion of authority over *all* powers that oppress people and stand in the way of the coming kingdom of God, including Rome. It is speculative but plausible that the townspeople encountered the healed man with fear and begged Jesus to leave the region out of concern that Jesus's public ridicule of the Roman military might stir up trouble with Rome.

Fourth and more straightforwardly, Jesus's healing might be interpreted as a *relational* healing. This man was ostracized from his community, lived among the dead, and related to others only in the context of fear, confrontation, and violence. But at the end of the story, he is "clothed and in his right mind" and reintegrated into the community from which he had been ostracized. Though he asked to follow Jesus to the other side of the sea of Galilee, Jesus told him to "go home to your friends, and tell them how much the Lord has done for you, and what mercy he has shown you." Some have even observed that because the Decapolis on the eastern side of the Sea of Galilee was a predominantly gentile area, this man—the man who had the legion, the man who was ostracized, the man who had been forcibly restrained and greeted with fear—became the first missionary to the gentiles.[5]

What kind of healing, then, was Jesus's healing of the man in the tombs? While we may want to assign this episode as a medical, spiritual, political, *or* relational healing, the gospel refuses these divisions. Jesus's healing was broader and deeper than the way that healing is often understood in modern health care. It was medical, spiritual, political or liberatory, *and* relational. Jesus refuses any reductionistic approach to healing and calls us to a wider view.[6]

Each of these four dimensions of healing, though, can be understood as a movement from oppression to freedom and from control to wonder. Whatever his past experiences or actions, at the outset of the story, the Gerasene man finds himself bound in complex systems of control. He was controlled by shackles and chains. He resisted and escaped control by breaking the chains and yet remained controlled by the legion of unclean spirits, bruising himself with stones even though he was physically stronger than anyone else around him. Jesus healed him by controlling the unclean spirits.

5. Pheme Perkins, "Mark," in *New Interpreter's Bible* (Nashville: Abingdon, 1994), 8:584–85.

6. For an account of the healing of the Gerasene man that emphasizes its cosmic, political, and relational dimensions in conversation with the contemporary opioid use crisis in the United States, see Brett McCarty, "Salvation and Health in Southern Appalachia: What the Opioid Crisis Reveals about Health Care and the Church," *Christian Bioethics* 29 (2023): 221–34.

And yet at the end of this story, the central narrative is not about control. It is rather about freedom and agency. The people from the surrounding area found the man not naked and tormented but clothed and *sōphrōn*, which in Greek connotes wisdom, sound-mindedness, and freedom that comes from within (Mark 5:15). After Jesus refuses the man's request to follow him to the other side of the sea, he reenters the life of the community from which he was ostracized, "[proclaiming] in the Decapolis how much Jesus had done for him" (5:20). And everyone, the gospel tells us, was left in a state of marvel, amazement, and wonder (*ethaumazon*) (5:20). The healing of the man in the tombs was, in all of its dimensions, a movement from an economy of control to an economy of wonder.

Modern mental health care, particularly when it operates within the machine metaphor, is dominated by an economy of control. Ann, whose story we encountered in the introduction, speaks of the challenges of growing up "in a kind of shame-laced society, and a home where it was just not cool to not have control over yourself."[7] Patients seek help when they feel out of control, or—as in the case of the man in the tombs—when they are judged by others to be uncontrollable. Clinicians seek to control symptoms and to help patients control their unwanted experiences and behaviors. Many critics of psychiatry charge that this control of symptoms can easily extend to the control of human bodies and lives. To be sure, control is an important good and brings important benefits. But what would it mean for modern mental health care, like those who surrounded the healed Gerasene man, to move from postures of control to postures of wonder?

The Paradox of Control

Control is an important good within modern mental health care. People often seek mental health treatment when they are facing unbearable suffering or when they feel that they can no longer direct the course of their lives. Often people feel betrayed by their bodies and minds and so find it natural to split self from symptoms and to understand unwanted experience and behavior as something that is "not me" and needs to be controlled.

Responding to this desire, control is central to the way pharmaceutical companies market medications. A recent advertisement for a new medica-

---

7. Personal interview, June 3, 2022.

tion for ADHD in children promises, "Less chaos, More control."[8] Another advertisement for a medication for tardive dyskinesia (a movement disorder sometimes caused by long-term treatment with antipsychotics) encourages clinicians to "help your adult patients with tardive dyskinesia (TD) Take. Control."[9] A client-oriented self-help book by two eminent psychotherapy researchers is titled *Controlling Your Drinking*.[10]

There are times when the first aim of mental health care should be the establishment of control. When persons are tormented by hallucinations or gripped by delusions that are making it dangerous for them to navigate the world, it is good to use medication to bring these experiences under control. When persons are depressed to the point that they are contemplating suicide or unable to engage in basic life activities, or having frequent panic attacks that prevent them from leaving home, it is good to seek treatment to bring these experiences under control. Helping patients establish and maintain control over experiences and behaviors that threaten their safety and well-being is a core part of the work that I do as a psychiatrist.

Control is also deeply important for survivors of trauma. As noted in the last chapter, Judith Herman states that experiences and events are traumatic when "they overwhelm the ordinary systems of care and connection that give people a sense of control, connection, and meaning."[11] Post-traumatic stress is the lingering experience of living in a world that has at one time (and often far more than once) been experienced as dangerous and uncontrollable. The ability to seek and to establish safety and control—not only control of the body's responses but control over the circumstances of one's life and relationships—is a central part of trauma healing. Control over one's life and one's body helps to protect trauma survivors from violence and retraumatization.

Not just trauma survivors but *everyone* needs a basic sense of control in navigating life circumstances. As I argued in the last chapter when discussing the virtues of self-regulation, control is the seedbed of agency. Just as I am more capable of successful and purposeful action when at home in North Carolina, surrounded by familiar places and institutions where I belong, than

8. Advertisement for Qelbree (viloxazine) in the *American Journal of Psychiatry*, inside front cover, September 2021 issue.

9. Advertisement for Ingrezza (valbenazine) in *Psychiatric News*, Neurocrine Biosciences, May 2022, inside front cover.

10. William R. Miller and Ricardo F. Muñoz, *Controlling Your Drinking: Tools to Make Moderation Work for You*, 2nd ed. (New York: Guilford, 2013).

11. Judith Herman, *Trauma and Recovery: The Aftermath of Violence—from Domestic Abuse to Political Terror* (New York: Basic Books, 1997), 33.

I am when I visit California or New York, so are all of us more able to be the *principia* of our action when we have been able to establish basic levels of control of our bodies, our relationships, and our daily lives.

But pursuing control can also be dangerous. Control is a good, but it is not the *ultimate* good of mental health care. When pursued as an ultimate good, it can paradoxically diminish and thwart agency rather than promote it. There are three dangers that attend the pursuit of control as the highest good of mental health care.

First, the pursuit of control always entails recognition of an authority that has helped to establish and to maintain control. When mental health care is focused on control of symptoms or unwanted experiences and behaviors above all else, this naturally grants authority to whatever technology or system is credited with having achieved that control. A particular medication, and with it the systems of commercialization and distribution that make the medication possible, may be seen as indispensable. A particular form of psychotherapy, and with it the mental health leaders most responsible for developing and promoting that form of therapy, may be seen as authorities not only on the particular therapeutic technique but on life as a whole. Ways of seeing human experience such as self-body dualism or self-symptom dualism may be regarded as the only ways to avoid stigma and promote recovery.

Submitting to authority for a time in order to gain control of a difficult situation is necessary in human life. But to the extent that our lives revolve around gaining and maintaining control, we will serve the authority that has delivered control to us. Deferring to that authority, we will begin to understand ourselves through the lens of that authority, interpreting our own experience in a way that is amenable to being guided and helped by that authority. Deeply wanting to be helped by a medication, we might imagine ourselves and our bodies as broken or "chemically imbalanced." Deeply wanting to be helped by a trauma-focused psychotherapy, we might understand our experience through the framework of the *DSM* diagnosis of post-traumatic stress disorder (PTSD) and locate the source of our distress in a particular traumatic event. We may envision not just our problems but our *selves* in relation to the authorities that have delivered, or promise to deliver, control to us.

But then we have to ask, Toward what ends are we being formed, in submitting ourselves to these authorities? Nothing in mental health care is value neutral. Patients are always being shaped to value certain things and not others; to act in certain ways and not others; to relate to others in particular ways and not others. Even psychotherapy that aspires to be nondirective forms patients to be a certain kind of person—most of the time, a modern liberal self who discovers values and acts according to them.[12] Some forms of psychotherapy assume a clear vision of human flourishing that is the goal of care, to the extent that psychotherapy can be understood as analogous to religious formation and training.[13] But other forms of therapy, especially medication, are commodities that can point to a wide variety of ends, depending on who is promoting and using them in a market economy. All of this raises the question, Who decides who needs controlling, or what needs to be controlled? The quest for control can all too easily just reinforce prevailing social norms about respectability or productivity.

The need to be vigilant about the ends toward which we are directed when pursuing control was made clear in a *New York Times* opinion essay that was published soon after the US Food and Drug Administration (FDA) approved the neurosteroid brexanolone (trade name Zulresso) for postpartum depression, the first drug to be specifically approved by the FDA for this condition. Postpartum depression is indeed a major source of suffering for many women at a critical period for mothers and infants alike and can be associated not only with the suffering of major depressive disorder but also with challenges in mother-infant bonding and maternal suicide. It would seem that any pharmacological treatment of postpartum depression would be an unqualified good. But Elisa Albert and Jennifer Block argue that while brexanolone may help some women, it is important not to understand postpartum depression as a chemical or hormonal problem requiring a chemical or hormonal solution. They point out that postpartum depression is more common in countries with high income inequality, high maternal and child mortality, and a prioritization of work—all of which characterize the United States. They argue that postpartum depression is worsened by the lack of support given to new mothers and parents in the United States. They observe that because brexanolone is an injection-only drug that must be administered in a hospital setting and costs several tens of thousands of dollars per treatment, it is likely to be more available to those with wealth and good health benefits. And they argue that beyond its accessibility and affordability, clinical promotion of brexanolone may further burden individual mothers and deflect attention from the kinds of social supports that all new mothers need:

> In an article for the National Women's Health Network, one of the few watchdog groups that shun industry funding, two researchers wrote that

12. James Mumford, "Therapy beyond Good and Evil," *New Atlantis* 68 (2022): 28–38.
13. Don Browning and Terry Cooper, *Religious Thought and the Modern Psychologies*, 2nd ed. (Minneapolis: Fortress, 2000).

if Zulresso becomes the go-to fix for postpartum depression, "the onus of treatment will remain where it's always been, on individual mothers— hardly a revolution in postpartum care."

If insurers are willing to throw down tens of thousands of dollars for a mother's mental health, we can think of some alternatives that might have a better cost-benefit ratio: Six months paid leave. A live-in doula and a private sleep-training coach. Weekly massages and pelvic-floor rehab sessions. Relocation to a commune in the Bahamas.

In the meantime, we fear that Zulresso is just a stopgap, and yet another instance of pathologizing a very sane reaction to our very insane culture.[14]

Albert and Block echo many other critics of psychiatry and mental health care who argue that in its promise of control, often framed in medical language as control of medical problems, mental health care may intentionally or unintentionally transmit dominant neoliberal cultural values of productivity, competition, independence, and consumption. In chapter 1, we encountered Linda Blum's sociological observations that mothers of children with disabilities often feel implicit and explicit pressure to accept medication for their children in order to facilitate their participation in resource-strapped educational systems,[15] Joseph Davis's observation that the "neurobiological imaginary" discourages deep reflection on the inner life and encourages flat, productivity-oriented ways of describing unwanted emotion,[16] and Bruce Rogers-Vaughn's critique of counseling that only adjusts clients to living in a neoliberal political and economic order without engaging the root problems.[17] To this, we might add Jeffrey Bishop's, M. Therese Lysaught's, and Andrew Michel's argument that the practices and deployment of contemporary neuroscience are deeply bound up in neoliberal ways of thinking, and that neuroscience does not so much discover truths about human morality as

14. Elisa Albert and Jennifer Block, "It Will Take More Than a $34,000 Drug to Stop Postpartum Depression," *New York Times*, March 24, 2019, https://www.nytimes.com /2019/03/24/opinion/postpartum-depression-zulresso.html. The authors are quoting Sophie Krensky and Olivia Shannon, "A New Treatment for Postpartum Depression: Boon or Bane?," National Women's Health Network, March 20, 2019, https://nwhn.org/a-new-treat ment-for-postpartum-depression-boon-or-bane/.

15. Linda F. Blum, *Raising Generation Rx: Mother Kids with Invisible Disabilities in an Age of Inequality* (New York: New York University Press, 2015).

16. Joseph E. Davis, *Chemically Imbalanced: Everyday Suffering, Medication, and Our Troubled Quest for Self-Mastery* (Chicago: University of Chicago Press, 2020).

17. Bruce Rogers-Vaughn, *Caring for Souls in a Neoliberal Age* (New York: Palgrave Macmillan, 2016).

reflect prevailing economic and moral assumptions.[18] We might also engage Jonathan Metzl's argument that traditional twentieth-century gender norms that were often reflected in mid-century psychoanalysis were not challenged but rather continued in the rise of psychopharmacology. The rise of psychopharmacology, Metzl argues, should not be read as a scientific story alone but rather as the "product of multiple, interrelated discourses, each one of which comes to inform the other."[19]

Control, then, is a good, but it is not the highest good, and pursuit of control for its own sake leads us to defer to the authorities that we understand to have enabled us to establish and to maintain control. How, then, might Thomas Aquinas help us make sense of the possibilities and limits of control, and the way that control should be pursued?

Aquinas holds that humans are by nature the kind of creatures who act for ends that we perceive to be good, and that human actions take their identity by what they are *for*. Part of the answer to the question of control has already been given in chapter 6, related to Aquinas's discussion of *beatitudo*, participation in blessing. Lower-order goods such as wealth, honors, and pleasure are genuine goods, but pursuing them for their own sake, as one's highest good, will lead to neither *beatitudo* nor genuine freedom. Given that modern neoliberal economic orders place the pursuit of these lower-order goods, particularly wealth and pleasure, at the center of human decision making, then it is no surprise from a Thomistic perspective that rates of depression, anxiety, and substance-use problems are on the rise in a culture dominated by the pursuit of lower-order goods. But framing this as a problem of individual choices and individual risk factors, as modern mental health care tends to do, only reinforces the problem, because it ignores the systemic and structural forces that have led us to understand ourselves as individuals to begin with. Accepting lower-order goods as the highest goods invites structures of death-dealing power to operate in us and through us without our conscious awareness. Furthermore, modern mental health care practices that focus only on reducing the subjective distress of individuals or on meeting the consumer choices of individuals, without consideration of higher-order goods, can easily become a cipher for these systems and structures of power.

---

18. Jeffrey P. Bishop, M. Therese Lysaught, and Andrew A. Michel, *Biopolitics after Neuroscience: Morality and the Economy of Virtue* (London: Bloomsbury Academic, 2022).

19. Jonathan Michael Metzl, *Prozac on the Couch: Prescribing Gender in the Era of Wonder Drugs* (Durham, NC: Duke University Press, 2003), 18.

CHAPTER 9

For Aquinas, because God is the good that all seek, and because only the pursuit of God as one's highest end can enable true participation in blessing, the solution of the paradox of control is to pursue union with God and not to pursue lower-order goods such as wealth, honor, pleasure, or even physical and mental health as one's highest good. But this answer, even if it is true, is too simple. How does one avoid being deceived by religious communities and authorities who represent themselves as avenues to God but who are consumed by economies of control? Furthermore, what does union with God look like for those who are struggling with mental health problems while doing their best to make it in a complex world? What does it mean to pursue God as one's highest good for a veteran who is just returning from war and tormented by post-traumatic memories? What does it mean to pursue God as one's highest good for a college student who feels immobilized by anxiety, two weeks before final exams? What does it mean to pursue God as one's highest good for a single mother of three children who is working two jobs and still struggling to pay rising rent?

Fortunately, Aquinas does not leave readers only with a general affirmation to pursue God. As reviewed in detail in chapters 7 and 8, he offers a detailed picture of the journey toward agency and freedom in God in his description of intellect, will, emotion, the virtues, and the gifts of the Holy Spirit. While even Aquinas's most ardent readers would not embrace all of his prescriptions, his broad picture of the human as wayfarer in need of virtues and gifts for a successful journey remains compelling.

In addition to his teaching on the virtues and gifts, Aquinas offers an additional framework for understanding how humans might pursue life in the world while also orienting ourselves to God as our highest good. Following an established tradition in ancient and medieval thought, he describes two characteristic forms of human life: the active life (*vita activa*) and the contemplative life (*vita contemplativa*). The active life—far more familiar to most of us—is the arena in which humans pursue various forms of productive activity: farming, parenting, teaching, shopping, cleaning, and so on. The active life is a positive good, essential for human life and for the pursuit of *beatitudo*. But the active life cannot stand alone. It both enables and is sustained by a very different form of life, the contemplative life, which is characterized not by productive economic activity but by "holy leisure," by rest and enjoyment in God and in the truths of God. The active life is *for* the contemplative life. Control is *for* wonder, love, and praise.

I will first examine Aquinas's teaching on the active life, showing that even on its own terms, it offers a compelling account of agency as a central good of mental health care. Then I will examine Aquinas's teaching on the contemplative life and show how both action and contemplation are important human goods and central to *beatitudo*. Finally, I will consider the shape of a mental health care that is ordered to the goods of contemplation.

The Active Life

The active life is the life that most of us, most of the time, live in the world. It is the life devoted to various forms of productive activity—to building, serving, teaching, cultivating, and nurturing. The active life, Aquinas says, "provides for the necessities of the present life by means of well-ordered activity" (*STh* IIaIIae q. 179 a. 2 *ad3*). It is *not* a life devoted to pleasure, the *vita voluptuosa*, which for Aquinas is a form of life shared with the animals (*STh* IIaIIae q. 179 a. 2 *ad1*).

Aquinas holds that the active life is good. First, it is good because God's creation is good and needs care and love. As humans, we depend on each other for nurture and care. As I write this paragraph, I am sitting on the porch of a lovely Franciscan retreat center in the hills of central North Carolina, enjoying the warm sunshine of a cool spring day. It is a beautiful and holy place, a space that is given to prayer and contemplation. But my time here is possible only because of the careful, skilled productive activity of many people. Most immediately, I am indebted to the kind retreat center hosts who greet visitors, prepare meals, clean the rooms, and maintain the buildings. But I am also indebted to the workers who cleared the land, blazed the graveled trails, and built the buildings, to those who operated the gas station from which I purchased gasoline for my journey, and to many others. All of these people, as they fulfilled these roles, were devoted to the active life. The active life is a way that we serve each other and cultivate our common life as human beings—including forms of life that make contemplation possible. The active life is good because through it we love our neighbors and love God *by* loving our neighbors. Aquinas states that in contrast to the contemplative life, which seeks to devote itself to God alone,

> the active life, which ministers to our neighbor's needs, belongs directly to the love of one's neighbor. And just as out of charity we love our neighbor for God's sake, so the services we render our neighbor redound to God, according to Matthew 25:40, *What you have done . . . to one of these my least brethren, you did it to me.* (*STh* IIaIIae q. 188 a. 2 *resp.*)

For Aquinas, we love God in part by loving others, and this God-directed love of others happens within the active life.

Second, the active life is good because it is in the context of the active life that the virtues of acting (the moral virtues) are developed, tended, and displayed. Aquinas agrees with Aristotle that what we do shapes who we become: we become just by the doing of just actions, courageous by doing brave things, temperate by caring rightly for ourselves in the face of temptation, and so on. Virtue therefore requires action, and the active life is the seedbed and field of the moral virtues. Indeed, the active life is largely the life that Aquinas lived as a busy Dominican friar, teacher, and scholar, and he strongly defended the role of the active life among members of religious orders (*STh* IaIIae q. 188 a. 2). Aquinas is also quick to point out that Jesus himself, in his preaching and teaching, lived the active life—though, to be sure, Christ's active life was "built on abundance of contemplation" (*STh* IIIa q. 40 a. 1 *ad2*). The active life is the testing ground on which we are able to develop the intellectual and moral virtues necessary for "quieting and directing the internal passions of the soul" and therefore preparing the way for contemplation. Quoting Gregory the Great, Aquinas affirms that "those who wish to hold the fortress of contemplation must train in the camp of action" (*STh* IaIIae q. 182 a. 3 *resp.*).

Not surprisingly, considering "mental health" through the perspective of Aquinas's treatment of the active life looks similar to the account of mental health given by his treatment of the virtues and gifts. Pursuing a healthy active life requires that one orient one's life not to the pursuit of pleasure (the *vita voluptuosa*) but to the pursuit of meaningful and engaging activity. Correlatively, the central good of the active life is not subjective well-being but rather agency, the capacity to be the seat of one's action and to pursue goals that are meaningful. A healthy active life would focus on the cultivation of the virtues of knowing and acting as pathways to agency. It would also focus on social connectedness and relationships, both because agency emerges within these relationships and because a central part of the active life is the concrete expression of love for others. From the perspective of the active life, mental health names a life that is connected, purposive, and constructive of the common good.

It follows from this that if the active life is a goal, mental health care would depart significantly from the machine metaphor. First, it would focus not primarily on symptoms but on agency—on whether and how someone is able to act freely as the *principium*, or originator, of his or her action, and to navigate effectively in the world. Second, because the active life happens in the context of a social whole, a vision of mental health care focused on the active life would foreground the material and social conditions of someone's life and focus on how to effectively appraise and to navigate these conditions rather than to assume that mental health problems somehow spring primarily from inside the brain circuits of an individual. It would focus not on inside-out models of mental illness, where mental illness springs from the inside of a person, but rather on outside-in models, where mental health challenges arise as contextual problems in navigating complex social realities (see chapter 3). This is to say that mental health care pointing to the active life would focus on justice as a primary good and virtue. Third, mental health care focused on the active life would place primary weight on the development, cultivation, and sustenance of the moral virtues as constitutive of flourishing—not in a way that is moralistic or judgmental but in a way that understands that with virtue comes freedom to live justly and joyfully in a fragmented and complex world.

The Contemplative Life

A vision of mental health care focused on the active life already resists the individualistic, dualistic, technicist, commodified forms that modern mental health care can sometimes take. We may want to stop there and to hold out the active life as the goal of mental health care. But this would not satisfy Aquinas. For Aquinas the active life, as good as it is, is not the highest or the best form of life. The active life both points to and is sustained by a higher and deeper form of life, the contemplative life (*vita contemplativa*).

Aquinas's discussion of the kinds of ends that will deliver true participation in blessing (*beatitudo*; see chapter 6) points to the importance of the contemplative life. In discussing the goods in which *beatitudo* consists, he specifically argues that many common goals of human action—wealth, honor, fame, glory, power, bodily health, pleasure, or any other good of life—do not themselves constitute *beatitudo* (*STh* IaIIae q. 2). The goods pursued within the active life, that is, are good but not ultimately satisfying. Indeed, happiness cannot consist in any created good, because "nothing can bring the will of [humans] to rest except the universal good," which is God (*STh* IaIIae q. 2 a. 8 *resp.*). For Aquinas, the ultimate end of humanity—what humans and all human action are for—is God, the one who can so satisfy our desires that there is nothing left to desire. Among all goods, God is uniquely enough. Therefore, because *beatitudo* is found ultimately in God, contemplative activity, not inquiry about the created world or the angels, provides the highest form of happiness (*STh* IaIIae q. 3 aa. 5–7). In fact, perfect happiness consists in contemplating, viewing, the essence of God (*STh* IaIIae q. 3 a. 8). And so true *beatitudo*, true participation in blessing, requires that we seek not only the active life but also the contemplative life.

What, then, is the essence of the contemplative life, and why is it important? It is an affirmation that our modes of productive doing and being—our serving, our teaching, our building, even our caring and nurturing—are not the sum total and end of our existence. The contemplative life emphatically proclaims that a culture that values productivity, efficiency, and consumption above all else is ultimately self-consuming and does not have the last word. There is a "more" to our existence, beyond our productive labor. And this "more" has to do with the fact that above all, God is love, and that love, not productivity, is the most powerful force in the cosmos. To participate in the contemplative life is to see God in and through all things, and to find ourselves drawn more deeply toward love of God and toward love of God's good creatures—including ourselves and all those who are around us.

Aquinas quotes Gregory the Great to say that "the contemplative life is to cling with our whole mind to the love of God and our neighbor, and to desire nothing beside our Creator" (*STh* IIaIIae q. 180 a. 1 *sed contra*). Indeed, for Thomas and Gregory, the contemplative life "consists in the love of God, inasmuch as through loving God we are aflame to gaze on [God's] beauty" (*STh* IIaIIae q. 180 a. 1 *resp.*). Reflecting on Thomas's formulation, Josef Pieper comments that contemplation in its fullest sense occurs "when love is directed toward the infinite divine appeasement which courses through all reality from the ultimate ground of reality."[20]

But this loving gaze at God's beauty allows us to see beauty in all other creatures as well. Reflecting on Aquinas's description of the contemplative life, Josef Pieper remarks,

> A man drinks at last after being extremely thirsty, and, feeling refreshment permeating his body, thinks and says, "What a glorious thing is fresh water!" Such a man, whether he knows it or not, has already taken a step toward that "seeing of the beloved object" which is contemplation. How splendid is water, a rose, a tree, an apple, a human face—such exclamations can scarcely be spoken without also giving tongue to an assent and affirmation which extends beyond the object praised and touches upon the origin of

20. Josef Pieper, *Happiness and Contemplation*, trans. Richard and Clara Winston (South Bend: Saint Augustine's, 1998), 81.

the universe. Who among us has not suddenly looked into his child's face, in the midst of the toils and troubles of everyday life, and at that moment "seen" that everything which is good, is loved and lovable, loved by God! Such certainties all mean, at bottom, one and the same thing: that the world is plumb and sound; that everything comes to its appointed goal; that in spite of all appearances, underlying all things is—peace, salvation, *gloria*; that nothing and no one is lost; that "God holds in his hand the beginning, middle, and end of all that is." Such nonrational, intuitive certainties of the divine base of all that is can be vouchsafed to our gaze even when it is turned toward the most insignificant-looking things, if only it is a gaze inspired by love. That, in the precise sense, is contemplation.[21]

On its face, this formulation sounds dangerously naive and shortsighted. The world is, after all, full of suffering. It rarely seems "plumb and sound." Truthful contemplation surely would focus attention not on the world as "in spite of all appearances, . . . peace, salvation, *gloria*" but on the messy brokenness of the world as we find it. Pieper recognizes this objection but refuses its premises. Contemplation, he argues, requires "consent to the world as a whole," and "no one who thinks of the world as at bottom unredeemable can accept the idea that contemplation is the supreme [human] happiness." But this "consent to the world as a whole," this affirmation of the fundamental goodness and soundness of creation, does not entail a refusal to face evil. Indeed, "the happiness of contemplation is not a comfortable happiness."[22] It is, rather, to see Christ—Christ's life, Christ's passion, Christ's resurrection—at the world's root:

> Earthly contemplation means to the Christian, we have said, this above all: that behind all that we directly encounter the Face of the incarnate Logos becomes visible. This is not meant in any gnostic and mythical sense. Rather, we mean something simultaneously superhistorical and historical. The historical element is this: that the Face of the Divine Man bears the marks of a shameful execution. Contemplation does not ignore the "historical Gethsemane," does not ignore the mystery of evil, guilt and its bloody atonement. The happiness of contemplation is a true happiness, indeed the supreme happiness, but it is founded upon sorrow.[23]

21. Pieper, *Happiness and Contemplation*, 84–85; quoting Plato, *Laws* 715e.
22. Pieper, *Happiness and Contemplation*, 106–7.
23. Pieper, *Happiness and Contemplation*, 108.

The essence of contemplation, then, is to see God in and through all things; to be able to look on the world and on each of its creatures with affirmation and love of the goodness of existence; to be able to see, in and through evil and sorrow, a love that is stronger and more tenacious than death.

How, according to Aquinas, does one cultivate the contemplative life? First, it turns out that while the moral virtues of prudence, justice, courage, and self-regulation pertain primarily to the active life, they are necessary also for the contemplative life. They prepare the way for it. As noted above, Aquinas approvingly quotes Gregory the Great that "those who wish to hold the fortress of contemplation must first of all train in the camp of action" (*STh* IIaIIae q. 182 a. 3 *sed contra*). So the practices by which we live in the everyday world turn out to be important for being able to see beyond, through the world to the goodness of God in all things.

Important as the moral virtues are for disposing us to the contemplative life, though, they are not its essence. Aquinas specifies that the contemplative life is ultimately about the intellect's extending itself, insofar as is possible in this life, to God and to the truths of God. Because consideration of God and the things of God does not come easily to us—as material creatures, we are not like the angels, who can perceive God by simple apprehension—a certain training of the intellect is also required for the contemplative life. This training of the intellect is the second building block of the contemplative life. In part, for Aquinas, this involves the cultivation of the virtues of knowing (the intellectual virtues), such as the capacity to reason clearly from principles (*STh* IIaIIae q. 180 a. 3 *resp.*). Partly it involves the ability to notice and to attend to our interior life as we seek wisdom and knowledge.[24] But Aquinas is most specific about practices required for the contemplative life when he reflects on Hugh of Saint Victor's statement that the contemplative life requires prayer, reading, and meditation. Humans, Aquinas states, reach the knowledge of truth not only through personal study and effort but through receiving what is true from others. The contemplative life, therefore, requires the practice of prayer, that we may open ourselves to receiving what is true from God. It also requires the practices of careful listening to the spoken word of others (*auditus*) and of reading (*lectio*), that we might open ourselves to the truth of

---

24. Quoting Richard of Saint Victor, who distinguishes between contemplation, meditation, and cogitation, Aquinas notes that "contemplation is the soul's clear and free dwelling upon the object of its gaze; meditation is the survey of the mind while occupied in searching for the truth; and cogitation is the mind's glance which is prone to wander" (*STh* IIaIIae q. 180 a. 3 *ad1*). These medieval contemplative practices resonate in some ways with modern mindfulness practices.

God as it is passed on to us by others. Finally, having received truth from God and from others, in the practice of meditation (*meditatio*), we apply ourselves to the truth received.

Third, Aquinas argues that while the contemplative life ultimately aims at God as its object, nonetheless as sensible, bodily creatures, we build capacity for contemplation by attending not just to God but to the created world, insofar as created things reflect God's truth and beauty and can point the way to God:

> Since, however, God's effects show us the way to the contemplation of God Himself, according to Rom. 1:20, "The invisible things of God . . . are clearly seen, being understood by the things that are made," it follows that the contemplation of the divine effects also belongs to the contemplative life, inasmuch as [humans are] guided thereby to the knowledge of God. Hence Augustine says that "in the study of creatures we must not exercise an empty and futile curiosity, but should make them the stepping-stone to things unperishable and everlasting." (*STh* IIaIIae q. 180 a. 4 *resp.*)[25]

As Pieper makes clear above, the contemplative life is not simply an opportunity to contemplate God but also to contemplate all things in God, and God in all things.

For all of this, however, the contemplative life is not entirely a matter of human effort. Like the life of faith in general, our capacity to see God and all things in God comes to us as gift, in the theological virtue of charity. Charity, as described in previous chapters, is God's love, given to us, by which we are able to love God and all things in return; and so the love that draws us to God is in fact given from God and is not of us. "The love whereby God is loved out of charity," Aquinas says, "surpasses all love. Hence it is written: 'O taste and see that the LORD is sweet' (Ps. 33:9 [ET 34:8])" (*STh* IIaIIae q. 180 a. 7 *resp.*).

The Activity of Rest: What Contemplation Makes Possible

The contemplative life is for Aquinas a form of rest—a restful activity that anticipates the active rest that will come when we see God in all of God's glory in the eschaton, when there is nothing left to desire. But it is a rest that makes possible certain forms of activity.

---

25. Aquinas is quoting Augustine, *True Religion* 24.

First, the contemplative life makes possible *play*—nonproductive, joyful exploration of created life. Just as developmental psychologists have long recognized that children need time and space for play, so also adults, including adults with mental illness and *all of us*, need time and space for play—not just play that is focused on external goods, like becoming physically fit or fitting into a social group, but play that encourages and enables creativity.

Second, the contemplative life is embodied by and makes possible practices of Sabbath. Just as God finished the productive activity of creation, including the creation of humans, on the sixth day, and then on the seventh day, "God finished the work that he had done, and he rested on the seventh day, . . . [and] blessed the seventh day and hallowed it" (Gen. 2:2-3), so also Sabbath is for us a commandment and call not to allow the world of productive labor and efficient control to define our lives. It is a call to actively rest in God's restful activity.[26]

Third, the contemplative life makes possible genuine celebration and festivity. We live in a culture of what Josef Pieper calls "artificial holidays"—holidays that promote or even are wholly founded on productive control. Artificial holidays, Pieper writes, "[point] to the claim that man, especially in the exercise of his political power, is able to bring about his own salvation as well as that of the world." But Pieper argues in contrast to this that true festivity emerges from the capacity to see beyond the busyness of productive labor to the fundamental beauty and goodness of creation and to respond in love to that beauty and goodness. The "inner structure of real festivity," Pieper argues, is shown most precisely in a formulation attributed to John Chrysostom, "*Ubi caritas gaudet, ibi est festivitas*, 'Where love rejoices, there is festivity.'" Festivity is a response of joy to the goodness of existence: it is "to live out, for some special occasion and in an uncommon manner, the universal assent to the world as a whole." The festivity enabled by contemplation renders us "in tune with the world."[27]

The Contemplative Life and Mental Health Care

While for Aquinas the active life challenges the reductive foundations of the machine metaphor of mental health, the contemplative life displays a radical

26. Abraham Joshua Heschel, *The Sabbath: Its Meaning for Modern Man* (New York: Farrar, Strauss & Giroux, 1951); Norman Wirzba, *Living the Sabbath: Discovering the Rhythms of Rest and Delight* (Grand Rapids: Brazos Press, 2006); Marva J. Dawn, *Keeping the Sabbath Wholly: Ceasing, Resting, Embracing, Feasting* (Grand Rapids: Eerdmans, 1989).

27. Josef Pieper, *In Tune with the World: A Theory of Festivity*, trans. Richard and Clara Winston (South Bend: Saint Augustine's, 1965), 23, 30, 62.

and incommensurable alternative to it. If life in its richest and fullest dimension involves the capacity to open oneself to the fundamental goodness and beauty of God and of the creation and to respond in love to that apprehension, and if this is the animating core of *beatitudo*, then any form of care that is adequate to who humans are must open space for wonder. To walk with and to care for humans in any setting, and especially in a mental health care setting, is to care for wayfarers whose hearts are yearning for connection to what is true and good and beautiful. Any form of mental health care that construes bodies and brains as machines to be tweaked or titrated, or complex experiences as merely symptoms to be controlled, will leave its practitioners and patients unsatisfied. It may be technically successful, but it will leave us unsatisfied and longing for more.

Because humans are not machines but rather wayfarers longing for God, it is wholly unsurprising that many of the most successful psychotherapeutic models within mental health care, including some that ardently present themselves as evidence based and scientific, invite participants into some form of contemplation. These models often draw explicitly from traditions of mystical or religious contemplation, and their founders and creators frequently draw on profound personal mystical and spiritual experiences. Dialectical behavior therapy (DBT), for example, is a widely accepted and celebrated treatment for borderline personality disorder and is helpful for people who struggle with strong and unpredictable swings of emotion, persistent feelings of emptiness, and challenges navigating complex interpersonal situations. Mindfulness practices, derived mostly from Zen meditative techniques, are a core component of DBT. The founder of DBT, psychologist Marsha Linehan, makes clear that DBT is a rigorously tested and empirically supported treatment for borderline personality disorder. But the seeds of it grew from a profound spiritual experience in Linehan's own life. Years after DBT became a mainstream treatment in modern mental health care, Linehan disclosed that as a teen she had been hospitalized for a total of twenty-six months in an inpatient psychiatric hospital for chronic suicidal thoughts and severe emotional dysregulation. As a young adult, she continued to struggle and also continued to turn to her Catholic faith. In her mid-twenties, she found profound healing while praying in the chapel of a Catholic retreat center in Chicago. A 2011 *New York Times* report described her story:

> "One night I was kneeling in there, looking up at the cross, and the whole place became gold—and suddenly I felt something coming toward me," she said. "It was this shimmering experience, and I just ran back to my room

and said, 'I love myself.' It was the first time I remember talking to myself in the first person. I felt transformed."[28]

Like DBT, mindfulness-based stress reduction (MBSR) is a widely used individual and group psychotherapeutic practice for anxiety, pain, and stress that is in essence a rendering of Zen Buddhist principles within the language and structure of contemporary, secular, western medicine.[29] MBSR has been found to be as effective for common anxiety disorders as the serotonin-active medication escitalopram.[30] Its founder, Jon Kabat-Zinn, states that MBSR "was developed as one of a possibly infinite number of skillful means for bringing the dharma into mainstream settings."[31] Kabat-Zinn reflects that MBSR grew out of his own spiritual wondering, as a molecular biology graduate student at MIT, "'what is my job with a capital J,' my 'karmic assignment' on the planet, so to speak."[32] He became deeply engaged in yoga and Zen meditation practice and carried these questions into a position at the newly formed University of Massachusetts Medical School in 1976. He describes how his "karmic assignment" then unfolded:

On a two-week vipassanā retreat at the Insight Meditation Society (IMS) in Barre, Massachusetts, in the Spring of 1979, while sitting in my room one afternoon about Day 10 of the retreat, I had a "vision" that lasted maybe 10 seconds. I don't really know what to call it, so I call it a vision. It was rich in detail and more like an instantaneous seeing of vivid, almost inevitable connections and their implications. It did not come as a reverie or a thought stream, but rather something quite different, which to this day I cannot fully explain and don't feel the need to.

I saw in a flash not only a model that could be put in place, but also the long-term implications of what might happen if the basic idea was sound

28. Benedict Carey, "Expert on Mental Illness Reveals Her Own Fight," *New York Times*, June 23, 2011, https://www.nytimes.com/2011/06/23/health/23lives.html. Linehan recounts the story in somewhat more detail in Marsha Linehan, *Building a Life Worth Living: A Memoir* (New York: Random House, 2021), 101–5.

29. Jon Kabat-Zinn, *Full Catastrophe Living: Using the Wisdom of Your Body and Mind to Face Stress, Pain, and Illness*, 15th anniversary ed. (New York: Delta, 2009), 12–13.

30. Elizabeth A. Hoge et al., "Mindfulness-Based Stress Reduction vs. Escitalopram for the Treatment of Adults with Anxiety Disorders: A Randomized Clinical Trial," *JAMA Psychiatry* 2022, https://doi.org/10.1001/jamapsychiatry.2022.3679.

31. Jon Kabat-Zinn, "Some Reflections on the Origins of MBSR, Skillful Means, and the Trouble with Maps," *Contemporary Buddhism* 12 (2011): 281.

32. Kabat-Zinn, "Some Reflections," 286.

and could be implemented in one test environment—namely that it would spark new fields of scientific and clinical investigation, and would spread to hospitals and medical centers and clinics across the country and around the world, and provide right livelihood for thousands of practitioners. Because it was so weird, I hardly ever mentioned this experience to others. But after that retreat, I did have a better sense of what my karmic assignment might be. It was so compelling that I decided to take it on wholeheartedly as best I could.[33]

What are Christians to make of this? Christians can affirm the efforts of many modern forms of psychotherapy, including DBT, MBSR, and loving-kindness meditation, to encourage participants to a stance of attentiveness and wonder that challenges the machine metaphor. This stance is central to the contemplative life. But Christian teaching on the contemplative life would also affirm that the ultimate good of meditative and mindfulness practice is not the emptying of the self and its desires. Rather, meditative and mindfulness practices for the Christian lead naturally to prayer, and as such, they seek a positive good, namely, union with God and participation in God's love. In a letter to Catholic bishops likely written by Josef Ratzinger before his elevation to the papacy, the Congregation for the Doctrine of the Faith articulated this distinction:

> Christian prayer is always determined by the structure of the Christian faith, in which the very truth of God and creature shines forth. For this reason, it is defined, properly speaking, as a personal, intimate and profound dialogue between man and God. It expresses therefore the communion of redeemed creatures with the intimate life of the Persons of the Trinity. This communion, based on Baptism and the Eucharist, source and summit of the life of the Church, implies an attitude of conversion, a flight from "self" to the "You" of God. Thus Christian prayer is at the same time always authentically personal and communitarian. It flees from impersonal techniques or from concentrating on oneself, which can create a kind of rut, imprisoning the person praying in a spiritual privatism which is incapable of a free openness to the transcendental God. Within the Church, in the legitimate search for new methods of meditation it must always be borne in mind that the essential element of authentic Christian prayer is

33. Kabat-Zinn, "Some Reflections," 287.

the meeting of two freedoms, the infinite freedom of God with the finite freedom of man.[34]

For Christians, the contemplative life is not a technique for altering mood or reducing stress, nor is self-emptying a good to be pursued for its own sake. Rather, it is a set of practices by which we are invited to attend to God and to all things in God.

That said, the experiences of Linehan and Kabat-Zinn affirm that mental health care that takes the contemplative life seriously will seek not only the cultivation of agency but also the cultivation of love. Just as apprehension of finite created goods engenders love, which then leads to desire for what is loved (see chapter 7), even more does contemplation of God, the ultimate and highest good, engender love for God and for all things in God. Rejecting the machine metaphor's focus on control, and exceeding the active life's focus on agency, the contemplative life encourages the growth of love in those who pursue it and helps us to train our loves. Aquinas's description of the contemplative life teaches us to ask, in our practice of and engagement in mental health care, not just, "Am I growing in agency and freedom?" but also, "Am I growing in love?"

Grounded in love, mental health care that takes the contemplative life seriously will not be shy about seeking joy. In Aquinas's system, joy is love's rest, the consummation of the union of lover with what is loved (*STh* IaIIae q. 31 a. 3). In his prayer "For the Attainment of Heaven," Aquinas asks God to grant him

> that life without death
> and that joy without sorrow
> > where there is
> > the greatest freedom
> > unconfined security
> > secure tranquility
> > delightful happiness
> > happy eternity
> > eternal blessedness
> > the vision of truth and praise, O God. (*STh* IaIIae q. 31 a. 3)

---

34. "Letter to the Bishops of the Catholic Church on Some Aspects of Christian Meditation," Congregation for the Doctrine of the Faith, October 15, 1989. While the document does not name the forms of prayer that it is opposing, it most likely was addressing concerns about the centering prayer method of Fr. Thomas Keating.

The "joy without sorrow" that Aquinas prays for is marked by a progressive reinforcement of freedom, security, happiness, and participation in blessing.

Mental health care that takes the contemplative life seriously will be characterized by the cultivation and training of love and the pursuit of joy, but this does not mean that such mental health care will lead to joy or will *feel* joyful all of the time. It will not. Sometimes it will be characterized by suffering and lament, or by the determination of clinician and patient alike simply to make it through. The point of Christian teaching on the contemplative life, though, is not that it will always feel joyful. Indeed, the literature of Christian contemplation is full of descriptions of how hard it can be—not least in the context of *acedia*, the "noonday demon" described by early monastic writers Evagrius of Pontus and John Cassian and often interpreted as a possible analogue of depression, in which monks were beset by an intense restlessness and desire to escape from their contemplative form of life.[35] Mental health care modeled on contemplation may sometimes be a plodding road, but it aims at joy.

This discussion of the contemplative life may seem to be far too philosophical, theoretical, and even mystical to be of much relevance to modern mental health professionals, but this is not the case. Even clinicians who are deeply engaged in the neurosciences are increasingly calling for a more holistic, contemplative view of the mind and of mental health care. In *The Master and His Emissary: The Divided Brain and the Making of the Western World*, for example, psychiatrist and literary scholar Iain McGilchrist argues that the two hemispheres of the brain, the left and the right, are associated with different ways of taking up with the world. The left hemisphere-congruent way of engaging the world operates in what we might speak of as a "spotlight" approach. It is focused on grasping, categorizing, and naming things. It analyzes, distinguishes, picks apart, looks closely and narrowly. The left hemisphere operates in a mode of analysis and control. It specializes in denotative language, artifice, and critical distance. It sorts experience into discrete episodes and engages in sequential analysis. It seeks an enclosed self-consistency, security, and prioritizes linear rationality. Because our language centers are in the left hemisphere, our left-brain ways of operating are privileged in our language. Indeed, McGilchrist characterizes the left hemisphere as in control of the three Ls—language, logic, and linearity—that are central to discursive argument. In its critical and logical distancing, it promotes a disenchanted inhabitation of the world.[36]

---

35. Andrew Crislip, "The Sin of Sloth or the Illness of the Demons? The Demon of Acedia in Early Christian Monasticism," *Harvard Theological Review* 98 (2005): 143-69.

36. Iain McGilchrist, *The Master and His Emissary: The Divided Brain and the Making of the Western World* (New Haven: Yale University Press, 2009).

The right hemisphere, by contrast, operates in what we might call a "flood-light" fashion. It is attentive to context, to breadth, to taking in the whole rather than isolated parts. It takes in experience in its immediate and "un-preconceived freshness," rather than in its categorization or its re-presentation in symbol and language.[37] It attends to things in their uniqueness, allowing experience simply to be rather than to force it into categories. If the left hemisphere attends to the rhythm of music, the right hemisphere attends to its melody, timbre, and harmony. It is the right hemisphere that is primarily associated with our experiences of beauty, and of transcendence, and of nonjudgmental awareness of the world. Eschewing enclosure, it also encourages enchantment and empathy.[38]

Both the left and the right hemispheres are deeply important for human flourishing, McGilchrist argues, and need each other. But he charges that Western philosophy and culture since Plato, including Western Christian philosophy, have privileged left-hemisphere ways of taking up with the world, which emphasizes categorization, linearity, analysis, and control. The left hemisphere, he argues, has come to be the master when it better operates as the emissary of the right brain.[39]

McGilchrist's advocacy for right-hemisphere ways of engaging the world are echoed in some ways by Daniel Siegel and other writers within interpersonal neurobiology. As discussed in chapter 6, Siegel understands mental health primarily in terms of integration, specifically integration of different parts of the brain. In his trade book *Mindsight*, he speaks of nine domains of integration. The first eight are the integration of consciousness (regulation of emotion and clear decision making), horizontal integration (left and right brain), vertical integration (brain and body), memory integration (past, present, and future), narrative integration (life as a coherent story), state integration (attention to basic human needs), interpersonal integration (flexible, realistic relationships), and temporal integration (acceptance of human finitude and mortality). This is followed by a ninth domain of integration, transpiration, an "integration of integration" in which "the boundaries of 'self' become wide open. Transpiration is how we dissolve our somehow confining sense of an 'I' and become part of an expanded identity, a 'we' larger than even

37. Iain McGilchrist, "Can the Divided Brain Tell Us Anything about the Ultimate Nature of Reality?," lecture to the Spirituality Interest Group of the Royal College of Psychiatrists, 2011, https://www.rcpsych.ac.uk/docs/default-source/members/sigs/spirituality-spsig/iain-mcgilchrist-can-the-divided-brain-tell-us-anything-about-the-ultimate-nature-of-reality.pdf.

38. McGilchrist, *Master and His Emissary*.

39. McGilchrist, *Master and His Emissary*.

our interpersonal relationships."[40] In the work of McGilchrist and Siegel, neuroscience itself gestures to a posture of wonder.

From Control to Wonder

The man in the tombs had long lived in an economy of control. At the beginning of the story, the unclean spirits seemed to be in control; they controlled the man and protested and rejected Jesus's efforts to cast them out. But Jesus, controlling the demons, restored the man to a place of control that he could not previously imagine and that he did not know that he wanted. Jesus's healing left him free, "clothed and in his right mind" and sitting before Jesus, with agency and a charge to tell his story to others (Mark 5:15). With the demons controlled, the man was free to seek Jesus and to participate in Jesus's ministry and life, and in doing so to invite all who were around him into a space of amazement and wonder.

The Gerasene man may or may not have had what we would now call a mental illness, but his story is relevant for modern mental health care. As in his story, control of symptoms (or unwanted experience and behavior) is often an important first step. But the goal of mental health care cannot *end* in control. If control is pursued for its own sake, mental health care will ultimately become a trap rather than a liberator.

The Gerasene man's story teaches us, rather, that while control is a good, it is not our highest good. We find our deepest fulfillment not in control but in love, wonder, praise, and rest, insofar as all of these are directed toward God as our highest end. For Christians, this begins with the affirmation that our lives are about more than control; that beyond the suffering of the present, God is present and is love; and that the calling of our lives is to grow into deeper and fuller lovers of God and of the beautiful and holy people and things that God has made.

In the light of this, we are able to ask ourselves, In our practices of caring and receiving care, are we growing in love for God and for God's good creatures? If the answer is no, we have some work to do. But if the answer is yes, then we are following the footsteps of the haunted Gerasene man who, liberated from the powers that controlled him, was freed for a life of mission, and left all who saw him in wonder.

---

40. Daniel Siegel, *Mindsight: The New Science of Personal Transformation* (New York: Bantam Books, 2011), 256.

From Fixing to Attending

We Journey Together, Awaiting a Feast

> Search me, O God, and know my heart;
> test me, and know my thoughts.
> See if there is any hurtful way in me,
> and lead me in the way everlasting.[1]
>
> *—Psalm 139:23-24*

> And he said to them, "What are you discussing with each
> other while you walk along?"
>
> *—Luke 24:17a*

We meet the two disciples on the road. They are weary and sad. They have followed Jesus through the countryside and into Jerusalem. They have seen him welcomed by an expectant crowd. They have seen him challenge the religious leaders whose power was centered in the temple. They watched as he was arrested, convicted in an unjust mob trial, and executed in a grisly, inhumane way. The trauma inflicted on Jesus's body is now lodged in theirs. On top of this, some women visited the tomb where Jesus was buried on the day following the Sabbath and found Jesus's body missing. They claimed that they had seen angels who told them that Jesus was alive. But whether because these disciples did not trust traumatized women, or did not trust themselves, or did not dare to hope, or all of these things, this word did not take away their sadness and grief. They had hoped that Jesus, this "prophet mighty in deed and word before God and all the people," would set Israel free, but the

---

1. The NRSV supplies "hurtful" as an alternative translation for the Hebrew *otseb*.

imperial Romans and their vassal authorities have violently reaffirmed their rule (Luke 24:19-21). They are walking together, away from the site of trauma, toward Emmaus.

Then a man comes near to them and begins to walk with them. "What are you discussing with each other while you walk along?" he asks (24:17). They tell him the story and context as they understand it.

What happened next may be surprising to those with modern therapeutic sensibilities. As far as we know, the man does not lament with them or take time to validate their sadness and grief. We do not know whether he speaks to them gently or sternly. Perhaps his tone holds a measure of both. We do know that he accuses them of not reasoning clearly with their minds and not allowing their hearts (their whole selves, including emotions) to believe and to trust the words of their own prophets that indicated that the Liberator's glory and rule would come not through triumphant political and military conquest but rather by suffering (24:25-26).[2] He then leads them in a study of Scripture, "beginning with Moses and all the prophets" (24:27). And he continues to walk alongside them.

Perhaps the two disciples, Cleopas and his companion, enjoyed the man's company and were intrigued by his deep knowledge of the law and the prophets. Perhaps they were simply bound by deep-seated norms of hospitality. But when they came near to Emmaus and the man walked ahead of them as if he were going on, they "urged him strongly" to stay with them (24:29).[3] The man went in to stay with them, went to the table with them, and "took bread, blessed and broke it, and gave it to them" (24:30). Their eyes were opened. They recognized him, not just as someone they knew about but as someone they knew in a deep and personal way. They recognized him as Jesus.

As a Christian with multiple graduate degrees who teaches at a medical school and a seminary, I am always humbled by the story of these two weary, traumatized, wandering disciples. If anyone had access to the right information and the right educational resources, they did. They probably knew Jesus personally. They were in Jerusalem on the week of his conviction and execution. They heard firsthand testimony of his reported resurrection. They walked many miles

---

2. The Greek word that the NRSV renders "foolish," *anoētos*, connotes a failure to properly use *nous*, mind or reason.

3. The Greek here, *parabiazomai*, suggests strong persuasion that borders on coercion. In the New Testament, it is used only here and in Acts 16:15, when after her baptism Lydia "prevailed" on Paul and his traveling companions to stay at her home. There is also a lovely and ironic parallel between the disciples' strong insistence that Jesus stay (abide, remain) with them and the Johannine Jesus's persistent admonition to the disciples to abide and remain in him (John 15:1-11).

with Jesus on the road, with *Jesus himself* leading them in a study of Scripture. Jesus was their Bible study leader! And yet they did not recognize him as Jesus. In fact, the text says that "their eyes were kept from recognizing him" (24:16).

Like the deaf man of Mark 7 whose ears needed to be opened by Jesus (Mark 7:31–37), their eyes needed to be opened. How did this opening happen? Not simply through impartation of information. Not through the study of Scripture alone. Not simply by being rebuked for their dullness of mind and slowness of heart. It happened, rather, because Jesus continued to walk with them, carefully and patiently talking with them about things that he would have already expected them to know. It happened because they invited him not just to walk with them but to stay (remain, abide) with them for the evening. It happened because Jesus, transforming from guest to host, took bread, blessed and broke it, and gave it to them—just as, perhaps, he had done with them only three evenings before with a larger group of disciples, though to them that would have been quite literally a lifetime ago. They knew him, not in the study of Scripture, not in abstract debate, not even when he was walking alongside them, but "in the breaking of the bread" (Luke 24:35).

Tables of Knowledge and Love

What kind of knowledge is healing for those who live with mental health problems? Mental health clinicians, and especially psychiatrists, tend to place a lot of weight on the importance of accurate, valid, and reliable diagnosis. The whole project of the *DSM*, psychiatry's diagnostic table, hinges on faith that reliable and valid diagnoses will lead to innovative and effective treatments for specific mental disorders.[4] Clinical diagnosis is a way of knowing that runs deep in the practice of medicine, at least since the time of Hippocrates. In Greek, the word *diagnōsis* connotes a practice of discerning or distinguishing. It is related to the verb *diaginōskō*, "to distinguish" or "to determine," and from there to the root word *gnōsis*, "knowledge," and the prefix *dia-*, which connotes "between" and also "thoroughly" and "entirely."[5] In the Greek, diagnosis is *knowledge of* or *knowledge about*, perhaps even *comprehensive* knowledge of or about.

---

4. As described in chapter 1, the NIMH RDoC project, though rejecting the *DSM* taxonomy, is just an extension of this quest for reliable and valid psychiatric diagnoses that lead to innovative and effective treatments.

5. *Online Etymology Dictionary*, s.v. "diagnosis (n.)," https://www.etymonline.com/word/diagnosis.

The machine metaphor traffics in this kind of abstract knowledge about. To the extent that human experience and behavior can be abstracted as symptoms, symptoms can be grouped into diagnoses. The point of mental health care is then to apply interventions to these diagnoses that have been shown in controlled studies to reduce symptoms. In this way, psychiatry churns along as a self-reinforcing system. Mental health clinicians and researchers (especially psychiatrists), as the authors and custodians of diagnosis and the designers and implementers of interventions, maintain our authority. People with mental health challenges, to the extent that they are conditioned to interpret unwanted experience and behavior through the language of diagnosis—especially if this is reinforced by self-body dualism, the assumption that what's wrong is enclosed in the body and therefore a medical or neurobiological problem—accede to clinicians' and researchers' authority even if they are uncomfortable with it. Politicians and policymakers readily attribute a variety of complex social ills such as gun violence, homelessness, and veteran suicide to mental illness (read: inside-out, internal problems of individuals) and thereby burnish the status and authority of clinicians and researchers. Patients and advocacy groups insist that people are not their diagnoses, that no one is an alcoholic or a schizophrenic, and clinicians respond by enforcing person-first language; but in truth, this association of illness with identity is probably inevitable in a system that places so much value in diagnostic "knowledge about." If the most important thing that I as a clinician know about persons is that they have schizophrenia, and if that concept stands at the very center of how I interact with them and what treatments I recommend to them, it will hardly be a surprise if these patients feel like I am treating them primarily as schizophrenics.

Interestingly, though, neither the Greek word *diagnōsis* nor its cognate verb *diaginōskō* are frequently used in the New Testament. In each case, they describe legal or juridical decisions rendered by Roman or Jewish authorities. In Acts 25, the Roman governor Porcius Festus tells the vassal king Agrippa that the imprisoned Paul has appealed "to be kept in custody for the decision [*diagnōsis*] of his Imperial Majesty" (i.e., the Roman emperor; Acts 25:21). Shortly before that, a group of Paul's enemies asked the chief priests and elders to "give notice now to the tribune to bring him down to you, as though you were going to determine [*diaginōskein*] his case more exactly" (Acts 23:15 RSV). The governor Felix later promises Paul that when he is joined by a Roman tribune named Lysias, "I will decide [*diagnōsomai*] your case" (Acts 24:22). In the New Testament, diagnosis is a form of knowing, but it is a formal, impersonal decision made by those in authority.

The knowledge that counts in Scripture and Christian faith, and certainly the kind of knowledge that heals, is not this diagnostic knowledge about. It is, rather, *personal* knowledge that connotes familiarity, intimacy, and love. It is knowledge that implies not only knowing another but also being known (Gal. 4:9; 1 Cor. 8:3). The disciples at Emmaus did not simply diagnose the presence of Jesus. They did not just know *about* him. Rather, they *recognized* and *knew* him in a personal and visceral way. The table where Jesus broke and blessed the bread was not a diagnostic table concerned with abstract *knowledge-about* but a table of communion, eucharistic blessing, and knowing in which they saw Jesus and each other in intimate ways that could not be abstracted in concepts or encapsulated in words. It was a table not of *knowledge-about* but of *knowledge-in-relation* (see figure 5). They associated his presence and then his absence with a burning in their hearts (Luke 24:32). They knew him and were known by him. And having recognized him, they did not stay alone in Emmaus. They did not continue to walk away from the site of Jesus's and their trauma. Rather, immediately after supper, they left and returned the seven miles to Jerusalem (possibly in the dark) to join the other disciples in amazement and wonder. Knowing Jesus, known by Jesus, they were led into community and communion with each other.

Resisting the Machine Metaphor

As she has navigated depression, Ann says that a quotation from Parker Palmer, in which Palmer reflects on his own depression, has been meaningful for her:

> The human soul doesn't want to be advised or fixed or saved. It simply wants to be witnessed—to be seen, heard and companioned exactly as it is. When we make that kind of deep bow to the soul of a suffering person, our respect reinforces the soul's healing resources, the only resources that can help the sufferer make it through.[6]

Palmer is not a Thomist, and he is speaking here not of the soul's desire for God but of his experience of well-meaning friends who tried to fix the situation and to reason and cajole him out of depression and yet only made his isolation

---

6. Parker Palmer, "The Gift of Presence, the Perils of Advice," *On Being* (blog), April 27, 2016, https://onbeing.org/blog/the-gift-of-presence-the-perils-of-advice/.

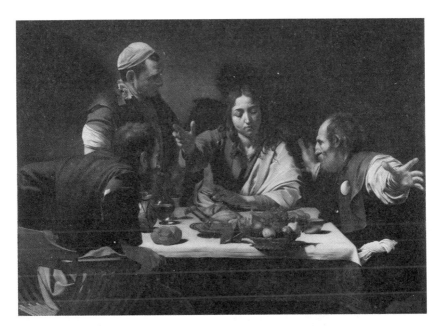

Figure 5. Caravaggio, *Supper at Emmaus*, 1601, National Gallery, London

and suffering more intense. But there is nevertheless considerable resonance between Palmer's Quaker spirituality and Aquinas's teaching that humans, though wounded by original sin, are made in the image of God, known and loved by God, and created for freedom. There is also resonance with Aquinas's teaching that this freedom comes most clearly and sustainably not through following external precepts of law but through growth in capacity to know what is true and to love and to act toward what is good and genuinely freeing. The best that any clinician, pastor, or friend can do when accompanying someone with depression or other mental health problems is to patiently nurture these capacities for knowledge and love. While Aquinas advocated for a holistic, multidimensional approach to treating what we would now call depression, including contemplation of truth and bodily practices like sleep and baths, Aquinas like Palmer understood that healing occurs in empathic, connected relationships:

> Since sorrow has a depressing effect, it is like a weight whereof we strive
> to unburden ourselves: so that when a man sees others saddened by his
> own sorrow, it seems as though others were bearing the burden with him,
> striving, as it were, to lessen its weight; wherefore the load of sorrow be-

comes lighter for him: something like what occurs in the carrying of bodily burdens. [Also,] when a man's friends condole with him, he sees that he is loved by them, and this affords him pleasure. (STh IaIIae q. 38 a. 3 resp.)

Ann describes how a group of friends provided this kind of empathic, connected support at a critical period in her own life:

I think immediately of three friends who were with me when I had a major emotional meltdown at a women's retreat. These three . . . were right there with me, present, not judging at all, as I had this major emotional meltdown. Laying exhausted on the floor. They just held me. Then after that, one of the speakers for that retreat pulled me aside and she said, "You understand, this is just the door opening. And now, you've got to go through this door and deal with this shit that's kind of coming, bubbling up and all this. What comes next is going to be harder."

These three friends pledged to meet with me. All four of us met together every week, for I don't know, two years. I would just go and sit with them and they would pray and I would cry and we would laugh. Sometimes we'd eat lunch, and then I knew I could come back and do it the next week. That was my group.

I could just be me. I wasn't getting judged and I wasn't getting fixed. I was just being embraced and trusted that I was doing my own work. Sometimes, I would talk about it. They never really even asked me questions. They just drew alongside and didn't try to fix me. They rejoiced when it looked like I was making progress. It was a real blessed time.[7]

As wayfarers, *viatores*, in this life, we travel alongside one another, loving and bearing up (and, all too often, wounding) one another. We do not fix, tweak, manage, or solve one another. We do not save one another: Christians believe that only God does that, even as we are granted the opportunity to participate in God's healing and saving work.

At its best, mental health care is a vital set of practices of caring for and traveling with wayfarers who are on the way to God. It is at its best not when it is viewed as an industrial process of providing technical means to achieve prespecified ends but as an organic process of tending to the needs of living human creatures who are always growing, always seeking safety and nurture, always on the way. It is at its best when it focuses not on helping workers

7. Personal interview, June 3, 2022.

and consumers streamline themselves to the demands of a neoliberal economic order and its demands for productivity, efficiency, and consumption but when it is rooted in a vision of participation in blessing (*beatitudo*) that exceeds and often contradicts this order and that beckons to a vision of what is true and good that brings freedom and the capacity to resist structures of injustice and dehumanization.

The pull of the machine metaphor in modern psychiatry and mental health care is strong. In our modern, industrialized, medicalized culture, it is hard not to see bodies as machines, illness as symptoms, therapy as technology, healing as symptom reduction, and care as quantifiable and commodifiable units of production. All of these are ways of seeing, perceiving, and describing human persons, human experience and behavior, and the promise and possibility of treatment. These ways of perceiving and speaking are not always bad. As I have argued in previous chapters, there are times when it is useful, for a time and in a certain context, to frame symptoms as separate from the self, illness as lodged in the body, and medications and other technologies as ways to reduce symptoms. But it is dangerous for the machine metaphor to be made synonymous with care. When this happens, policymakers, insurers, and health systems are authorized and emboldened to further mechanize and industrialize the work that "mental health providers" are expected to do. Treatment success becomes identified more with what can be measured on validated symptom scales than with what any particular person identifies as healing and transformative. The guardians of psychiatric diagnosis and of psychiatric research and development (the American Psychiatric Association, academic medical centers, pharmaceutical companies, and those who hold copyright on manual-based psychotherapy protocols) grow in wealth and power. Meanwhile, patients and clinicians alike are all too often left with a nagging suspicion that amidst all of the protocols and all of the technology, something deep and fundamental—the attention, care, and love that makes it possible to regard human beings in all of their beauty, dignity, and messy complexity—is missing.

This book is not intended to offer a set of policy prescriptions for fixing what is broken in modern mental health care (an image that itself would simply reproduce the machine metaphor). Though I value teaching in a well-regarded medical school and have deep respect for how hard my department works to train excellent psychiatrists, psychologists, and other mental health clinicians, I do not believe that the answer will come through educational tweaks such as the addition of courses on spirituality, narrative medicine, or whole-person care to mental health training curricula. Academic medical centers are far too formed in the practices of the machine metaphor for such modifications to be transformative.[8] But I believe that there is profound value in encouraging both students and practicing clinicians to take time and effort to root themselves in sustaining communities of moral thought and practice that are capable of grounding the work that they do in something other than the machine metaphor.[9] Like Aristotle and Aquinas, I believe that the best form of training comes through committed, concrete, practical mentorship in which wise practitioners who are open about their own moral commitments form students and colleagues in the art of good mental health care.[10] I believe that in the pluralistic world of modern health care, students and practitioners might turn to any number of traditions, including religious traditions, to build capacity for resisting the machine metaphor and for caring well and holistically for their patients.[11] I am also confident that Christian faith offers tremendous resources for this task. Inhabiting traditions of thought and practice that are many times older than modern psychology, psychiatry, and medicine, Christian clinicians can engage with each other and with these traditions, preferably in community, to ask foundational questions about the ends and goals of their practice and to encourage each other in knowledge and in love.[12] Even more importantly, Christian clinicians can contribute to, participate in, and learn from the work of the church, which is the site in

8. Jeffrey P. Bishop, *The Anticipatory Corpse: Medicine, Power, and the Care of the Dying* (Notre Dame: University of Notre Dame Press, 2011).

9. Warren A. Kinghorn, Matthew D. McEvoy, Andrew Michel, and Michael Balboni, "Professionalism in Modern Medicine: Does the Emperor Have Any Clothes?," *Academic Medicine* 82 (2007): 40–45.

10. Warren A. Kinghorn, "Medical Education as Moral Formation: An Aristotelian Account of Medical Professionalism," *Perspectives in Biology and Medicine* 53 (2010): 87–105.

11. We have seen in prior chapters how Zen Buddhist practice has been influential for innovative psychotherapy practitioners and researchers such as Jon Kabat-Zinn, Daniel Siegel, and Marsha Linehan, with Linehan also drawing from Benedictine Christian spirituality. In a different context, Muslim psychiatrists such as Rania Awaad draw deeply on Islamic history and thought to reduce barriers between high-quality mental health care and Muslim populations in the United States and around the world. See, for example, Rania Awaad and Sara Ali, "A Modern Conceptualization of Phobia in al-Balkhi's 9th Century Treatise: Sustenance of the Body and Soul," *Journal of Anxiety Disorders* 37 (2016): 89–93; Rania Awaad, Danah Elsayed, and Hosam Helal, "Holistic Healing: Islam's Legacy of Mental Health," Yaqeen Institute, https://yaqeeninstitute.org/read/paper/holistic-healing-islams -legacy-of-mental-health.

12. This is the core of our formation work with health professions students, practicing clinicians, and others with vocations to health care within the Theology, Medicine, and Culture Initiative at Duke Divinity School; see Brett McCarty and Warren Kinghorn, "The 'Why' of Healthcare: Theological Imagination and the Moral Formation of Healthcare

which "the wisdom of God in its rich variety might . . . be made known to the rulers and authorities in the heavenly places" (Eph. 3:10). For Christians the church, and not the clinic, is the community that is most likely to offer in its life a meaningful alternative to the machine metaphor.[13]

Engaging Mental Health Care with the Journey in View

With this in mind, what are practical steps that clinicians and those who seek mental health care can take to resist the machine metaphor and to travel well together as wayfarers? I conclude with five recommendations that lead to ways of seeing, discerning, and acting differently in the world of mental health care. These five recommendations are rooted within the Christian vision at the heart of this book but can also apply to mental health care in more pluralistic and secular settings.

First, as Ann's story communicates so clearly, *don't travel alone.* People facing mental health problems all too often encounter stigma from others, which implies, "This is your problem, yours alone. If it becomes public, you will be judged." This external guard of stigma is often accompanied by the internal guard of shame, which says, "If others knew the truth about me, I would be ostracized." But it is at just these times that the consolation, counsel, and company of other wayfarers is most valuable and most needed.

Second, *keep the journey in view and the end in mind.* The primary question for a clinician to ask someone who presents for mental health care is not, What's wrong or broken with you? but rather, From where have you traveled? Where are you trying to go? Do you know how to get there? And what, if anything, is getting in the way? The primary question for a person seeking care to ask of a new clinician is not, How can you fix me? but rather, Would you walk alongside me, witnessing my journey, and helping me to find my way?

Third, *pay attention to whom and what we love.* Sometimes painful emotions associated with mental illness mean nothing except that the body or brain is

Practitioners," presentation at the annual meeting of the Society for the Study of Christian Ethics, London, United Kingdom, September 2019.

13. There are now a number of high-quality resources from a diverse set of perspectives on how churches can constructively support people with mental health problems. See, for example, "The Sanctuary Course," Sanctuary Mental Health Ministries, https://sanctuarymentalhealth.org/sanctuary-course/, and the work of Pathways to Promise, https://www.pathways2promise.org. The church has an opportunity and call to be a site of hospitality, advocacy and institution building, personal transformation and healing, justice seeking, storytelling and support, friendship and being known, and Sabbath rest.

not working as it should. But most of the time, even our most uncomfortable emotions can help us to understand whom or what we love and therefore why we are angry, sad, anxious, or distressed. The primary question we might ask about distressing emotion is not, How can I make this go away? but rather, What, if anything, are my feelings telling me about my loves? What do I want or need to do to respond to those loves? How can I become a wiser and deeper lover of God, of others, and of myself? The answers to these questions will go a long way in determining whether medications or other technical interventions to modify emotional states are a good idea.

Fourth, *always ask, What is needed, right now, for the journey?* Sometimes the answers are the same as the answers that the machine metaphor would give. Often what is needed is medication or a structured course of psychotherapy. Sometimes what's needed is inpatient hospitalization. Sometimes what's needed is electroconvulsive therapy (ECT). But to travel with wayfarers is to remain open to the answers that the machine metaphor doesn't deliver. Perhaps what's most needed is not technology but time and space to grieve, to rest, to seek safety, to connect with others, to play, and to discover one's path and vocation.

Fifth and finally, *remain open to wonder and surprise.* The machine metaphor prescribes control, rewards control, and is reinforced by the pursuit of control. Control is a good thing when life has been uncontrollable. But there are limits to the pursuit of control, and to travel with wayfarers is to be always alert to the burning in our hearts (Luke 24:32) that points beyond control to a posture of discovery and wonder.

Seeing and Knowing in Wonder

The machine metaphor casts the body and mind as machine, behavior and experience as symptoms, therapy as technology, and diagnosis as *knowledge-about.* I conclude by describing four ways that the image of the wayfarer helps both clinicians and those who seek mental health care to see and to know differently.

From duality to unity. First, if humans are not machines but wayfarers, then clinicians and those who seek care are invited to move beyond every form of dualism, especially dualism of self and symptoms and dualism of self and body, and to see each human being as a unified *nephesh,* an embodied soul. At times, it will be appropriate to assure people that they are not their experiences and behaviors (self-symptom dualism) or that particular things in their body and brain are happening *to* them (self-body dualism), or both. These are helpful *temporary* strategies for reducing shame and for fostering agency. But this temporary, strategic externalization of symptoms and body must not become permanent. The goal is that people would be able to live in and through their experiences, and in and through their bodies, and not to regard either as perpetual enemies.

From individual to relational experience. The image of the wayfarer affirms that we journey through the world as individuals. Each human being is a unique person. Each of our bodies is configured differently, with its own strengths and vulnerabilities. Each of us makes our own decisions and seeks to become the originator (*principium*) of our own actions. But neither our successes and joys nor our challenges and sufferings are ours alone. We are originally and always persons in relation, creatures of earth who love, grow, and find ourselves in relationship. When things are going wrong in the life of a wayfarer, it is important not only to look at the person experiencing the challenges (the inside-out model) but also and especially to look at the physical, relational, and communal ecosystem in which they are traveling (the outside-in model). Often the problems felt by individuals, and all too often blamed on individuals, originate in these broader contexts and will be resolved only when these broader contexts are addressed.

From fixing to attending. Ann's husband Dave, reflecting on his experiences trying to help his wife and children navigate mental health challenges, writes,

> For many years, I labored under the assumption that I was supposed to, that I COULD, fix my family members, that I could solve their problems (if only they would listen to me). It took a longlonglong time to recognize: you fix broken appliances and you solve crossword puzzles, but in no way am I equipped OR CALLED to do either with my family and friends.[14]

Just as Dave could not fix his family members, neither can clinicians fix those who seek our care, no matter how hard we try. We do not fix our patients, because our patients are not machines. As those who are ourselves on a journey, we travel with other wayfarers, attending to them and to their needs, always asking *with* them, "What is needed, right now, for the journey?"

From wayfaring to feasting. As important as the image of the wayfarer is to human life and to my argument in this book, it is also important to remember that the journey is not the destination. We do not know what the disciples on

---

14. Address at a congregational gathering, May 1, 2016.

the road to Emmaus intended as the goal of their journey. Perhaps they simply wanted to get out of Jerusalem, away from the site of execution and violence and the other anxious, grieving disciples. Perhaps they were seeking to meet loved ones who cared about them and were worried about them. Perhaps they needed a simpler, quieter place to grieve. We do not know. But whatever they were expecting, they received more. They expected a meal with a fellow traveler who was an interesting conversation partner. They received Jesus himself. They expected bread to nourish their bodies after an afternoon's walk. They received a eucharistic feast. They expected a retreat from a discouraging and perplexing world. They received a summons to reenter that world with a message of hope and resurrection.

Aquinas knew also that the journey is not the destination. He longed, as a wayfarer or *viator*, to become a *comprehensor*, one who would by God's grace participate in an eternal vision of God's glory.

> I see no wounds, as Thomas did
> But I profess you God above.
> Draw me deeply into faith,
> into Your hope, into Your love. . . .
>
> Jesus, Whom now I see enveiled,
> What I desire, when will it be?
> Beholding Your fair face revealed
> Your glory shall I be blessed to see. [15]

The journey of the Christian wayfarer has a destination, and it is a feast.

15. Thomas Aquinas, "*Adoro Te Devote, Latens Deitas* (Devoutly I Adore You, Hidden Deity)," in *The Aquinas Prayer Book: The Prayers and Hymns of St. Thomas Aquinas*, trans. and ed. Robert Anderson and Johann Moser (Manchester, NH: Sophia Institute Press, 2000), 68–71. The epigraph of this hymn notes that Aquinas would pray these verses while elevating the host at the altar, longing for the full vision of the Christ whose body he was breaking.

Acknowledgments

It is fitting that a book like this, written with the image of the wayfarer at its center, would itself be a kind of travelogue. Though a different document in nearly every respect, it is rooted in my doctoral dissertation work at Duke Divinity School under the direction of Stanley Hauerwas and supported by Keith Meador, Reinhard Hütter, Allen Verhey, Paul Griffiths, and many other capable teachers and mentors. Stanley introduced me to Aquinas's virtue theory and served as a patient, incisive, and encouraging mentor, and Stanley and Keith taught me to ask critical questions of medicine and psychiatry while also embracing the good and joy of caring well for patients. Reinhard modeled for me a careful and deep respect for Aquinas's theology and metaphysics (and should not be held responsible for Thomistic shortcomings in this book). Allen and Paul, in their different ways, taught me the value of theology formed by love and done in the service of the church. I am grateful to each of them.

This book is also rooted in my study and work as Faculty Scholar in the Program on Medicine and Religion at the University of Chicago from 2013 to 2015, funded by the John Templeton Foundation. I am grateful to Dan Sulmasy, Farr Curlin, Susan Hazlett, Dan Blazer, and fellow scholars John Hardt, Lydia Dugdale, Aasim Padela, Abraham Nussbaum, Amy DeBaets, Elena Salmoirago-Blotcher, and Michael Balboni for helping me to think through what was then a project on Aquinas, human flourishing, and the virtues. I am grateful to Roy and Laura Nichol for their support during this time of a conference in Houston focused on past and present Christian innovations in mental health care.

Since 2015, the book has grown alongside me, in open windows for writing, as I've worked as a psychiatrist at the Durham VA Medical Center, have jointly taught at Duke University School of Medicine and Duke Divinity School, and have worked to build the Theology, Medicine, and Culture Initiative (TMC) at Duke Divinity School. I'm grateful to a thoughtful group of scholars and practitioners who gathered in 2017 for a colloquium on Christian engagement with psychiatric medication, and to Peter McDonald and the McDonald Agape Foundation for encouraging and supporting me then and now. I'm grateful to Dan Blazer for his patient mentorship and persistent nudge for me to write. I'm also grateful to Duke Divinity School for a teaching leave in 2018–2019. I've been blessed to be surrounded by a wonderful group of TMC and Duke Divinity colleagues, including Brett McCarty, Sarah Jean Barton, Martha Carlough, Farr Curlin, Susan Eastman, Brewer Eberly, Rachel Meyer Gallagher, Heather Plonk, Victoria Yunez Behm, Stanley Hauerwas, Jan Holton, Maria Mugweru, Patrick Smith, Danielle Stulac, Carl Weisner, Wylin Wilson, Kavin Rowe, and Norman Wirzba, who have been encouragers, collaborators, and conversation partners along the way. Brett McCarty and Farr Curlin provided helpful editorial suggestions on a later version of the manuscript, and Reinhard Hütter generously pointed to some helpful Thomistic resources. A group of three colleagues in other disciplines and at other institutions provided critical encouragement and accountability for the writing process. My VA patients and my wonderful colleagues at the VA and Duke Psychiatry have taught me a great deal about what it means to travel with wayfarers, in good times and hard times.

The present form of this book emerged over several years in conversations about the difference that Christian faith makes for mental health, mental illness, and mental health care. I appreciate the patience and care of James Ernest at Eerdmans, who encouraged me to move Aquinas from the "front porch" to the "living room" of the book and to write about mental health in a way that was not simply an interpretation of Saint Thomas. I appreciate my friend and psychiatrist colleague Matt Rosa for a critical piece of advice that helped me to see the structure of the book. I am deeply grateful for many friends and colleagues who have spoken with me about their own personal and family experience of mental illness, including Ann and Dave and also Beth Cantrell. I'm grateful to many years of students at Duke Divinity School who have inspired me with their passion for integrating mental health and Christian faith, and for the many TMC students who have taught me so much about the difference that the gospel makes in health care. I'm also grateful for the many groups and organizations who hosted me for conversations and lectures that have become part of the content of this book, including the Society for Christian Psychology, Myers Park United Methodist Church (Charlotte, NC), the Center for Christianity and Scholarship, the North Carolina Study Center, the Veritas Forum, the American Association of Christian Counselors, Furman University, the International Association of Catholic Bioethicists, Centenary United Methodist Church, Matthews United Methodist Church, Tyndale University College and Seminary, Calvin Symposium on Worship, Hyde Park Institute,

Trinity Evangelical Divinity School, Chesterton House, Saddleback Church, Look Up Faith Conference on Mental Health (Fort Wayne, IN), Seminary of the Southwest, Christ Episcopal Church (Charlotte, NC), CMDA Psychiatry Section, the Center for Public Christianity, Baylor University, the Church of the Heavenly Rest (New York, NY), Signal Mountain Presbyterian Church (Chattanooga, TN), Trinity Church Princeton, Cedar Creek Church (Aiken, SC), University of Calgary, Salem Presbyterian Church (Winston-Salem, NC), and the Duke Center for Spirituality, Theology, and Health. I'm grateful to John Swinton, Eric Johnson, Curt Thompson, John Peteet, Andy Michel, Abraham Nussbaum, L. Gregory Jones, Charlotte vanOyen Witvliet, Harold Koenig, Bill Pearson, Matt Varnell, and Victor Shepherd for their friendship and critical encouragement to think and write theologically about mental health. I'm also grateful to participants in several conference sessions at the Conference on Medicine and Religion, the Society for Christian Ethics, the American Psychiatric Association, and the American Society for Bioethics and Humanities.

Above all, I'm grateful to Susan, Ava, and Mills, who have not only supported and patiently encouraged me through the difficult process of writing a book on borrowed time but also, in their love of me, helped me to understand, more deeply than I deserve, the meaning of grace and the love of God.

APPENDIX: AQUINAS, DISABILITY, AND THE *IMAGO DEI*

In chapter 5, I argue that all humans, regardless of capacity, are made in the image of God (*imago Dei*) and that this good news for those who live with mental health challenges. In this chapter I foreground John Kilner's interpretation of the *imago Dei* rather than that of Thomas Aquinas. But it is worthwhile to consider Aquinas's exposition of the *imago Dei* in *STh* Ia q. 93, along with ways that Aquinas can be defended against modern critics who charge that his account denies or devalues the image of God in persons with intellectual disability or serious mental illness.

The doctrine of the *imago* is very important for Aquinas's account of human beings: he affirms that humans are made in the image of God, presenting it near the end of his account of creation as the "end" (*finis*) or "term" (*terminus*) of the production of humans. The *imago Dei* is, in other words, the final cause of human creation, the template for the full realization of human nature. Aquinas centers Christ: following Scripture and Augustine, he affirms that Christ "is the perfect Image of God, reflecting perfectly that of which He is the image," and that while Christ bears this perfect image in an "identical nature" to the Father, other humans bear the image imperfectly, in an "alien nature" (*STh* Ia q. 93 *ad2*). Elsewhere he makes clear that while the Son "is the image," humans are "to the image" (*STh* Ia q. 35 a. 2 *ad3*). Also following Scripture, he affirms that the image is to be found in every human, including women (*STh* Ia q. 93 a. 4). Though he follows the traditional Irenaean distinction between image and likeness rather than Kilner's preferred distinction between image/likeness and glory, he offers a similar way to balance the affirmation that all humans are created in God's image and the affirmation that humans can grow into God's image by distinguishing three overlapping ways that the image of God is in humans: (a) by virtue of the natural aptitude for knowing and loving God, which is common to all humans; (b) by virtue of knowing and loving God actually and habitually but imperfectly, which is common to those in a state of grace in this life; and (c) by virtue of knowing and loving God perfectly, which is common only to the blessed in beatitude (*STh* Ia q. 93 a. 4). Humans, made in God's image, are called to union with God through knowledge and love.

Aquinas then affirms, following Augustine, that humans are not made in the image of the Son alone, but rather in the image of the whole Trinity, because the Son images the Father and because God said, "Let *us* make human-kind in *our* image," implying the Trinity (Gen. 1:26; *STh* Ia q. 93 a. 5). Also following Augustine, he affirms that the image of God is properly in humans as regards to what differentiates humans (the rational animal) from other creatures, which is the mind: "now the intellect or mind is that whereby the rational creature excels other creatures; wherefore this image of God is not found even in the rational creature except in the mind" (*STh* Ia q. 93 a. 6 *resp.*). He further accepts Augustine's pictures of the Trinity as lover, beloved, and loved and as mind, its knowledge of itself, and its love of itself. This leads him to assert that "first and chiefly, the image of the Trinity is to be found in the acts of the soul, that is, inasmuch as from the knowledge which we possess, by actual thought we form an internal word; and thence break forth into love" (*STh* Ia q. 93 a. 7 *resp.*). Because the image of God is found most properly in the acts of mind or soul, the human body bears not likeness of image but rather likeness to God by a trace (*vestigium*), just as other creatures also bear traces (or imprints) of the Trinity (*STh* Ia q. 93 a. 6 *resp.*). Because angels are non-corporeal creatures with an intellectual nature, by this reasoning the image of God is more perfect in angels than in humans, though there are certain accidental ways (such as the soul existing in the whole body as God exists in the whole world) that humans more properly image God than the angels (*STh* Ia q. 93 a. 3 *resp.*).

Some critics of Aquinas, including Kilner, charge that this account locates the image of God in human rationality and rational capacity in a way that po-tentially devalues or excludes people who live with intellectual disability and mental illness. A careful reading of Aquinas, though, shows that this is not necessarily the case. Contrary to Kilner's assertion, Aquinas does not locate the image of God in any particular person's capacity for or display of rational or discursive thought. Aquinas clearly affirms that the intellectual faculty of the soul—and therefore the *imago*—is imparted directly by God in creation and is found in all human beings regardless of capacity (*STh* Ia q. 90 a. 3; Ia q. 93 a. 4 *resp.*). Aquinas was well aware of persons with what would now be called intellectual disability or serious mental illness (he frequently refers to them as *amentes* or *furiosi*) and consistently affirms that such persons are endowed with the intellectual faculty of the soul even if the enactment of these powers is hindered by bodily impediment (*impedimentum corporale*). He affirms that such persons should be recognized as fully human, should be treated with dignity (*STh* IIaIIae q. 75 a. 2 *resp.*), and should be baptized "in the faith of the church" (*STh* IIIa q. 68 a. 12). In addition, when the display of rationality is hindered, God grants special graces: the Holy Spirit, for instance, gives baptized *amentes* the habit of wisdom, which is a marker of participation in Christ (*STh* IIaIIae q. 45 a. 5 *ad3*; q. 45 a. 6 *resp.*).

Additionally, Aquinas's affirmation that the *imago Dei* is to be found chiefly in the knowing and loving acts of the soul does not entail that persons with intellectual disability somehow image God in a way that is inferior to those with culturally valued linguistic and cognitive abilities. While making clear that they are ultimately the same power, Aquinas distinguishes between intellect (*intellectus*), which is the capacity to understand and to apprehend intelligible truth immediately, and reason (*ratio*), which is the capacity to advance from one known thing to another (*STh* Ia q. 79 a. 8). He also states that the image of the Trinity is in the soul most perfectly as it pertains to the soul's knowledge of *God*, not of other creatures: "thus the image of God is found in the soul according as the soul turns to God, or possesses a nature that enables it to turn to God" (*STh* Ia q. 93 a. 8 *resp.*). It follows, then, that a person with limited rational or cognitive capacity who is fully open to God (for example, in worship, or in open-hearted attention to the graces present in everyday life) may in fact be displaying the *imago Dei* more vividly than someone whose immediate apprehension of God is clouded by other rational pursuits. Aquinas seems to affirm this when he observes that persons with intellectual disability (*idiotae*), who while praying can attend to God but cannot understand either the words spoken or their sense, are in fact doing that which is most necessary in prayer (*STh* IIaIIae q. 83 a. 13 *resp.*).

On a formal level, therefore, Aquinas can be defended against his disability-conscious critics. But I highlight Aquinas's account in this appendix, rather than in the body of chapter 5, because I am not persuaded that Augustine's and Aquinas's location of the *imago* primarily in the acts of mind and soul follows necessarily from the witness of Scripture, because on a practical and pastoral level it is difficult to understand and to communicate this teaching in a way that does not reinforce intellectualist hierarchies of value, and because with Kilner I long for an explicitly christological account of the *imago Dei* when this is mostly *implicit* in Aquinas' account.

For a detailed overview of Aquinas's account of disability, see Miguel J. Romero, "Aquinas on the *corporis infirmitas*: Broken Flesh and the Grammar of Grace," in *Disability in the Christian Tradition: A Reader*, ed. Brian Brock and John Swinton (Grand Rapids: Eerdmans, 2012), 101–51. For more context on Thomas's teaching on the *imago Dei*, see D. Juvenal Merriell, CO, "Trinitarian Anthropology," in *The Theology of Thomas Aquinas*, ed. Rik van Nieuwenhove and Joseph Wawrykow (Notre Dame: University of Notre Dame Press, 2005), 123–42; Michael A. Dauphinais, "Loving the Lord Your God: The *Imago Dei* in Saint Thomas Aquinas," *Thomist* 63 (1999): 241–67; Montague Brown, "*Imago Dei* in Thomas Aquinas," *Saint Anselm Journal* 10 (2014): 1–11; Craig A. Boyd, "Participation Metaphysics, the *Imago Dei*, and the Natural Law in Aquinas' Ethics," *New Blackfriars* 88 (2007): 274–87; and especially Ian A. McFarland, "When Time Is of the Essence: Aquinas and the *Imago Dei*," *New Blackfriars* 82 (2001): 208–23.

Bibliography

Albert, Elisa, and Jennifer Block. "It Will Take More Than a $34,000 Drug to Stop Postpartum Depression." *New York Times*. March 24, 2019. https://www.nytimes.com/2019/03/24/opinion/postpartum-depression-zulresso.html.

American Psychiatric Association. *Diagnostic and Statistical Manual of Mental Disorders*. 3rd ed. [*DSM-III*]. Washington, DC: American Psychiatric Association, 1980.

———. *Diagnostic and Statistical Manual of Mental Disorders*. 4th ed. [*DSM-IV*]. Washington, DC: American Psychiatric Association, 1994.

———. *Diagnostic and Statistical Manual of Mental Disorders*. 5th ed. [*DSM-5*]. Washington, DC: American Psychiatric Association, 2013.

———. *Diagnostic and Statistical Manual of Mental Disorders*. 5th ed. rev. [*DSM-5-TR*]. Washington, DC: American Psychiatric Association, 2022.

Andreasen, Nancy C. *The Broken Brain: The Biological Revolution in Psychiatry*. New York: Harper & Row, 1984.

Aquino Ferreira, Lucas Fortaleza de, Fábio Henrique Queiroz Pereira, Ana Maria Luna Neri Benevides, and Matias Carvalho Aguiar Melo. "Borderline Personality Disorder and Sexual Abuse: A Systematic Review." *Psychiatry Research* 262 (2018): 70–77.

Aristotle. *De Anima (On the Soul)*. Translated by Hugh Lawson-Tancred. New York: Penguin Books, 1986.

Ashley, Benedict M. *Healing for Freedom: A Christian Perspective on Personhood and Psychotherapy*. Arlington, VA: Institute for the Psychological Sciences Press, 2013.

———. *The Way toward Wisdom: An Interdisciplinary and Intercultural Introduction to Metaphysics*. Notre Dame: University of Notre Dame Press, 2006.

"Assertive Community Treatment: The Evidence (DHHS Pub. No. SMA-08-4344)." Substance Abuse and Mental Health Services Administration. Rockville, MD: Center for Mental Health Services, Substance Abuse and Mental

Health Services Administration, US Department of Health and Human Services, 2008. https://www.samhsa.gov/.

Augustine, *On Genesis*. Translated by Edmund Hill, OP. Hyde Park, NY: New City Press, 2002.

Awaad, Rania, and Sara Ali. "A Modern Conceptualization of Phobia in al-Balkhi's 9th Century Treatise: Sustenance of the Body and Soul." *Journal of Anxiety Disorders* 37 (2016): 89–93.

Awaad, Rania, Danah Elsayed, and Hosam Helal. "Holistic Healing: Islam's Legacy of Mental Health." Yaqeen Institute. https://yaqeeninstitute.org/read/paper/holistic-healing-islams-legacy-of-mental-health.

Bakermans-Kranenburg, Marian, and Marinus H. van IJzendoorn. "The First 10,000 Adult Attachment Interviews: Distributions of Adult Attachment Representations in Clinical and Non-clinical Groups." *Attachment and Human Development* 11 (2009): 223–63.

Baranyi, Gergő, Martín Hernán Di Marco, Tom C. Russ, Chris Dibben, and Jamie Pearce. "The Impact of Neighbourhood Crime on Mental Health: A Systematic Review and Meta-analysis." *Social Science and Medicine* 282 (2021): https://doi.org/10.1016/j.socscimed.2021.114106.

Bauerschmidt, Frederick Christian. *Thomas Aquinas: Faith, Reason, and Following Christ*. New York: Oxford University Press, 2013.

Bayer, Ronald. *Homosexuality and American Psychiatry: The Politics of Diagnosis*. Princeton: Princeton University Press, 1981.

Beck, Aaron T., A. John Rush, Brian F. Shaw, and Gary Emery. *Cognitive Therapy of Depression*. New York: Guilford, 1979.

Benjamin, Ludy T. "A History of Clinical Psychology as a Profession in America (and a Glimpse of Its Future)." *Annual Review of Clinical Psychology* 1 (2005): 1–30.

Berry, Wendell. *Another Turn of the Crank*. Berkeley: Counterpoint, 1995.

———. *Sex, Economy, Freedom, and Community: Eight Essays*. New York: Pantheon, 1992.

Bishop, Jeffrey P. *The Anticipatory Corpse: Medicine, Power, and the Care of the Dying*. Notre Dame: University of Notre Dame Press, 2011.

———. "Of Minds and Brains and Cocreation: Psychopharmaceuticals and Modern Technological Imaginaries." *Christian Bioethics* 24 (2018): 224–45.

———. "Technics and Liturgics." *Christian Bioethics* 26 (2020): 12–30.

Bishop, Jeffrey P., M. Therese Lysaught, and Andrew A. Michel. *Biopolitics after Neuroscience: Morality and the Economy of Virtue*. London: Bloomsbury Academic, 2022.

Bishop, Tara F., Matthew J. Press, Salomeh Keyhani, and Harold Alan Pincus,

"Acceptance of Insurance by Psychiatrists and the Implications for Access to Mental Health Care." *JAMA Psychiatry* 71 (2014): 176–81.

Black, Daniel. *Embodiment and Mechanisation: Reciprocal Understandings of Body and Machine from the Renaissance to the Present*. Burlington, VT: Ashgate, 2014.

Blazer, Dan. *The Age of Melancholy: "Major Depression" and Its Social Origins*. New York: Routledge, 2005.

Bloom, Harold, ed. *William Shakespeare's Hamlet*. New York: Bloom's Literary Criticism, 2009.

Blum, Linda F. *Raising Generation Rx: Mothering Kids with Invisible Disabilities in an Age of Inequality*. New York: New York University Press, 2015.

Bobik, Joseph. *Aquinas on Matter and Form and the Elements: A Translation and Interpretation of the* De Principiis Naturae *and the* De Mixtione Elementorum *of St. Thomas Aquinas*. Notre Dame: University of Notre Dame Press, 1998.

Boorse, Christopher. "Health as a Theoretical Concept." *Philosophy of Science* 44 (1977): 542–73.

——. "On the Distinction between Disease and Illness." *Philosophy and Public Affairs* 5 (1975): 49–68.

——. "What a Theory of Mental Health Should Be." *Journal of the Theory of Social Behavior* 6 (1976): 61–84.

——. "Wright on Functions." *Philosophical Review* 85 (1976): 70–86.

Bowlby, John. *Attachment and Loss*. Vol. 1, *Attachment*. New York, Basic Books, 1969.

Boyd, Craig A. "Participation Metaphysics, the *Imago Dei*, and the Natural Law in Aquinas' Ethics." *New Blackfriars* 88 (2007): 274–87.

Bradburn, Norman M. *The Structure of Psychological Well-Being*. Chicago: Aldine, 1969.

Brennan, Robert Edward. *Thomistic Psychology: A Philosophic Analysis of the Nature of Man*. New York: Macmillan, 1941.

Brock, Brian C. *Christian Ethics in a Technological Age*. Grand Rapids: Eerdmans, 2010.

Brown, Montague. "*Imago Dei* in Thomas Aquinas." *Saint Anselm Journal* 10 (2014): 1–11.

Browning, Don, and Terry Cooper. *Religious Thought and the Modern Psychologies*. 2nd ed. Minneapolis: Fortress, 2000.

Buchman-Wildbaum, Tzipi, Zsolt Unoka, Robert Dudas, Gabriella Vizin, Zsolt Demetrovics, and Mara J. Richman. "Shame in Borderline Personality Disorder: Meta-analysis." *Journal of Personality Disorders* 35, supp. A (2021): 149–61.

Cacioppo, Stephanie, Angela J. Grippo, Sarah London, Luc Goossens, and John T. Cacioppo. "Loneliness: Clinical Import and Interventions." *Perspectives on Psychological Science* 10 (2015): 238–49.

Calahan, Susannah. *The Great Pretender: The Undercover Mission That Changed Our Understanding of Madness.* New York: Grand Central, 2019.

Cândea, Diana-Mirela, and Aurora Szentagotai-Tăta. "Shame-Proneness, Guilt-Proneness, and Anxiety Symptoms: A Meta-analysis." *Journal of Anxiety Disorders* 58 (2018): 78–106.

Cannon, Walter B. "The James-Lange Theory of Emotions: A Critical Examination and an Alternative Theory." *American Journal of Psychology* 39 (1927): 106–24.

Carey, Benedict. "Expert on Mental Illness Reveals Her Own Fight." *New York Times.* June 23, 2011. https://www.nytimes.com/2011/06/23/health/23lives.html.

Carroll, Aaron E. "The Real Reason the U.S. Has Employer-Sponsored Health Insurance." *New York Times.* September 5, 2017. https://www.nytimes.com/2017/09/05/upshot/the-real-reason-the-us-has-employer-sponsored-health-insurance.html.

Caspi, Avshalom, Karen Sugden, Terrie E. Moffitt, Alan Taylor, Ian W. Craig, HonaLee Harrington, Joseph McClay et al. "Influence of Life Stress on Depression: Moderation by a Polymorphism in the 5-HTT Gene." *Science* 301 (2003): 386–89.

Cates, Diana Fritz. *Aquinas on the Emotions: A Religious-Ethical Inquiry.* Washington, DC: Georgetown University Press, 2009.

Cessario, Romanus, Craig Steven Titus, and Paul C. Vitz, eds. *Philosophical Virtues and Psychological Strengths: Building the Bridge.* Manchester, NH: Sophia Institute Press, 2013.

Clarke, W. Norris, SJ. *Person and Being: The Aquinas Lecture, 1993.* Milwaukee: Marquette University Press, 1993.

Coblentz, Jessica. *Dust in the Blood: A Theology of Life with Depression.* Collegeville, MN: Liturgical Press, 2022.

Coleman, Monica. *Bipolar Faith: A Black Woman's Journey with Depression and Faith.* Minneapolis: Fortress, 2016.

Collicutt, Joanna. "Jesus and Madness." In *The Bible and Mental Health,* edited by Christopher C. H. Cook and Isabelle Hamley, 34–53. London: SCM, 2020.

Compton, Michael T., and Ruth S. Shim, eds. *The Social Determinants of Mental Health.* Washington, DC: American Psychiatric, 2015.

Cook, Christopher C. H. "The Gerasene Demoniac." In *The Bible and Mental Health: Towards a Biblical Theology of Mental Health,* edited by Christopher C. H. Cook and Isabelle Hamley, 141–56. London: SCM, 2020.

Crislip, Andrew. "The Sin of Sloth or the Illness of the Demons? The Demon of Acedia in Early Christian Monasticism." *Harvard Theological Review* 98 (2005): 143–69.

Crossley, Nick. "Prozac Nation and the Biochemical Self: A Critique." In *Debating Biology: Sociological Reflections on Health, Medicine, and Society*, edited by Simon J. Williams, Lynda Birke, and Gillian A. Bendelow, 245–58. New York: Routledge, 2003.

Culverhouse, R. C., N. L. Saccone, A. C. Horton, Y. Ma, K. J. Anstey, T. Banaschewski, M. Burmeister et al. "Collaborative Meta-analysis Finds No Evidence of a Strong Interaction between Stress and 5-HTTLPR Genotype Contributing to the Development of Depression." *Molecular Psychiatry* 23 (2018): 133–42.

Cunningham, Katherine C., Stefanie T. LoSavio, Paul A. Dennis, Chloe Farmer, Carolina P. Clancy, Michael A. Hertzberg, Nathan A. Kimbrel, Patrick S. Calhoun, and Jean C. Beckham. "Shame as a Mediator between Posttraumatic Stress Disorder Symptoms and Suicidal Ideation among Veterans." *Journal of Affective Disorders* 243 (2019): 216–19.

Curlin, Farr A., Shaun V. Odell, Ryan E. Lawrence, Marshall H. Chin, John D. Lantos, Keith G. Meador, and Harold G. Koenig. "The Relationship between Psychiatry and Religion among U.S. Physicians." *Psychiatric Services* 58 (2007): 1193–98.

Curlin, Farr, and Christopher Tollefsen. *The Way of Medicine: Ethics and the Healing Profession*. Notre Dame: University of Notre Dame Press, 2021.

Curtin, S. C., M. F. Garnett, and F. B. Ahmad. "Provisional Numbers and Rates of Suicide by Month and Demographic Characteristics: United States, 2021." National Center for Health Statistics. Vital Statistics Rapid Release 24. September 2022. https://dx.doi.org/10.15620/cdc:120830.

Cuthbert, Bruce N. "Research Domain Criteria: Toward Future Psychiatric Nosologies." *Dialogues in Clinical Neuroscience* 17 (2015): 89–97.

Damasio, Antonio. *The Feeling of What Happens: Body and Emotion in the Making of Consciousness*. San Diego: Harvest, 1999.

Daniels, Anthony M., and J. Allister Vale. "Did Sir Winston Churchill Suffer from the 'Black Dog'?" *Journal of the Royal Society of Medicine* 111 (2018): 394–406.

Dauphinais, Michael A. "Loving the Lord Your God: The *Imago Dei* in Saint Thomas Aquinas." *Thomist* 63 (1999): 241–67.

Davies, Brian, ed. *Thomas Aquinas: Contemporary Philosophical Perspectives*. New York: Oxford University Press, 2002.

Davis, Joseph E. *Chemically Imbalanced: Everyday Suffering, Medication, and Our Troubled Quest for Self-Mastery*. Chicago: University of Chicago Press, 2020.

Dawn, Marva J. *Keeping the Sabbath Wholly: Ceasing, Resting, Embracing, Feasting.* Grand Rapids: Eerdmans, 1989.

Dearing, Ronda L., Jeffrey Stuewig, and June Price Tangney. "On the Importance of Distinguishing Shame from Guilt: Relations to Problematic Alcohol and Drug Use." *Addictive Behaviors* 30 (2005): 1392–1404.

Decker, Hannah. *The Making of DSM-III°: A Diagnostic Manual's Conquest of American Psychiatry.* New York: Oxford University Press, 2013.

DeCrane, Susanne E. *Aquinas, Feminism, and the Common Good.* Washington, DC: Georgetown University Press, 2004.

"Deinstitutionalization: A Psychiatric 'Titanic.'" *Frontline.* https://www.pbs.org /wgbh/pages/frontline/shows/asylums/special/excerpt.html.

Demos, E. Virginia, ed. *Exploring Affect: The Selected Writings of Silvan S. Tomkins.* Cambridge: Cambridge University Press, 1995.

"Depression and Other Common Mental Disorders: Global Health Estimates." World Health Organization, 2017. http://apps.who.int/iris/bitstream /handle/10665/254610/WHO-MSD-MER-2017.2-eng.pdf.

Descartes, René. *Discourse on the Method of Rightly Conducting the Reason and Seeking Truth in the Sciences.* Translated by John Veitch. In *The Rationalists.* New York: Anchor, 1960.

———. *The Passions of the Soul.* Translated by Stephen H. Voss. Indianapolis: Hackett, 1989.

DeYoung, Patricia A. *Understanding and Treating Chronic Shame: A Relational/ Neurobiological Approach.* New York: Routledge, 2015.

DeYoung, Rebecca Konyndyk, Colleen McCluskey, and Christina Van Dyke. *Aquinas's Ethics: Metaphysical Foundations, Moral Theory, and Theological Context.* Notre Dame: University of Notre Dame Press, 2009.

Diener, Ed. "Subjective Well-Being." *Psychological Bulletin* 95 (1984): 542–75.

———. "Subjective Well-Being: The Science of Happiness and a Proposal for a National Index." *American Psychologist* 55 (2000): 34–43.

Dixon, Thomas. *From Passions to Emotions: The Creation of a Secular Psychological Category.* Cambridge: Cambridge University Press, 2003.

Dulmus, Catherine, and Carolyn Hilarski. "When Stress Constitutes Trauma and Trauma Constitutes Crisis: The Stress-Trauma-Crisis Continuum." *Brief Treatment and Crisis Intervention* 3 (2003): 27–35.

Dunne, Joseph. *Back to the Rough Ground: "Phronesis" and "Techne" in Modern Philosophy and in Aristotle.* Notre Dame: University of Notre Dame Press, 1993.

Eberl, Jason. *The Nature of Human Persons: Metaphysics and Bioethics.* Notre Dame: University of Notre Dame Press, 2020.

Elliott, Carl. *Better Than Well: American Medicine Meets the American Dream.* New York: Norton, 2003.

Elwyn, Glyn, Dominick Frosch, Richard Thomson, Natalie Joseph-Williams, Amy Lloyd, Paul Kinnersley, Emma Cording et al. "Shared Decision Making: A Model for Clinical Practice." *Journal of General Internal Medicine* 27 (2012): 1361–67.

Felitti, Vincent J., Robert F. Anda, Dale Nordenberg, David F. Williamson, Alison M. Spitz, and Valerie Edwards. "Relationship of Childhood Abuse and Household Dysfunction to Many of the Leading Causes of Death in Adults: The Adverse Childhood Experiences (ACE) Study." *American Journal of Preventive Medicine* 14 (1998): 245–58.

Ferngren, Gary. *Medicine and Health Care in Early Christianity.* Baltimore: Johns Hopkins University Press, 2009.

Feser, Edward. "Nature versus Art." *Edward Feser* (blog). April 30, 2011. http://edwardfeser.blogspot.com/2011/04/nature-versus-art.html.

Finnegan-Hosey, David. *Christ on the Psych Ward.* New York: Church, 2018.

Flanagan, R. J., J. Lally, S. Gee, R. Lyon, and S. Every-Palmer. "Clozapine in the Treatment of Refractory Schizophrenia: A Practical Guide for Healthcare Professionals." *British Medical Bulletin* 135 (2020): 73–89.

Fonagy, Peter, Gyorgy Gergely, Elliot L. Jurist, and Mary Target. *Affect Regulation, Mentalization, and the Development of the Self.* New York: Other, 2002.

Fosha, Diana. *The Transforming Power of Affect: A Model for Accelerated Change.* New York: Basic Books, 2000.

Foster, Adriana, James Gable, and John Buckley. "Homelessness in Schizophrenia." *Psychiatric Clinics of North America* 35 (2012): 717–34.

Foucault, Michel. *Madness and Civilization: A History of Insanity in the Age of Reason.* Translated by Richard Howard. New York: Vintage Books, 1965.

Fowers, Blaine. *Virtue and Psychology: Pursuing Excellence in Ordinary Practices.* Washington, DC: American Psychological Association, 2005.

Freud, Sigmund. *The Ego and the Id*, translated by James Strachey, 1–66. In *The Standard Edition of the Complete Psychological Works of Sigmund Freud*, vol. 19. London, Hogarth, 1966.

——. *The Standard Edition of the Complete Psychological Works of Sigmund Freud.* Vol. 1, *Pre-Psychoanalytic Publications and Unpublished Drafts (1886–1899).* London: Hogarth, 1966.

Fulford, K. W. M. "Facts/Values: Ten Principles of Values-Based Medicine." In *The Philosophy of Psychiatry: A Companion*, ed. Jennifer Radden, 205–34. New York: Oxford University Press, 2004.

——. "'What Is (Mental) Disease?': An Open Letter to Christopher Boorse." *Journal of Medical Ethics* 27 (2001): 80–85.

Fulton, Jessica J., Patrick S. Calhoun, H. Ryan Wagner, Amie R. Schrya, Lauren P. Hair, Nicole Feeling, Eric Elbogen, and Jean C. Beckham. "The Prevalence of Posttraumatic Stress Disorder in Operation Enduring Freedom/Operation Iraqi Freedom (OEF/OIF) Veterans: A Meta-analysis." *Journal of Anxiety Disorders* 31 (2015): 98–107.

"FY 2022 Budget—Congressional Justification." National Institute of Mental Health. https://www.nimh.nih.gov/about/budget/fy-2022-budget-congressional-justification.

Galderisi, Silvana, Andreas Heinz, Marianne Kastrup, Julian Beezhold, and Norman Sartorius. "Toward a New Definition of Mental Health." *World Psychiatry* 14 (2015): 231–33.

Gariépy, Geneviève, Helena Honkaniemi, and Amelie Quésnel-Vallée. "Social Support and Protection from Depression: Systematic Review of Current Findings in Western Countries." *British Journal of Psychiatry* 209 (2016): 284–93.

Gaukroger, Stephen. *Descartes: An Intellectual Biography.* Oxford: Clarendon, 1995.

George, Linda K., Dan G. Blazer, Dana C. Hughes, and Nancy Fowler. "Social Support and the Outcome of Major Depression." *British Journal of Psychiatry* 154 (1989): 478–85.

Gilbert, Paul. "What Is Shame? Some Core Issues and Controversies." In *Shame: Interpersonal Behavior, Psychopathology, and Culture,* ed. Paul Gilbert and Bernice Andrews, 3–38. New York: Oxford University Press, 1998.

Gilson, Etienne. *The Christian Philosophy of St. Thomas Aquinas.* Translated by L. K. Shook. Notre Dame: University of Notre Dame Press, 1994.

Glebkin, Vladimir. "A Socio-Cultural History of the Machine Metaphor." *Review of Cognitive Linguistics* 11 (2013): 145–62.

Goffman, Erving. *Asylums: Essays on the Social Situations of Mental Patients and Other Inmates.* Piscataway, NJ: Aldine Transaction, 2007.

——. *Stigma: Notes on the Management of Spoiled Identity.* Englewood Cliffs, NJ: Prentice-Hall, 1963.

Goleman, Daniel. *Emotional Intelligence: Why It Can Matter More Than IQ.* New York: Bantam Books, 1995.

Gordon, Daniel Joseph. *The Passion of Love in the "Summa Theologiae" of Thomas Aquinas.* Washington, DC: Catholic University of America Press, 2023.

Greenberg, J. R., and Stephen A. Mitchell. *Object Relations in Psychoanalytic Theory.* Cambridge: Harvard University Press, 1983.

Greenberg, Leslie S., and Jeanne C. Watson. *Emotion-Focused Therapy for Depression*. Washington, DC: American Psychological Association, 2006.

Greene-McCreight, Kathryn. *Darkness Is My Only Companion: A Christian Response to Mental Illness*. Grand Rapids: Brazos, 2015.

Grenz, Stanley J. *Theology for the Community of God*. Grand Rapids: Eerdmans, 2000.

Grob, Gerald N., "Origins of *DSM-I*: A Study in Appearance and Reality." *American Journal of Psychiatry* 1991 (148): 421–31.

Gushee, David. *The Sacredness of Human Life: Why an Ancient Biblical Vision Is Key to the World's Future*. Grand Rapids: Eerdmans, 2013.

Hales, Craig M., Jennifer Servais, Crescent B. Martin, and Dafna Kohen. "Prescription Drug Use among Adults Aged 40–79 in the United States and Canada (NCHS Data Brief, no. 347)." Centers for Disease Control and Prevention. Hyattsville, MD: National Center for Health Statistics, 2019. https://www.cdc.gov/nchs/products/databriefs/db347.htm#:~:text=Nearly%207%20in%2010%20adults,and%2018.8%25%20in%20Canada.

Harrington, Anne. *Mind Fixers: Psychiatry's Troubled Search for the Biology of Mental Illness*. New York: Norton, 2019.

Hatfield, Gary. "The *Passions of the Soul* and Descartes' Machine Psychology." *Studies in History and Philosophy of Science* 38 (2007): 1–35.

Hayes, Steven C., Kirk D. Strosahl, and Kelly G. Wilson. *Acceptance and Commitment Therapy: An Experiential Approach to Behavior Change*. New York: Guilford, 1999.

Healy, Nicholas. *Thomas Aquinas: Theologian of the Christian Life*. Burlington, VT: Ashgate, 2003.

Heath, Elaine. *Healing the Wounds of Sexual Abuse: Reading the Bible with Survivors*. Grand Rapids: Brazos, 2019.

Herman, Judith Lewis. "Posttraumatic Stress Disorder as a Shame Disorder." In *Shame in the Therapy Hour*, ed. Ronda L. Dearing and June Price Tangney, 261–75. Washington, DC: American Psychological Association, 2011.

———. *Trauma and Recovery: The Aftermath of Violence—from Domestic Abuse to Political Terror*. New York: Basic Books, 1997.

Heschel, Abraham Joshua. *The Sabbath: Its Meaning for Modern Man*. New York: Farrar, Strauss & Giroux, 1951.

Hesse, Erik. "The Adult Attachment Interview: Protocol, Method of Analysis, and Empirical Studies." In *Handbook of Attachment: Theory, Research, and Clinical Applications*, ed. Jude Cassidy and Philip R. Shaver, 552–98. New York: Guilford, 2008.

Hoge, Elizabeth A., Eric Bui, Mihriye Mete, Mary Ann Dutton, Amanda W.

Baker, and Naomi M. Simon. "Mindfulness-Based Stress Reduction vs. Escitalopram for the Treatment of Adults with Anxiety Disorders: A Randomized Clinical Trial." *JAMA Psychiatry* 2022. https://doi.org/10.1001/jamapsychiatry.2022.3679.

Horwitz, Allan V. *DSM: A History of Psychiatry's Bible.* Baltimore: Johns Hopkins University Press, 2021.

Howard, David M., Mark J. Adams, Toni-Kim Clarke, Jonathan D. Hafferty, Jude Gibson, Masoud Shirali, Jonathan R. I. Coleman et al. "Genome-Wide Meta-analysis of Depression Identifies 102 Independent Variants and Highlights the Importance of the Prefrontal Brain Regions." *Nature Neuroscience* 22 (2019): 343–52.

Hunt, Morton. *The Story of Psychology.* New York: Doubleday, 1993.

Hütter, Reinhard. *Bound for Beatitude: A Thomistic Study in Eschatology and Ethics.* Washington, DC: Catholic University of America Press, 2019.

———. *Dust Bound for Heaven: Explorations in the Theology of Thomas Aquinas.* Grand Rapids: Eerdmans, 2012.

Insel, Thomas R. *Healing: Our Path from Mental Illness to Mental Health.* New York: Penguin Books, 2022.

———. "Transforming Diagnosis." National Institute of Mental Health. April 29, 2013. https://psychrights.org/2013/130429NIMHTransformingDiagnosis.htm.

Insel, Thomas R., and Bruce N. Cuthbert. "Brain Disorders? Precisely: Precision Medicine Comes to Psychiatry." *Science* 348 (2015): 499–500.

———. "Research Domain Criteria (RDoC): Toward a New Classification Framework for Research on Mental Disorders." *American Journal of Psychiatry* 167 (2010): 748–50.

"Issue Brief: Parity." Mental Health America. https://www.mhanational.org/issues/issue-brief-parity.

Jahoda, Marie. *Current Concepts of Positive Mental Health: A Report to the Staff Director, Jack R. Ewalt.* Joint Commission on Mental Illness and Health Monograph Series 1. New York: Basic Books, 1958.

James, William. *The Principles of Psychology.* 2 vols. Mineola, NY: Dover, 1950.

———. "What Is an Emotion?" *Mind* 34 (1884): 188–205.

Johnson, Eric. *Foundations for Soul Care: A Christian Psychology Proposal.* Downers Grove, IL: InterVarsity Press, 2007.

Jones, David Stedman. *Masters of the Universe: Hayek, Friedman, and the Birth of Neoliberal Politics.* Princeton: Princeton University Press, 2014.

Kabat-Zinn, Jon. *Full Catastrophe Living: Using the Wisdom of Your Body and Mind to Face Stress, Pain, and Illness.* 15th anniversary ed. New York: Delta, 2005.

———. "Some Reflections on the Origins of MBSR, Skillful Means, and the Trouble with Maps." *Contemporary Buddhism* 12 (2011): 281–306.

Kandel, Eric. "A New Intellectual Framework for Psychiatry." *American Journal of Psychiatry* 155 (1998): 457–69.

Karen, Robert. *Becoming Attached: First Relationships and How They Affect Our Capacity to Love.* New York: Oxford University Press, 1998.

Keller, Evelyn Fox. "Whole Bodies, Whole Persons? Cultural Studies, Psychoanalysis, and Biology." In *Subjectivity: Ethnographic Investigations*, ed. João Biehl, Byron Good, and Arthur Kleinman, 352–61. Berkeley: University of California Press, 2007.

Kelsey, David. *Eccentric Existence: A Theological Anthropology.* 2 vols. Louisville: Westminster John Knox, 2009.

Kendell, R. E., J. E. Cooper, A. J. Gourlay, J. R. M. Copeland, L. Sharpe, and B. J. Gurland. "Diagnostic Criteria of American and British Psychiatrists." *Archives of General Psychiatry* 25 (1971): 123–30.

Kessler, Ronald C., Patricia Berglund, Olga Demler, Robert Jin, Doreen Koretz, Kathleen R. Merikangas, A. John Rush, Ellen E. Walters, and Philip S. Wang. "The Epidemiology of Major Depressive Disorder: Results from the National Comorbidity Survey Replication (NCS-R)." *JAMA* 289 (2003): 3095–3105.

Kessler, Ronald C., Patricia Berglund, Olga Demler, Robert Jin, Kathleen R. Merikangas, and Ellen E. Walters. "Lifetime Prevalence and Age-of-Onset Distributions of DSM-IV Disorders in the National Comorbidity Survey Replication." *Archives of General Psychiatry* 62 (2005): 593–60.

"Key Substance Use and Mental Health Indicators in the United States: Results from the 2016 National Survey on Drug Use and Health (HHS Publication No. SMA 17-5044, NSDUH Series H-52)." Substance Abuse and Mental Health Services Administration. Rockville, MD: Center for Behavioral Health Statistics and Quality, Substance Abuse and Mental Health Services Administration, 2017. https://www.samhsa.gov/data/.

Kilner, John. *Dignity and Destiny: Humanity in the Image of God.* Grand Rapids: Eerdmans, 2015.

Kim, Sangmoon, Ryan Thibodeau, and Randall S. Jorgensen. "Shame, Guilt, and Depressive Symptoms: A Meta-analytic Review." *Psychological Bulletin* 137 (2011): 68–96.

King, Martin Luther, Jr. *Where Do We Go from Here: Chaos or Community?* Boston: Beacon, 1968.

Kinghorn, Warren A. "The Biopolitics of Defining 'Mental Disorder.'" In *Making the DSM-5: Concepts and Controversies*, ed. Joel Paris and James Phillips, 47–61. New York: Springer, 2013.

——. "Medical Education as Moral Formation: An Aristotelian Account of Medical Professionalism." *Perspectives in Biology and Medicine* 53 (2010): 87–105.

——. "Medicating the Eschatological Body: Psychiatric Technology for Christian Wayfarers." ThD diss., Duke University, 2011.

——. "The Politics of Virtue: An Aristotelian-Thomistic Engagement with the VIA Classification of Character Strengths." *Journal of Positive Psychology* 12 (2017): 436–46.

——. "Presence of Mind: Thomistic Prudence and Contemporary Mindfulness Practices." *Journal for the Society of Christian Ethics* 35 (2015): 83–102.

Kinghorn, Warren A., Matthew D. McEvoy, Andrew A. Michel, and Michael Balboni. "Professionalism in Modern Medicine: Does the Emperor Have Any Clothes?" *Academic Medicine* 82 (2007): 40–45.

Kinghorn, Warren A., and Abraham M. Nussbaum. *Prescribing Together: A Relational Guide to Psychopharmacology*. Arlington, VA: American Psychiatric Association, 2021.

Kinser, D. Dixon. "Reimagining Relationship: What Autism Reveals about What It Means to Relate to God." DMin thesis, Duke University, 2021.

Kirk, Stuart A., and Herb Kutchins. *The Selling of DSM: The Rhetoric of Science in Psychiatry*. New York: Aldine de Gruyter, 1992.

Kline, Nathan S. *From Sad to Glad: Kline on Depression*. Rev. and updated ed. New York: Ballantine Books, 1974.

Kraepelin, Emil. *Clinical Psychiatry: A Text-Book for Students and Physicians*. Translated by A. Ross Diefendorf. New York: Macmillan, 1912.

Krensky, Sophie, and Olivia Shannon. "A New Treatment for Postpartum Depression: Boon or Bane?" National Women's Health Network. March 20, 2019. https://nwhn.org/a-new-treatment-for-postpartum-depression-boon-or -bane/.

Kvaale, Erlend P., William H. Gottdiener, and Nick Haslam. "Biogenetic Explanations and Stigma: A Meta-analytic Review of Associations among Laypeople." *Social Science and Medicine* 96 (2013): 95–103.

Kvaale, Erlend P., Nick Haslam, and William H. Gottdiener. "The 'Side Effects' of Medicalization: A Meta-analytic Review of How Biogenetic Explanations Affect Stigma." *Clinical Psychology Review* 33 (2013): 782–94.

Laing, R. D. *The Divided Self*. New York: Pantheon Books, 1960.

La Mettrie, Julian Offray. *Man a Machine*. Chicago: Open Court, 1912.

LaPine, Matthew. *The Logic of the Body: Retrieving Theological Psychology*. Bellingham, WA: Lexham, 2020.

LeDoux, Joseph. *The Emotional Brain: The Mysterious Underpinnings of Emotional Life*. New York: Simon & Schuster, 1996.

"Letter to the Bishops of the Catholic Church on Some Aspects of Christian Meditation." Congregation for the Doctrine of the Faith. October 15, 1989.

Lewis, Helen Block. "Shame and Guilt in Neurosis." *Psychoanalytic Review* 58 (1971): 419–38.

Lewis, Michael. *Shame: The Exposed Self*. New York: Free Press, 1992.

Linehan, Marsha. *Building a Life Worth Living: A Memoir*. New York: Random House, 2021.

———. *Cognitive Behavioral Treatment for Borderline Personality Disorder*. New York: Guilford, 1993.

Lombardo, Nicholas. *The Logic of Desire: Aquinas on Emotion*. Washington, DC: Catholic University of America Press, 2011.

Luhrmann, T. M. *Of Two Minds: The Growing Disorder in American Psychiatry*. New York: Knopf, 2000.

———. "'The Street Will Drive You Crazy': Why Homeless Psychotic Women in the Institutional Circuit in the United States Often Say No to Offers of Help." *American Journal of Psychiatry* 165 (2008): 15–20.

MacIntyre, Alasdair. *Dependent Rational Animals: Why Human Beings Need the Virtues*. Chicago: Open Court, 2001.

Madden, James D. *Mind, Matter, and Nature: A Thomistic Proposal for the Philosophy of Mind*. Washington, DC: Catholic University of America Press, 2013.

Mallo, C. Jason, and David L. Mintz. "Teaching All the Evidence Bases: Reintegrating Psychodynamic Aspects of Prescribing into Psychopharmacology Training." *Psychodynamic Psychiatry* 13 (2008): 13–38.

Marcus, Joel. *Mark 1–8: A New Translation with Introduction and Commentary*. New York: Doubleday, 2000.

Marmodoro, Anna, and Ben Page. "Aquinas on Forms, Substances and Artifacts." *Vivarium* 54 (2016): 1–21.

Maynard, Merryn, Lesley Andrade, Sara Packull-McCormick, Christopher M. Perlman, Cesar Leos-Toro, and Sharon I. Kirkpatrick. "Food Insecurity and Mental Health among Females in High-Income Countries." *International Journal of Environmental Research in Public Health* 15 (2018): 1424.

McCabe, Herbert. *The Good Life: Ethics and the Pursuit of Happiness*. New York: Continuum, 2005.

———. *On Aquinas*. Edited by Brian Davies. London: Continuum, 2009.

McCarty, Brett. "Salvation and Health in Southern Appalachia: What the Opioid Crisis Reveals about Health Care and the Church." *Christian Bioethics* 29 (2023): 221–34.

McCarty, Brett, and Warren Kinghorn. "The 'Why' of Healthcare: Theological Imagination and the Moral Formation of Healthcare Practitioners." Presentation at the annual meeting of the Society for the Study of Christian Ethics, London, United Kingdom, September 2019.

McFarland, Ian. "When Time Is of the Essence: Aquinas and the *Imago Dei.*" *New Blackfriars* 82 (2001): 208–23.

McGilchrist, Iain. "Can the Divided Brain Tell Us Anything about the Ultimate Nature of Reality?" Lecture to the Spirituality Interest Group of the Royal College of Psychiatrists, 2011. https://www.rcpsych.ac.uk/docs/default-source/members/sigs/spirituality-spsig/iain-mcgilchrist-can-the-divided-brain-tell-us-anything-about-the-ultimate-nature-of-reality.pdf.

———. *The Master and His Emissary: The Divided Brain and the Making of the Western World.* New Haven: Yale University Press, 2009.

Mead, George Herbert. *Mind, Self, and Society: From the Standpoint of a Social Behaviorist.* Edited by Charles W. Morris. Chicago: University of Chicago Press, 1962.

"Mental Health." World Health Organization. July 8, 2022. https://www.who.int/features/factfiles/mental_health/en/.

"The Mental Health Parity and Addiction Equity Act (MHPAEA)." Centers for Medicare and Medicaid Services. https://www.cms.gov/CCIIO/Programs-and-Initiatives/Other-Insurance-Protections/mhpaea_factsheet.

Merriell, D. Juvenal, CO. "Trinitarian Anthropology." In *The Theology of Thomas Aquinas,* edited by Rik van Nieuwenhove and Joseph Wawrykow, 123–42. Notre Dame: University of Notre Dame Press, 2005.

Metzl, Jonathan Michael. *Prozac on the Couch: Prescribing Gender in the Era of Wonder Drugs.* Durham, NC: Duke University Press, 2003.

Miller, William R., and Ricardo F. Muñoz. *Controlling Your Drinking: Tools to Make Moderation Work for You.* 2nd ed. New York: Guilford, 2013.

Milne-Edwards, Henri. *Outlines of Anatomy and Physiology.* Boston: Little & Brown, 1841.

Miner, Robert. *Thomas Aquinas on the Passions: A Study of* Summa Theologiae *1a2ae 22–48.* New York: Cambridge University Press, 2009.

Mintz, David L., and David F. Flynn. "How (Not What) to Prescribe: Nonpharmacologic Aspects of Psychopharmacology." *Psychiatric Clinics of North America* 35 (2012): 143–65.

Mitchell, Stephen A., and Margaret J. Black. *Freud and Beyond: A History of Modern Psychoanalytic Thought.* New York: Basic Books, 1995.

Mojtabai, Ramin, and Mark Olfson. "National Patterns in Antidepressant Treatment by Psychiatrists and General Medical Providers: Results from the

National Comorbidity Survey Replication." *Journal of Clinical Psychiatry* 69 (2008): 1064–74.

Moncrieff, Joanna, Ruth E. Cooper, Tom Stockmann, Simone Amendola, Michael P. Hengartner, and Mark A. Horowitz. "The Serotonin Theory of Depression: A Systematic Umbrella Review of the Evidence." *Molecular Psychiatry* 28 (2023): 3243–56.

Moore, Thomas J., and Donald R. Mattison. "Adult Utilization of Psychiatric Drugs and Differences by Sex, Age, and Race." *JAMA Internal Medicine* 177 (2017): 274–75.

Mumford, James. "Therapy beyond Good and Evil." *New Atlantis* 68 (2022): 28–38.

Nathanson, Donald. *Shame and Pride: Affect, Sex, and the Birth of the Self*. New York: Norton, 1992.

"National College Health Assessment." American College Health Association. https://www.acha.org/NCHA/ACHA-NCHA_Data/Publications_and _Reports/NCHA/Data/Publications_and_Reports.aspx?hkey=d5fb767c -d15d-4efc-8c41-3546d92032c5.

National Committee for Mental Hygiene and Committee on Statistics, American Psychiatric Association. *Statistical Manual for the Use of Hospitals for Mental Diseases*. 10th ed. Utica, NY: State Hospitals Press, 1942.

Newman, Andy, Nate Schweber, and Chelsia Rose Marcius. "Decades Adrift in a Broken System, Then Charged in a Death on the Tracks." *New York Times*, February 5, 2022. https://www.nytimes.com/2022/02/05/nyregion/martial -simon-michelle-go.html.

Newton, William. "Why Aquinas's Metaphysics of Gender Is Fundamentally Correct: A Response to John Finley." *Linacre Quarterly* 87 (2020): 198–205.

Nussbaum, Martha C. *Upheavals of Thought: The Intelligence of Emotions*. New York: Cambridge University Press, 2001.

Palmer, Parker. "The Gift of Presence, the Perils of Advice." *On Being* (blog). April 27, 2016. https://onbeing.org/blog/the-gift-of-presence-the-perils -of-advice/.

Pasnau, Robert. *Thomas Aquinas on Human Nature: A Philosophical Study of* Summa Theologiae *Ia 75–89*. New York: Cambridge University Press, 2002.

Pattison, Stephen. *Shame: Theory, Therapy, Theology*. Cambridge: Cambridge University Press, 2000.

PDM Task Force. *Psychodynamic Diagnostic Manual*. Silver Spring, MD: Alliance of Psychoanalytic Organizations, 2006.

Perkins, Pheme. "Mark." In *New Interpreter's Bible*. Vol. 8. Nashville: Abingdon, 1994.

Peterson, Christopher, and Martin Seligman. *Character Strengths and Virtues: A Handbook and Classification*. New York: Oxford University Press, 2004.

Phillips, Susan D., Barbara J. Burns, Elizabeth R. Edgar, Kim T. Mueser, Karen W. Linkins, Robert A. Rosenbeck, Robert E. Drake, and Elizabeth C. McDonel Herr. "Moving Assertive Community Treatment into Standard Practice." *Psychiatric Services* 52 (2001): 772–79.

Pieper, Josef. *Faith, Hope, Love*. San Francisco: Ignatius, 1997.

———. *The Four Cardinal Virtues: Prudence, Justice, Fortitude, Temperance*. Notre Dame: University of Notre Dame Press, 1966.

———. *Happiness and Contemplation*. Translated by Richard and Clara Winston. South Bend: Saint Augustine's, 1998.

———. *In Tune with the World: A Theory of Festivity*. Translated by Richard and Clara Winston. South Bend: Saint Augustine's, 1965.

———. *The Silence of St. Thomas: Three Essays*. 3rd ed. South Bend: Saint Augustine's, 1999.

Pinckaers, Servais. *Morality: The Catholic View*. Translated by Michael Sherwin, OP. South Bend: Saint Augustine's, 2003.

———. *The Sources of Christian Ethics*. Translated by Mary Thomas Noble. Washington, DC: Catholic University of America Press, 1995.

Pires, Gabriel Natan, Andreia Gomes Bezerra, Sergio Tufik, and Monica Levy Andersen. "Effects of Acute Sleep Deprivation on State Anxiety Levels: A Systematic Review and Meta-analysis." *Sleep Medicine* 24 (2016): 109–18.

Porter, C., J. Palmier-Claus, A. Branitsky, W. Mansell, H. Warwick, and F. Varese. "Childhood Adversity and Borderline Personality Disorder: A Metaanalysis." *Acta Psychiatrica Scandinavica* 141 (2020): 6–20.

Porter, Jean. *Justice as a Virtue: A Thomistic Perspective*. Grand Rapids: Eerdmans, 2016.

"Public Policy Platform of the National Alliance on Mental Illness." National Alliance on Mental Illness. 12th ed. December 2016. https://www.nami.org /Advocacy/Policy-Platform

Radden, Jennifer. "Thinking about the Repair Manual: Technique and Technology in Psychiatry." In *Philosophical Perspectives on Technology and Psychiatry*, ed. James Phillips, 263–78. New York: Oxford University Press, 2009.

Rambo, Shelly. *Resurrecting Wounds: Living in the Afterlife of Trauma*. Waco, TX: Baylor University Press, 2017.

Rashed, Mohammed Abouelleil. *Madness and the Demand for Recognition: A Philosophical Inquiry into Identity and Mental Health Activism*. New York: Oxford University Press, 2019.

Reimers, Adrian J. *The Soul of the Person: A Contemporary Philosophical Psychology.* Washington, DC: Catholic University of America Press, 2006.

Reinders, Hans. "Life's Goodness: On Disability, Genetics, and 'Choice.'" In *Theology, Disability, and the New Genetics: Why Science Needs the Church*, ed. John Swinton and Brian Brock, 163–81. London: T&T Clark, 2007.

———. *Receiving the Gift of Friendship: Profound Disability, Theological Anthropology, and Ethics.* Grand Rapids: Eerdmans, 2008.

Ridgely, M. S., H. H. Goldman. "Mental Health Insurance." In *Handbook on Mental Health Policy in the United States*, ed. D. A. Rochefort, 341–62. Westport, CT: Greenwood, 1989.

Roberts, Robert C. *Emotion: An Essay in Aid of Moral Psychology.* New York: Oxford University Press, 2003.

Robins, Eli, and Samuel B. Guze. "Establishment of Diagnostic Validity in Mental Illness: Its Application to Schizophrenia." *American Journal of Psychiatry* 106 (1970): 107–11.

Robins, L. N., and Darryl A. Regier, eds. *Psychiatric Disorders in America: The Epidemiologic Catchment Area Study.* New York: Free Press, 1991.

Rogers, Adam. "Star Neuroscientist Tom Insel Leaves the Google-Spawned Verily for . . . a Startup?" *Wired.* May 11, 2017. https://www.wired.com/2017/05/star-neuroscientist-tom-insel-leaves-google-spawned-verily-startup.

Rogers-Vaughn, Bruce. *Caring for Souls in a Neoliberal Age.* New York: Palgrave Macmillan, 2016.

Romero, Miguel J. "Aquinas on the *corporis infirmitas*: Broken Flesh and the Grammar of Grace." In *Disability in the Christian Tradition: A Reader*, edited by Brian Brock and John Swinton, 101–51. Grand Rapids: Eerdmans, 2012.

Rosenhan, D. L. "On Being Sane in Insane Places." *Science* 1973 (179): 250–58.

Rota, Michael. "Substance and Artifact in Thomas Aquinas." *History of Philosophy Quarterly* 21 (2004): 241–59.

Roth, Alisa. *Insane: America's Criminal Treatment of Mental Illness.* New York: Basic Books, 2018.

Ryan, Richard M., and Edward L. Deci. "On Happiness and Human Potentials: A Review of Research on Hedonic and Eudaimonic Well-Being." *Annual Review of Psychology* 52 (2001): 141–66.

Ryff, Carol D. "Happiness Is Everything, or Is It? Explorations on the Meaning of Psychological Well-Being." *Journal of Personality and Social Psychology* 57 (1989): 1069–81.

Ryff, Carol D., and Corey Lee M. Keyes. "The Structure of Psychological Well-Being Revisited." *Journal of Personality and Social Psychology* 69 (1995): 719–27.

Ryff, Carol D., and Burton H. Singer. "Know Thyself and Become What You Are: A Eudaimonic Approach to Psychological Well-Being." *Journal of Happiness Studies* 9 (2008): 13–39.

Sadler, John. *Values and Psychiatric Diagnosis*. New York: Oxford University Press, 2005.

"The Sanctuary Course." Sanctuary Mental Health Ministries. https://sanctuarymentalhealth.org/sanctuary-course/.

Scarantino, Andrea, and Ronald de Sousa. "Emotion." *Stanford Encyclopedia of Philosophy*. September 25, 2018. https://plato.stanford.edu/entries/emotion/.

Scheff, Thomas J. *Being Mentally Ill: A Sociological Theory*. 3rd ed. Piscataway, NJ: Aldine Transaction, 1999.

Schore, Allan. *Affect Regulation and the Origin of the Self: The Neurobiology of Emotional Development*. New York: Routledge, 2016.

———. "Early Shame Experiences and Infant Brain Development." In *Shame: Interpersonal Behavior, Psychopathology, and Culture*, ed. Paul Gilbert and Bernice Andrews, 57–77. New York: Oxford University Press, 1998.

Scott, K. M., K. C. Koenen, A. King, and M. V. Petukhova. "Post-traumatic Stress Disorder Associated with Sexual Assault among Women in the WHO World Mental Health Surveys." *Psychological Medicine* 48 (2018): 155–67.

Scull, Andrew. *Desperate Remedies: Psychiatry's Turbulent Quest to Cure Mental Illness*. Cambridge: Belknap, 2022.

Seligman, Martin E. P. *Flourish: A Visionary New Understanding of Happiness and Well-Being*. New York: Free Press, 2011.

Sharpe, Katherine. "Bad Mothers and Single Women: A Look Back at Antidepressant Advertisements." *Huffington Post*. June 11, 2012. http://www.huffingtonpost.com/katherine-sharpe/antidepressant-advertising_b_1586830.html.

Shorter, Edward. *A History of Psychiatry: From the Era of the Asylum to the Age of Prozac*. New York: Wiley & Sons, 1997.

Siegel, Daniel. *The Developing Mind: How Relationships and the Brain Interact to Shape Who We Are*. 2nd ed. New York: Guilford, 2012.

———. *Mindsight: The New Science of Personal Transformation*. New York: Bantam, 2011.

Simeon, Daphne, and Frank Putnam. "Pathological Dissociation in the National Comorbidity Survey Replication (NCS-R): Prevalence, Morbidity, Comorbidity, and Childhood Maltreatment." *Journal of Trauma and Dissociation* (2022): 1–14. https://doi.org/10.1080/15299732.2022.2064580.

Singer, Mel. "Shame, Guilt, Self-Hatred and Remorse in the Psychotherapy of

Vietnam Combat Veterans Who Committed Atrocities." *American Journal of Psychotherapy* 58 (2004): 377–85.

Smith, S. G., J. Chen, K. C. Basile, L. K. Gilbert, M. T. Merrick, N. Patel, M. Walling, and A. Jain. *The National Intimate Partner and Sexual Violence Survey (NISVS): 2010–2012 State Report.* Atlanta: National Center for Injury Prevention and Control, Centers for Disease Control and Prevention, 2017.

Solomon, Robert C. "The Logic of Emotion." *Nous* 11 (1977): 41–49.

———. *The Passions: Emotions and the Meaning of Life.* 2nd ed. Indianapolis: Hackett, 1993.

Solms, Mark. *The Hidden Spring: A Journey to the Source of Consciousness.* New York: Norton, 2021.

———. "New Project for a Scientific Psychology: General Scheme." *Neuropsychoanalysis* 22 (2020): 1–35. https://doi.org/10.1080/15294145.2020.1833361.

Spitz, René. "Hospitalism." *Psychoanalytic Study of the Child* 2 (1946): 113–17.

Spitzer, Robert L., Janet B. W. Williams, and Andrew E. Skodol. "*DSM-III*: The Major Achievements and an Overview." *American Journal of Psychiatry* 137 (1980): 151–64.

Stump, Eleonore. *Aquinas.* New York: Routledge, 2003.

———. "Non-Cartesian Substance Dualism and Materialism without Reductionism." *Faith and Philosophy* 1995 (12): 505–31.

Styron, William. *Darkness Visible: A Memoir of Madness.* New York: Vintage, 1992.

Sullivan, Ezra. *Habits and Holiness: Ethics, Theology, and Biopsychology.* Washington, DC: Catholic University of America Press, 2021.

Sullivan, Harry Stack. *Conceptions of Modern Psychiatry.* Washington, DC: The William Alanson White Psychiatric Foundation, 1948.

Swinton, John. *Dementia: Living in the Memories of God.* Grand Rapids: Eerdmans, 2012.

———. *Finding Jesus in the Storm: The Spiritual Lives of Christians with Mental Health Challenges.* Grand Rapids: Eerdmans, 2020.

———. *Resurrecting the Person: Friendship and the Care of People with Mental Health Problems.* Nashville: Abingdon, 2000.

Szasz, Thomas S. "The Case against Psychiatric Coercion." *Independent Review* 1 (1997): 485–98.

———. *The Myth of Mental Illness: Foundations of a Theory of Personal Conduct.* Rev. ed. New York: Harper & Row, 1974.

———. *Psychiatry: The Science of Lies.* Syracuse, NY: Syracuse University Press, 2008.

———. "The Therapeutic State: The Tyranny of Pharmacracy." *Independent Review* 2001 (5): 485–521.

Tangney, June Price, and Ronda L. Dearing. *Shame and Guilt*. New York: Guilford, 2002.

Taylor, Charles. *A Secular Age*. Cambridge: Belknap, 2007.

———. *Sources of the Self: The Making of the Modern Identity*. Cambridge: Harvard University Press, 1989.

Tessman, Lisa. *Burdened Virtues: Virtue Ethics for Liberatory Struggles*. New York: Oxford University Press, 2005.

Thomas Aquinas. *The Aquinas Prayer Book: The Prayers and Hymns of St. Thomas Aquinas*. Translated and edited by Robert Anderson and Johann Moser. Manchester, NH: Sophia Institute Press, 2000.

———. *Commentary on the Gospel of John, Chapters 9–21*. Translated by Fr. Fabian R. Larcher, OP. Lander, WY: The Aquinas Institute for the Study of Sacred Doctrine, 2013.

———. *Summa Theologiae*. 61 vols. Cambridge: Cambridge University Press, 1964. Reprint, Cambridge: Cambridge University Press, 2006.

———. *Summa Theologica*. 5 vols. Translated by Fathers of the English Dominican Province. New York: Benziger, 1948. Reprint, Notre Dame: Christian Classics, 1981.

Thompson, Curt. *The Soul of Shame: Retelling the Stories We Believe about Ourselves*. Downers Grove, IL: InterVarsity Press, 2015.

Torrell, Jean-Pierre. *Aquinas' Summa: Background, Structure, and Reception*. Translated by Benedict M. Guevin. Washington, DC: Catholic University of America Press, 2005.

———. *Saint Thomas Aquinas*. Vol. 1, *The Person and His Work*. Rev. ed. Translated by Robert Royal. Washington, DC: Catholic University of America Press, 2005.

———. *Saint Thomas Aquinas*. Vol. 2, *Spiritual Master*. Translated by Robert Royal. Washington, DC: Catholic University of America Press, 2003.

Torrey, E. Fuller. *Out of the Shadows: Confronting America's Mental Illness Crisis*. New York: Wiley & Sons, 1997.

"Trend in Psychiatric Inpatient Capacity, United States and Each State, 1970 to 2014." National Association of State Mental Health Program Directors. August 2017. https://www.nri-inc.org/media/1319/tac-paper-10-psychiatric-inpatient-capacity-final-09-05-2017.pdf

Turner, Denys. *Thomas Aquinas: A Portrait*. New Haven: Yale University Press, 2013.

"2022 National Veteran Suicide Prevention Annual Report." Office of Mental Health and Suicide Prevention, Department of Veterans Affairs. September 2022. https://www.mentalhealth.va.gov/docs/data-sheets/2022/2022 -National-Veteran-Suicide-Prevention-Annual-Report-FINAL-508.pdf.

US Department of Health and Human Services. *Mental Health: A Report of the Surgeon General.* Rockville, MD: US Department of Health and Human Services, Substance Abuse and Mental Health Services Administration, Center for Mental Health Services, National Institutes of Health, National Institute of Mental Health, 1999.

"VA/DOD Clinical Practice Guideline for the Management of Posttraumatic Stress Disorder and Acute Stress Disorder." The Management of Posttraumatic Stress Disorder Work Group. 2017. https://www.healthquality.va.gov /guidelines/MH/ptsd/VADoDPTSDCPGFinal012418.pdf.

VanderWeele, Tyler J. "On the Promotion of Human Flourishing." *Proceedings of the National Academy of Sciences* 114 (2017): 8148–56.

Verhey, Allen. *Reading the Bible in the Strange World of Medicine.* Grand Rapids: Eerdmans, 2003.

"Vital Statistics Rapid Release Provisional Drug Overdose Death Counts." Centers for Disease Control and Prevention. https://www.cdc.gov/nchs/nvss/vsrr /drug-overdose-data.htm.

Vitz, Paul C., William J. Nordling, and Craig Steven Titus, eds. *A Catholic Christian Meta-model of the Human Person: Integration of Psychology and Mental Health Practice.* Sterling, VA: Divine Mercy University Press, 2020.

Wadell, Paul. *The Primacy of Love: An Introduction to the Ethics of Thomas Aquinas.* Eugene, OR: Wipf & Stock, 1992.

Wallin, David J. *Attachment in Psychotherapy.* New York: Guilford, 2007.

Wampold, Bruce E., and Zac E. Imel. *The Great Psychotherapy Debate: The Evidence for What Makes Psychotherapy Work.* 2nd ed. New York: Routledge, 2015.

Watson, John Broadus. "Psychology as the Behaviorist Views It." *Psychological Review* 20 (1913): 158–77.

Webb, Marcia. *Toward a Theology of Psychological Disorder.* Eugene, OR: Cascade Books, 2017.

Weissman, Myrna M., Bruce M. Livingston, P. J. Leaf, L. P. Florio, and C. I. Holzer. "Affective Disorders." In *Psychiatric Disorders in America: The Epidemiologic Catchment Area Study,* ed. L. N. Robins and Darryl A. Regier, 53–80. New York: Free Press, 1991.

White, Thomas Joseph, OP. *The Trinity: On the Nature and Mystery of the One God.* Washington, DC: Catholic University of America Press, 2022.

Wills, Richard W. *Martin Luther King Jr. and the Image of God.* New York: Oxford University Press, 2009.

Wilson, Mitchell. "*DSM-III* and the Transformation of American Psychiatry: A History." *American Journal of Psychiatry* 150 (1993): 399–410.

Wilson, Warner. "Correlates of Avowed Happiness." *Psychological Bulletin* 67 (1967): 294–306.

Wirzba, Norman. *From Nature to Creation: A Christian Vision for Understanding and Loving Our World*. Grand Rapids: Baker Academic, 2015.

———. *Living the Sabbath: Discovering the Rhythms of Rest and Delight*. Grand Rapids: Brazos, 2006.

Wittgenstein, Ludwig. *Philosophical Investigations*. Translated by G. E. M. Anscombe. Malden, MA: Blackwell, 2001.

Wood, Adam. *Thomas Aquinas on the Immateriality of the Human Intellect*. Washington, DC: Catholic University of America Press, 2020.

Wurmser, Leon. *The Mask of Shame*. Baltimore: Johns Hopkins University Press, 1981.

Yandell, Michael. "'Do Not Torment Me': The Morally Injured Gerasene Demoniac." In *Exploring Moral Injury in Sacred Texts*, ed. Joseph McDonald, 135–49. London: Kingsley, 2017.

Index

Note: Page numbers in italics refer to illustrations. Figures and tables are indicated by page numbers followed by *f* and *t*, respectively.